D1093062

How Gut and Brain Control Metabolism

Frontiers of Hormone Research

Vol. 42

Series Editor

Ezio Ghigo Turin

Co-Editors

Federica Guaraldi Turin
Andrea Benso Turin

How Gut and Brain Control Metabolism

Volume Editors

Patric J.D. Delhanty Rotterdam
Aart J. van der Lely Rotterdam

32 figures, 22 in color, and 3 tables, 2014

KARGER Basel · Freiburg · Paris · London · New York · Chennai · New Delhi · Bangkok · Beijing · Shanghai · Tokyo · Kuala Lumpur · Singapore · Sydney

Frontiers of Hormone Research
Founded 1972 by Tj.B. van Wimersma Greidanus, Utrecht
Continued by Ashley B. Grossman, Oxford (1996–2013)

Patric J.D. Delhanty, PhD
Department of Internal Medicine
Erasmus MC
Rotterdam, The Netherlands

Aart J. van der Lely, MD, PhD
Department of Internal Medicine
Erasmus MC
Rotterdam, The Netherlands

Library of Congress Cataloging-in-Publication Data

How gut and brain control metabolism / volume editors, Patric J.D. Delhanty, Aart J. van der Lely.
    p. ; cm. -- (Frontiers of hormone research ; vol. 42)
  Includes bibliographical references and indexes.
  ISBN 978-3-318-02638-2 (hard cover : alk. paper) -- ISBN 978-3-318-02639-9 (e-ISBN)
  I. Delhanty, Patric J. D., editor of compilation. II. Lely, Aart Jan van der., editor of compilation.
III. Series: Frontiers of hormone research ; v. 42. 0301-3073
  [DNLM: 1. Gastrointestinal Hormones--metabolism. 2. Brain--metabolism.
3. Neuropeptides--metabolism. 4. Receptors, Gastrointestinal Hormone--metabolism.
W1 FR946F v.42 2014 / WK 170]
  QP572.G35
  573.4'4--dc23
                                                                              2014004435

Bibliographic Indices. This publication is listed in bibliographic services, including Current Contents® and PubMed/MEDLINE.

© Copyright 2014 by S. Karger AG, P.O. Box, CH–4009 Basel (Switzerland)
www.karger.com
Printed in Germany on acid-free and non-aging paper (ISO 9706) by Kraft Druck, Ettlingen
ISSN 0301–3073
e-ISSN 1662–3762
ISBN 978–3–318–02638–2
e-ISBN 978–3–318–02639–9

Contents

Foreword

The ability of mammals to maintain 'constancy' has intrigued humans and has roused curiosity since antiquity. This includes the inherent communication between peripheral tissues and the brain. This is exemplified by brain-gut communication. Claude Bernard pioneered the field of brain-gut communication with an experiment that fascinated his contemporary physiologists. The experiment consisted in making a rabbit artificially diabetic following the piqûre, or puncture, of the floor of the fourth ventricle (ca. 1855). However, only in recent decades has there been significant progress in our understanding of the fundamental mechanisms underlying gut-brain communication.

This progress has been largely driven by the alarming increase in the incidence of obesity and diabetes in countries around the globe. Fortunately, largely as a result of the work of our expert colleagues in endocrinology, neuroanatomy, and genetics, we now recognize that a plethora of molecules and cellular events are involved in the communication between the brain and the gut. Furthermore, with the recent discovery of the regulatory effects of the gut microbiome on metabolic health, our understanding of gut-brain communication has reached a new level of complexity. There is also strong persuasive and emerging evidence that several potential anti-diabetic and anti-obesity pharmacological agents, not to mention weight loss surgery itself, can directly regulate the physiological processes underlying gut-brain interactions. Thus, many clinicians and researchers now acknowledge that identifying the pathways underlying the integration of neural and hormonal information arising from the gut is a true challenge that is necessary in the fight against obesity and diabetes.

Despite the aforementioned enormous advances, surprisingly, traditional textbooks in endocrinology or neurosciences do not deal at great length with gut-brain communication. The editors of this volume, who are renowned endocrinologists and scientists, have assembled a group of expert authors who now provide a comprehensive text that encompasses all of the recent advances in understanding the role of gut-brain interactions in metabolic functions. In this volume, the elegant work of several distinguished biologists is appropriately reflected as the intellectual underpinning of modern gut-brain medicine. We can only hope that this volume will inspire new research in the field of gut-brain communication.

Laurent Gautron, PhD
Joel K. Elmquist, DVM, PhD
Division of Hypothalamic Research
Department of Internal Medicine
UT Southwestern Medical Center at Dallas
Dallas, Tex., USA

Preface

The aim of this book is to explore specific topics related to gut-brain interactions in the control of systemic metabolism, providing an overview of the most recent findings in this field, and relating these findings to previous work. The chapters describe novel aspects of this interaction, including regulation of insulin sensitivity in the brain, the roles of smell and taste, the gut microbiome, and novel gut-derived neuropeptides in regulating metabolism via the brain. These topics have been subdivided into three sections. The first section, 'Aspects of metabolic interplay between the brain and the gut', includes chapters related to mechanisms of interactions between the gut and the brain including neural and gut biome interactions, the hypothalamic-gut axis, central insulin action, the impact of sleep patterns, the link with brown adipose tissue function, and Prader-Willi syndrome as an example of dysregulated gut-brain interaction. The second section deals specifically with 'Smell and taste'. This section includes chapters on taste receptors both on the tongue and in the gut and their important role in regulating metabolism via the brain. The final section, 'The role of neuropeptides in metabolism', includes chapters on how the gut communicates with the brain via short peptide hormones. Here, chapters on PYY, nutropoids and proghrelin-derived peptides cover some of the most recent developments in this field.

The connection between the gut and the brain is one of the most promising therapeutic targets for the treatment of obesity and metabolic syndrome. Obesity is a global problem not limited to Western society. There are few new medical treatments for metabolic syndrome, and one of the aims of this volume is to bring together reviews that could spark in the reader, both researcher and clinician, new ideas or approaches to tackle this difficult medical problem.

The editors gratefully thank all of the authors who contributed their time and effort to this volume and the staff at Karger who assisted with its timely completion.

Patric J.D. Delhanty, PhD
Aart J. van der Lely, MD, PhD
Department of Internal Medicine
Erasmus MC, Rotterdam, The Netherlands

Delhanty PJD, van der Lely AJ (eds): How Gut and Brain Control Metabolism.
Front Horm Res. Basel, Karger, 2014, vol 42, pp 1–28 (DOI: 10.1159/000358312)

Hormonal Control of Metabolism by the Hypothalamus-Autonomic Nervous System-Liver Axis

Andries Kalsbeek[a, b] · Eveline Bruinstroop[a] · Chun-Xia Yi[b] ·
Lars Klieverik[a] · Ji Liu[a] · Eric Fliers[a]

[a]Department of Endocrinology and Metabolism, Academic Medical Center, University of Amsterdam, and
[b]Hypothalamic Integration Mechanisms, Netherlands Institute for Neuroscience, Amsterdam, The Netherlands

Abstract

The hypothalamus has long been appreciated to be fundamental in the control and coordination of homeostatic activity. Historically, this has been viewed in terms of the extensive neuroendocrine control system resulting from processing of hypothalamic signals relayed to the pituitary. Through these actions, endocrine signals are integrated throughout the body, modulating a vast array of physiological processes. Our understanding of the responses to endocrine signals is crucial for the diagnosis and management of many pathological conditions. More recently, the control emanating from the hypothalamus over the autonomic nervous system has been increasingly recognized as a powerful additional modulator of peripheral tissues. However, the neuroendocrine and autonomic control pathways emanating from the hypothalamus are not separate processes. They appear to act as a single integrated regulatory system, far more subtle and complex than when each is viewed in isolation. Consequently, hypothalamic regulation should be viewed as a summation of both neuroendocrine and autonomic influences. The neural regulation is believed to be fine and rapid, whereas the hormonal regulation is more stable and widespread. In this chapter, we will focus on the hypothalamic control of hepatic glucose and lipid metabolism.   © 2014 S. Karger AG, Basel

Dual Control by the Biological Clock

A nice example of this dual control mechanism used by the hypothalamus is provided by the control of the biological clock over daily rhythms in hormone release. The mammalian biological clock resides in the suprachiasmatic nuclei (SCN) located in the anterior hypothalamus. We showed that the SCN uses its projections to both the neuroendocrine and pre-autonomic hypothalamic neurons for generating the daily rhythm in plasma corticosterone concentrations [1]. On the one hand the SCN uses its projections to the subparaventricular nucleus (subPVN) and the dorsomedial hypothalamus (DMH) to modulate the activity of the CRH neurons in the PVN and the subsequent release of ACTH from the pituitary, whereas on the other hand it uses its GABAergic and glutamatergic projections to the pre-autonomic neurons in the PVN to control the sensitivity of the adrenal cortex to the incoming ACTH signal. Another example was recently provided by the work on the circadian regulation of the osmoregulatory circuit [2].

Our investigations on the circadian control of plasma glucose concentrations also yielded more insight into the hypothalamic control mechanisms of glucose homeostasis. It turned out that the SCN uses its GABAergic and glutamatergic projections to the sympathetic pre-autonomic neurons in the PVN to control hepatic glucose production, and its GABAergic projections to the parasympathetic pre-autonomic neurons in the PVN to control the meal-induced insulin responses from the endocrine pancreas. In addition, these experiments provided evidence for an important role of the hypothalamic orexin, PACAP and VIP systems in the (circadian) control of hepatic glucose production [3].

Neuroanatomical Connections between Hypothalamus and Liver

The brain is a major energy-consuming organ, and it depends almost entirely on glucose as a substrate. It is therefore not surprising that the plasma glucose concentration is tightly controlled by an efficient and complex regulatory neural system. By some this elaborate regulatory system and its safeguard of brain glucose supply, even – if necessary – at the expense of other organ systems, has been phrased as the 'selfish brain'. The hypothalamus is a key component of this system. Next to the intrinsic hypothalamic control of glucose metabolism by the biological clock it has become clear that the hypothalamus also serves as an important relay center for (humoral) feedback information from the periphery, with important roles for hypothalamic leptin [4] and more recently insulin receptors [5, 6] as striking examples. The hypothalamus consists of different nuclei with distinct neuronal populations. The hypothalamic arcuate nucleus (ARC) is localized at the base of the hypothalamus where the blood-brain barrier is largely absent. Neurons in the ARC express a variety of nutrient and hormone receptors, including leptin, insulin and thyroid hormone receptors. In close proximity to the ARC are the ventromedial hypothalamus (VMH), DMH and lateral hypothalamus (LH), which are also known to be anatomically connected and functionally implicated in energy metabolism [7]. Located centrally in the hypothalamus, the PVN is believed to integrate a variety of signals both from within (ARC, VMH, SCN, LH) and outside the hypothalamus. The PVN integrates this information with signals from other brain regions, and uses several output pathways for the regulation of peripheral metabolism. One of these pathways is the classical neuroendocrine route via the median eminence to the anterior pituitary, which in turn regulates a variety of endocrine glands like the adrenal, gonads and thyroid. Another pathway arising from the PVN relays neural information from its pre-autonomic neurons to the autonomic nervous system (ANS). The neural connection between the brain and the liver consists of both branches of the ANS, i.e. the sympathetic and parasympathetic nervous system. Retrograde tracing studies have shown that sympathetic and parasympathetic connections to the liver originate from different brain regions in the hypothalamus and brainstem [7–9].

Sympathetic Nervous System
All sympathetic input to the liver is relayed via the sympathetic preganglionic cells in the lateral horn of the thoracic spinal cord. These cell bodies lie in the intermediolateral column (IML) and associated cell groups. In the hypothalamus, the pre-autonomic neurons in the PVN and LH send direct projections to the preganglionic neurons in the IML or project indirectly to the IML via brainstem circuits [10]. In the brainstem, central autonomic regions that show direct projections to the preganglionic motoneurons in the IML are the rostroventrolateral medulla, A5 region and the parapyramidal region (which can be separated into ventromedial medulla and raphe nucleus), which send direct projections to the IML. The IML in the spinal cord is connected via splanchnic nerves to the celiac ganglion innervating the liver. Sympathetic hepatic nerves innervate the liver through nerve bundles that accompany the large vessels in the liver hilus from where they penetrate to different extents into the acinus. Large species differences exist in the extent of sympathetic innervation of liver parenchyma [11] (fig. 1).

Sympathetic hepatic nerves can modulate hepatocyte function by direct action of their neurotransmitter noradrenaline on the α- and β-adrenergic receptors. Besides noradrenaline, sympathetic hepatic nerve endings may also release neuropeptides, such as NPY and galanin.

Parasympathetic Nervous System
The efferent parasympathetic autonomic signal is conveyed via preganglionic cells in the dorsal motonucleus of the vagus (DMV) in the brainstem. Tracing studies combining a sympathetic denervation of the liver with injection of a tracer confirm that many of the above-mentioned central autonomic nuclei (PVN, LH, A5, parapyramidal area) also contribute to the control of the parasympathetic function, although from separate neuronal populations, thus indicating a functional specialization [9]. The DMV via the vagal nerve directly connects to ganglion cells, without involvement of the spinal cord (fig. 2).

The right posterior subdiaphragmatic vagal nerve branches into the left and right hepatic branch proper and the ganglion cells concerned are located close to the liver. Postganglionic parasympathetic nerves mainly use acetylcholine as their neurotransmitter, although peptides (such as cholecystokinin) are also involved. Acetylcholine acts on two types of receptors, the muscarinic and nicotinic cholinergic receptors.

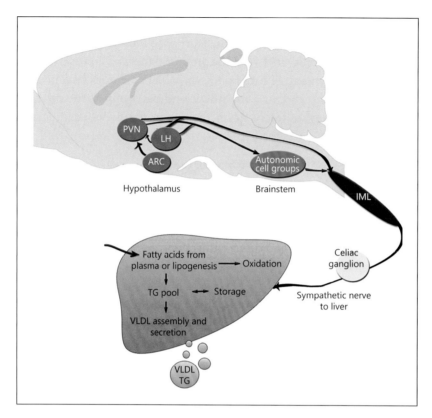

Fig. 1. Graphical representation of the efferent sympathetic connections between the brain and liver and a schematic representation of hepatic lipid metabolism.

Hypothalamic Control of Liver Metabolism via the Autonomic Nervous System

It is widely assumed that metabolic changes observed during metabolic and hormonal disorders such as type 2 diabetes, but also for instance thyrotoxicosis, Cushing's syndrome and menopause, are mediated via direct actions of insulin, thyroid hormone, cortisol and estrogen, respectively, on hormone receptors in peripheral organs such as the liver, muscle and adipose tissue. However, as will be shown in this chapter, the metabolic changes induced by insulin, thyroid hormone, glucocorticoids and estrogen are also partly mediated via the hypothalamus and the ANS. This concept is nicely illustrated by insulin, which is known to lower plasma glucose by facilitating glucose uptake in muscle and adipose tissue, as well as by inhibiting endogenous glucose production (EGP) in the liver. The latter effect is mediated by insulin's actions on several aspects of glucose metabolism including glycogenolysis and gluconeogenesis in the hepatocyte. At the turn of the century, however, it became clear that in rodents, EGP is inhibited by 40% upon low dose intracerebroventricular (ICV) infusion of insulin, and this occurs independently of circulating insulin concentrations [5, 6].

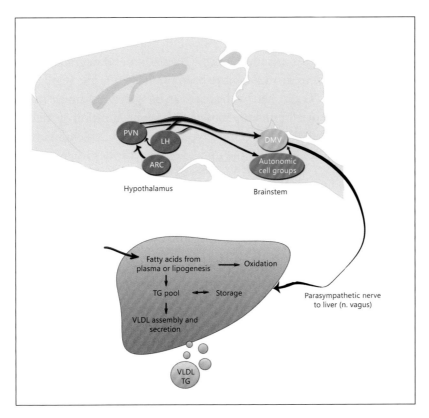

Fig. 2. Graphical representation of the efferent parasympathetic connections between the brain and liver and a schematic representation of hepatic lipid metabolism.

The pathway involved in this central effect of insulin on hepatic glucose metabolism has been partly unravelled, and involves insulin receptors in the ARC, hypothalamic potassium-dependent ATP channels, neuropeptidergic projections from the ARC to the PVN and autonomic output from the hypothalamus to the liver [5, 6, 12]. As indicated, this principle seems to hold not only for a glucoregulatory hormone such as insulin, but also other classic hormones such as estrogen, cortisol and thyroid hormone. In addition to carbohydrate metabolism, the hypothalamic-ANS-liver connection appears also to be involved in the control of lipid metabolism.

Physiologically, triglycerides represent the largest energy store in the body. The liver is a central organ in fatty acid and triglyceride metabolism, receiving two sources of fatty acids: hydrolysis of gut-derived triglycerides packed in chylomicrons during the postprandial period, and non-esterified fatty acids derived from lipolysis of adipose tissue during fasting conditions. Next to these sources of lipids, the liver is also capable of synthesizing fatty acids (de novo lipogenesis) from excess glucose. These fatty acids from different sources can be either used for oxidation within the liver, or assembled into triglycerides for storage or secretion from the liver into the plasma in VLDL particles (VLDL-TG). The regulation of VLDL-TG assembly and secretion is complex although several factors have been identified. Next to the availability of fatty acids, hormones (e.g. insulin) and the formation and degradation of ApoB, the major structural protein of VLDL, have been implicated in the regulation of VLDL-TG secretion. VLDL-TG secreted by the liver can be stored in adipose tissue or used as a source of energy by predominantly muscles. The concentration of triglycerides in plasma indicates the balance between triglycerides packed in chylomicrons or VLDL particles secreted by the liver and the uptake of triglycerides in peripheral tissues.

Insulin

One of the best known hypothalamic neuropeptidergic networks involved in the control of energy metabolism is represented by the NPY-containing neurons in the ARC with their projections to several hypothalamic brain areas, including the PVN. NPY is well known for its appetite-stimulating effects and, in fact, NPY is considered the most potent orexigenic neuropeptide known in mammals to date [13].

The first report on the glucoregulatory effects of the hypothalamic NPY system appeared in the mid-1990s when it was shown that ICV administration of NPY increases EGP in rats, probably by decreasing hepatic insulin sensitivity [14]. Later on, these results were confirmed in mice [15]. In view of the inhibitory effects of hypothalamic insulin receptors on hepatic glucose production [5, 6], the abundant expression of insulin receptors in the ARC, the inhibitory effect of insulin on NPY neuronal activity, and the effects of ICV NPY on sympathetic activity [16], we decided to test whether NPY could be the hypothalamic intermediate between the insulin receptors in the ARC and the pre-autonomic neurons in the PVN. Hereto we combined the euglycemic hyperinsulinemic clamp technique with the ICV administration of NPY, and performed these experiments in hepatic sympathetic-, hepatic parasympathetic- and hepatic sham-denervated rats. Our results confirmed that ICV NPY is able to (partially) block the inhibitory effects of peripheral hyperinsulinemia on hepatic glucose production, and also showed that selective denervation of hepatic sympathetic nerves blocks the effect of NPY on hepatic insulin sensitivity [12]. Therefore, the brain-mediated inhibitory effect of insulin on hepatic glucose production is probably effectuated via an inhibition of NPY neuronal activity in the ARC. Subsequently, the resulting diminished release of NPY will decrease the stimulatory input to the sympathetic pre-autonomic neurons in the PVN and thus reduce the sympathetic stimulation of hepatic glucose production. The results of Pocai et al. [17], however, showed that also the parasympathetic innervation of the liver is involved in the inhibitory effect of insulin on hepatic glucose production. This means that in addition to the effect of NPY on the sympathetic pre-autonomic neurons there is probably another neurotransmitter that is responsible for the transmission of insulin's effects in the ARC

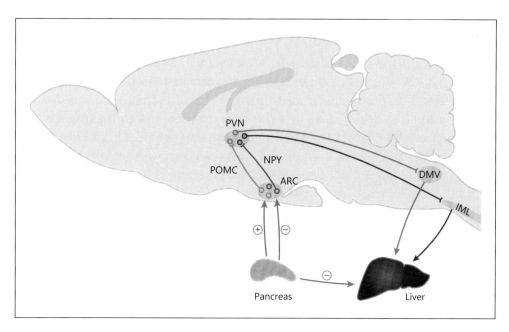

Fig. 3. Mid-sagittal view of the rat brain with a schematic representation of the hypothalamic connections involved in the inhibitory effects of circulating insulin on hepatic glucose production in addition to the direct inhibitory effects of insulin at the level of the liver. Increased insulin concentrations will inhibit the activity of the NPY neurons in the ARC. The resulting reduced release of NPY at the level of the pre-autonomic neurons in the PVN will also reduce the stimulatory effect of the hepatic sympathetic innervation glucose production. Next to a reduction of sympathetic hepatic input the increasing insulin levels most likely also cause a reduction of hepatic glucose production by increasing the parasympathetic input to the liver. In the current graph it is proposed that this involves the POMC-containing in the ARC, but this connection has not been proven yet.

to the parasympathetic pre-autonomic neurons in the PVN. Moreover, the effects of NPY also seem to be specific for glucose *production* as in none of the above-mentioned studies there was a significant effect on whole-body glucose *disposal* (fig. 3).

A few studies have shown that chronic ICV infusion of NPY, mimicking high levels of hypothalamic NPY in animal models of obesity, causes hypertriglyceridemia and lipogenesis in the liver even when animals are pair-fed [18]. Recently, Rojas et al. [19] showed that the hypothalamic effects of NPY signaling on hepatic VLDL-TG secretion via the Y1 receptor were dissociable from its effect on feeding via the Y2 receptor. Moreover, the effect on plasma triglycerides was abolished in adrenalectomized rats, but reappeared in adrenalectomized rats co-infused centrally with NPY and glucocorticoids. Interestingly, glucocorticoids have a strong effect on the arcuate NPY neurons as well [20]. Van den Hoek et al. [15] were the first to describe an acute stimulatory effect of NPY on VLDL-TG secretion, in mice. In this study, hyperinsulinemia decreased VLDL-TG secretion and this effect was abolished when the hyperinsulinemic clamp was combined with the ICV administration of NPY. This suggests that in the fed state the inhibitory effect of insulin on the activity of NPY neurons is responsible for the decrease in VLDL-TG secretion. No effects of NPY on VLDL-TG secretion were found in the basal state. More recently, however, Stafford et al. [21] showed that ICV administration of NPY in rats increased VLDL-TG in the postabsorptive state. The concomitant increase in liver MTP, ARF-1, and SCD-1 mRNA and the decrease of fatty acid synthase (FAS) mRNA suggested that the increased release of hypothalamic NPY causes a mobilization of stored triglycerides in the liver, whereas de novo fatty acid synthesis is inhibited. Moreover, after a longer fast, ICV administration of an Y1 antagonist decreased VLDL-TG secretion, suggesting a physiological role for the increased activity of hypothalamic NPY neurons in the ARC in the control of hepatic triglyceride secretion during fasting. Recently we showed that central NPY increases VLDL-TG secretion via the sympathetic branch of the ANS, as a selective hepatic sympathetic denervation completely blocked the stimulatory effect of ICV administered NPY [22]. Moreover, in that same study we also showed that an intact ARC and hepatic sympathetic innervation are necessary to maintain VLDL-TG secretion during fasting. Contrary to the effects of chronic insulin, acute infusion of peripheral insulin decreases VLDL-TG secretion. As this can be prevented by the ICV infusion of NPY, a central mechanism of insulin seems to be involved in the decreased VLDL-TG secretion [15]. Insulin infused into the mediobasal hypothalamus increases lipogenesis and suppresses lipolysis in white adipose tissue (WAT), which is mediated by the sympathetic nervous system (SNS), but no effects on the liver have been described so far [23]. In addition, ICV administered insulin has tissue-specific effects on the uptake of glucose and fatty acids [24]. It is not clear at present whether these central effects of insulin are also mediated via the NPY neurons in the ARC.

Previously it has been shown that NPY differentially regulates energy intake and energy expenditure in the PVN and LH [25], but together the findings above indicate that also within one hypothalamic nucleus the function of NPY is differentiated. The increased release of NPY during fasting from ARC neurons onto pre-autonomic PVN neurons stimulates the SNS to maintain hepatic glucose production as well as VLDL-TG secretion. Remarkably, a similar pathway has recently been described for the control of brown adipose tissue (BAT) activity, i.e. increased release of NPY from ARC-derived terminals results in a decreased expression of tyrosine hydroxylase in pre-autonomic, probably dopaminergic, neurons in the PVN and subsequently downregulation of uncoupling protein 1 (UCP1) expression and thermogenesis in BAT [26].

In addition to the orexigenic NPY/AgRP neurons, the ARC also contains a population of anorexigenic POMC/CART-containing neurons. The most important POMC-derived peptide with respect to feeding and metabolism is α-MSH. The reciprocally antagonistic function of the NPY/AgRP and POMC/CART cell populations is most clearly illustrated by the fact that AgRP acts as an endogenous antagonist of the melanocortin receptors 3 and 4 (MC3R, MC4R), for which α-MSH is the main endogenous agonist. MC signaling plays an important role in energy metabolism, as clearly evidenced by the fact that MC4R deficiency represents the commonest known mono-genic cause of human obesity [27]. Given the important and opposite effects of POMC and NPY neurons on energy homeostasis, the POMC neurons seemed to be good candidates for the missing parasympathetic link in the previous paragraph, i.e. the neurons in the ARC that are responsible for transmission of insulin's effects to the parasympathetic pre-autonomic neurons in the PVN, but the experimental evidence is ambiguous. Genetic deletion or reactivation of insulin receptors specifically on POMC neurons did not alter hepatic insulin sensitivity in a way that could be separated from its impact on energy expenditure [28]. On the other hand, when insulin receptors are selectively removed or reactivated specifically within AgRP neurons, hepatic insulin sensitivity is respectively impaired or improved [28]. In MC4R knockout mice, plasma insulin levels are increased and central administration of the α-MSH agonist MTII dose-dependently inhibits basal insulin release, but ICV administration of α-MSH or MTII enhances the action of insulin on both glucose uptake and production and transgenic overexpression of α-MSH leads to improved glucose metabolism. Moreover, the phenotype of the MC4R-deficient mice and humans, i.e. reduced heart rate and diastolic blood pressure in the face of severe obesity, is explained by a decreased sympathetic/parasympathetic balance [29]. Finally, recently Rossi et al. [30] used loxP-modified null Mc4r alleles (loxTB MC4R) to genetically dissect the specific role of MC signaling in sympathetic versus parasympathetic preganglionic neurons. This was achieved by either the general re-expression of MC4R in all cholinergic neurons including brainstem and spinal cord autonomic motoneurons (loxTB MC4R, ChAT-Cre), or by specifically re-expressing MC4Rs only in autonomic control neurons, including the parasympathetic motoneurons in the dorsal motonucleus of the vagus (loxTB MC4R and Phox2b-Cre), but excluding the sympathetic motoneurons in the spinal cord. Interestingly, reactivation of MC4R signaling in cholinergic neurons improved hyperinsulinemia and hyperglycemia, while re-expression of MC4R selectively in brainstem neurons only improved hyperinsulinemia. Specifically, they found improved efficiency of insulin-induced inhibition of hepatic glucose production following general re-expression of MC4R in cholinergic neurons, but not by specific re-expression in the vagal motoneurons. These observations nicely fit with our previous data [12], and the concept that activity of the sympathetic input to the liver is balanced by the NPY- and POMC-containing projections from the ARC. An increased NPY input to sympathetic pre-autonomic hypothalamic neurons reduces hepatic insulin sensitivity, whereas a reinstatement of MC signaling (derived from the ARC) onto sympathetic preganglionic neurons in the spinal cord increases hepatic insulin sensitivity. Surprisingly, however, α-MSH does not seem to be involved in the inhibitory effect of hypothalamic insulin on HGP, as co-administration of a melanocortin antagonist failed to block the decrease in HGP induced by hyperinsulinemia [6]. Blocking α-MSH signaling via ICV infusion of the melanocortin 3/4 receptor (MC3R/MC4R) antagonist SHU9119 has no effects on glucose metabolism, but ICV infusion of α-MSH itself has a clear stimulatory effect on EGP via gluconeogenesis which can be antagonized by SHU9119 [31].

It has been proposed that the hypothalamic MC3R/MC4R signaling pathway mediates the effect of systemic leptin on EGP [32]. Central administration of leptin has been proven to be involved in the autoregulation of hepatic glucose output, i.e. an increase in gluconeogenesis with a concomitant decrease in glycogenolysis without changing total glucose production. Recently, elegant experiments showed that the adenoviral-induced expression of leptin receptors in the ARC of leptin receptor knockout animals improves glucose tolerance via enhanced suppression of EGP [33]. The ARC-induced expression of the leptin receptor was associated with a reduced hepatic expression of G6Pase and phosphoenolpyruvate carboxykinase (PEPCK), but again, no significant changes in the insulin-stimulated whole-body glucose utilization were apparent. Moreover, the effects of hypothalamic leptin signaling on hepatic insulin sensitivity could be blocked by a selective hepatic vagotomy, providing further support for the idea that ARC projections to pre-autonomic neurons (in the PVN) are important for the transmission of the effect of leptin on EGP. Further supporting the involvement of POMC neurons in these effects are the observations that re-expression of leptin receptors specifically in POMC neurons improves glucose metabolism, whereas removal of both leptin and insulin receptors specifically from POMC neurons causes severe insulin resistance and increases HGP. Evidently more experiments are needed to unravel the precise hypothalamic pathways.

Contrary to the effect of chronic ICV administration of NPY, chronic blockade of the central melanocortin system does not change plasma levels of triglycerides and fatty acids, although it does increase circulating HDL cholesterol levels [34] and induce an obese phenotype. On the other hand, both chronic blockade of the melanocortin system in the agouti yellow mice and infusion of a melanocortin antagonist promote lipogenesis and lipid accumulation in liver with a possible role for SREB1c and PPAR-γ. MC4R knockout mice display increased levels of the lipogenic gene, FAS, as well as hepatic steatosis. In contrast, activation of the melanocortin system with leptin, MTII or NDP-MSH reduces the expression of lipogenic genes in the liver. Thus, although the melanocortin system seems to be involved in the control of hepatic lipid metabolism, its interaction with dietary factors and hormones such as insulin is still under debate. For instance, the significance of insulin's stimulating effect on the expression of lipogenic genes, such as SREBP1c and possibly PPAR-γ, is unclear at present, as the increased FAS expression and hepatic steatosis in MC4R knockout mice is abolished in pre-obese mice not displaying hyperinsulinemia. Likewise, the interpretation of two other observations in these mice: (1) increased hepatic lipogenesis and fat content is largely prevented by pair-feeding, and (2) acute blockade or activation of the central melanocortin system does not significantly alter VLDL-TG secretion, remains enigmatic [21].

Lam et al. [35] investigated the acute effects of ICV glucose on VLDL-TG secretion, to mimic a fed state only in the brain, while the rat is fasted. Acute ICV infusion of glucose lowered VLDL-TG secretion, which was prevented by a hepatic vagotomy. This indicates that the parasympathetic nervous system is involved in the central

Kalsbeek · Bruinstroop · Yi · Klieverik · Liu · Fliers

effects of glucose on VLDL-TG secretion. The authors proposed that the effect of ICV glucose on VLDL-TG secretion is mediated via lowered SCD1 activity and decreased oleyl-CoA levels. Recent studies in our laboratory have provided additional evidence for the involvement of the parasympathetic branch of the ANS in the control of VLDL-TG secretion. We found that postprandial plasma triglyceride concentrations were significantly elevated in parasympathetically denervated rats as compared to control rats, and that VLDL-TG production tended to be increased. Furthermore, in rats fed on a 6-meals-a-day schedule for several weeks, a parasympathetic denervation resulted in >70% higher plasma triglycerides during the day, whereas a sympathetic denervation had no effect [36]. These results show that abolishing the parasympathetic input to the liver results in increased plasma triglyceride levels during postprandial conditions.

Thyroid Hormone

Decades before the discovery and isolation of thyroxine (T_4), increased activity of the SNS was thought to play an important pathophysiological role in the syndrome characterized by goiter, exophthalmos and palpitations (i.e. the so-called 'Merseburger triad') that we now know as Graves' disease. This assumption was reflected by the treatment of severe thyrotoxicosis by resection of the cervical sympathetic chain in the second half of the 19th century, and by high spinal anesthesia or adrenal demedullation as a surgical alternative to thyroidectomy until the 1930s. After the successful isolation and synthesis of thyroid hormone and the subsequent development of anti-thyroid drugs, these treatment modalities were gradually abandoned. However, β-adrenergic blockers are still routinely used in the initial management of severe thyrotoxicosis.

Changes in SNS activity during hyperthyroidism have been assessed with various techniques. Plasma catecholamine concentrations were found to be typically low to normal, but more recent studies reported increased 24 h urinary excretion of noradrenaline even during mild hyperthyroidism. The measurement of catecholamines in plasma or urine does not allow for a distinction between catecholamines released from the adrenal medulla or from sympathetic nerve endings, nor between sympathetic activities in specific organs or tissues. For the latter purpose, the tissue efflux rate of tritiated noradrenaline after its systemic infusion became available, somewhat unexpectedly showing increased efflux from the adrenal glands in hypothyroid, rather than hyperthyroid rats [37]. In line, assessment of sympathetic nerve activity in muscle by microneurography in patients with hyper- and hypothyroidism showed a negative correlation of sympathetic activity with serum thyroid hormone concentrations [38]. By contrast, assessment of heart rate variability in thyrotoxic patients indicated sympathovagal imbalance with a shift to increased sympathetic and decreased vagal input to the heart [39]. Increased sympathetic tone in hyperthyroidism was also indicated by microdialysis experiments revealing increased glycerol (reflecting the rate of lipolysis) and noradrenaline concentrations in subcutaneous adipose tissue of hyperthyroid patients and opposite findings in hypothyroidism [40]. These findings suggested a direct relationship between sympathetic tone, thyroid hormone concentrations and lipolysis in adipose tissue. In sum, the relationship between SNS activity and thyroid state is rather complex, and points to differential effects depending on the organ and tissue studied. In recent years, studies on systemic and local regulation of thyroid hormone production and action have shed new light on the role of triiodothyronine (T_3) in body weight regulation, as well as glucose and lipid homeostasis [41]. Specifically, studies focusing on the interaction between thyroid hormone, the ANS and the liver, revealed an important role for the hypothalamus which may partly explain the differential effects of thyroid hormone on autonomic outflow to peripheral organs.

Thyroid Hormone Modulates Glucose Production via the Hypothalamus

While recent studies have reported subtle associations between serum thyroid hormone concentrations and parameters for insulin sensitivity even within the euthyroid range, overt thyrotoxicosis is associated with a broad range of alterations in metabolism and energy homeostasis. EGP, lipolysis and proteolysis are increased during thyrotoxicosis, providing the substrates needed for the concomitant increase in energy expenditure. Alterations in whole-body lipid metabolism are accompanied by tissue-specific changes in triglyceride-derived fatty acid uptake with increased uptake in muscle and heart, and decreased uptake in BAT [42]. The increase in EGP is facilitated by increased activities of hepatic gluconeogenic enzymes such as PEPCK and pyruvate carboxylase and by increased hepatic expression of the glucose transporter GLUT2. Although evidence from clinical studies is scarce, thyrotoxicosis has been reported to increase EGP in the basal state and to decrease hepatic insulin sensitivity in humans.

In view of the abundant expression of thyroid hormone receptors in the hypothalamic ARC and PVN [43] and the elucidation of the importance of neural pathways between the hypothalamus and the liver for the regulation of carbohydrate metabolism, we hypothesized a role for sympathetic and parasympathetic innervation of the liver in the pathogenesis of the metabolic effects of thyrotoxicosis. To investigate this, we first studied the effects of thyrotoxicosis on plasma glucose, EGP and hepatic insulin sensitivity using the stable isotope ($6,6\text{-}^2H_2$-glucose) dilution technique in freely moving rats. Thyrotoxic rats treated with T_4 released from osmotic minipumps exhibited a fourfold increase in plasma T_3 compared with euthyroid rats. In these rats, basal plasma glucose was increased while basal plasma insulin was unaffected. EGP was increased by 45% and correlated positively with plasma T_3. In addition, thyrotoxic rats showed an increased hepatic mRNA expression of PEPCK and of the

Kalsbeek · Bruinstroop · Yi · Klieverik · Liu · Fliers

T_3-responsive gene deiodinase type 1, supporting the thyrotoxic state of the hepato-cytes. During hyperinsulinemia, EGP decreased in all groups, but the suppression of EGP was 35% less in thyrotoxic rats, indicating hepatic insulin resistance.

In euthyroid rats, selective hepatic sympathetic or parasympathetic denervation did not affect glucose concentration, insulin concentration, or EGP. In thyrotoxic rats, however, the relative increase of EGP by thyrotoxicosis was smaller after a sympathetic denervation, while a selective hepatic parasympathectomy induced a marked increase in basal insulin concentration. This increase in insulin concentration was not accompanied by altered glucose concentration or EGP, indicating hepatic insulin resistance. Thus, changes in EGP and hepatic insulin sensitivity during thyrotoxicosis can be modulated by selective hepatic sympathetic and parasympathetic denervation, pointing to neurally mediated effects of thyroid hormone on glucose metabolism.

As a next step, we investigated if intrahypothalamic administration of thyroid hormone modulates hepatic glucose production via autonomic outflow from the hypothalamus. EGP was measured before and after bilateral microdialysis of T_3 for 2 h in the PVN. T_3 microdialysis in the PVN significantly increased plasma glucose and EGP compared to vehicle microdialysis. These effects were independent of plasma T_3, insulin, glucagon, and corticosterone. Furthermore, selective hepatic sympathectomy completely prevented the effect of T_3 microdialysis on EGP, indicating that stimulation of T_3-sensitive neurons in the PVN of euthyroid rats increases EGP via sympathetic projections to the liver [44]. Our findings may be relevant for the recent demonstration of altered hepatic glucose metabolism in mice expressing a mutant thyroid hormone receptor α_1, since these mice had been shown earlier to exhibit hypermetabolism due to an overactive SNS [45]. Taken together, we propose a novel central pathway for modulation of hepatic glucose metabolism by thyroid hormone (fig. 4). Currently it is not clear what the physiological role for the central effects of thyroid hormone is. It is tempting to speculate that the role of this neural regulatory loop is the fine-tuning of direct, peripheral effect of thyroid hormone on the hepatocyte.

Similar thyroid hormone-sensitive connections may exist between the PVN and organs such as the heart, BAT and the thyroid itself, which may explain the complex and differential nature of the effects of thyrotoxicosis on the SNS. Indeed there is convincing evidence that thyroid hormone signalling in the ARC may be responsible for the hyperphagia observed during thyrotoxicosis. Hyperthyroid rats exhibit a marked upregulation of AgRP and NPY mRNA expression in the ARC, as well as a downregulation of POMC mRNA. At the same time a significant upregulation of the hypothalamic mammalian target of rapamycin (mTOR) signalling pathway was observed [46]. Interestingly, mTOR co-localizes with the TR-α in PVN and ARC. Central administration of T_3 or genetic activation of thyroid hormone signalling in the ARC recapitulated the effects of thyrotoxicosis on feeding behavior, whereas central inhibition of the mTOR pathway in thyrotoxic rats with rapamycin reversed hyperphagia. Previously it had been shown that thyroxicosis decreases pAMPK activity in the VMH and that genetic inactivation of this enzyme in the VMH resulted in an increased activity

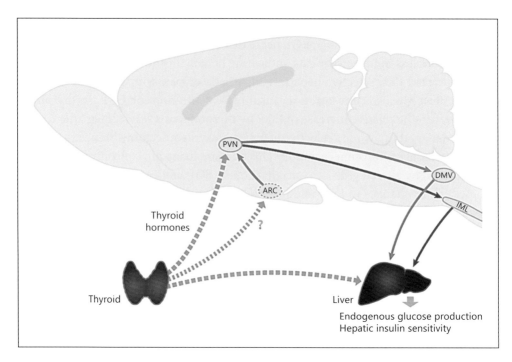

Fig. 4. Humoral and neural pathways for thyroid hormone to affect hepatic glucose metabolism. Sympathetic outflow from the hypothalamic PVN via the IML to the liver is represented in red, whereas parasympathetic outflow via the DMV to the liver is indicated in blue. Thyrotoxicosis results in increased EGP and reduced hepatic insulin sensitivity by thyroid hormone's effects on the liver. Administration of T_3 within the hypothalamic PVN increases hepatic glucose production, without affecting plasma concentrations of glucoregulatory hormones, and this effect can be blocked by a selective hepatic sympathectomy. After a selective hepatic parasympathectomy during systemic thyrotoxicosis, plasma insulin increases without affecting glucose production, indicating hepatic insulin resistance. Both sympathetic and parasympathetic outflow from the hypothalamic PVN to the liver modulates hepatic glucose metabolism. Although the blood-brain barrier is largely absent in the ARC and the ARC expresses thyroid hormone receptors, there are no data at present on the hepatic effects of T_3 administration to the ARC selectively.

of BAT [47]. However, the local changes in ARC thyroid hormone signalling did not seem to affect BAT thermogenic activity, i.e. no changes in BAT UCP1/3, PPAR-γ or PGC-1α/β expression. On the other hand, local administration of T_3 in the VMH did not cause hyperphagia but did activate the thermogenic program in BAT [46].

Thus a picture is unfolding in which changes in thyroid hormone signalling in specific hypothalamic nuclei are responsible for specific changes in energy metabolism. Thyroid hormone signalling in the PVN controls glucose metabolism, while in the VMH it modulates thermogenic BAT activity and in the ARC feeding behavior. Clearly, the picture is not complete yet because thyrotoxicosis increases ARC NPY expression, and increased ARC NPY expression increases BAT activity [26], but local T_3 administration in the ARC does not activate BAT [46]. So how does T_3 activate ARC

NPY expression during thyrotoxicosis? Since, in the study of Shi et al. [26] T_3 was administered systemically and not locally in the hypothalamus, one possibility is that the NPY neurons in the ARC are activated in an indirect manner by T_3 acting in the VMH. The future unravelling of selective TR-α- and TR-β-mediated hypothalamic effects on metabolism will be relevant for the further development of selective thyroid hormone analogues and for the interpretation of their effects.

Estrogen

Estradiol (E_2) plays a major role in the control of energy homeostasis, as is exemplified by the increased body weight in female rats after ovariectomy (OVX), which is reversible with E_2 replacement. Likewise, hormone replacement therapy reverses the development of obesity and metabolic dysfunctions in postmenopausal women. E_2's effects on energy homeostasis are thought to be mediated primarily through the hypothalamus, as direct injections of E_2 into the PVN, ARC or VMH effectively reduce food intake and body weight after OVX in rodents. A link between hypothalamic E_2 receptors, which are widely expressed in the hypothalamus [48], and energy expenditure was elegantly shown by the obese phenotype induced by selective silencing of estrogen receptor (ER)-α in VMH [49, 50]. Together with many more studies, these data have convincingly shown that reduced estrogen signaling in the hypothalamus increases body weight and is associated with impaired glucose tolerance and insulin resistance. Less clear is whether estrogen affects glucose metabolism directly or indirectly – by inducing obesity. When OVX rats are studied before the onset of obesity they exhibit higher glucose/insulin ratios (with decreased plasma insulin concentration) compared to intact rats, suggesting that OVX increases insulin sensitivity. This surprising finding thus indicates a direct obesity-independent effect of estrogen on glucose metabolism.

Considering that the hypothalamus plays a key role in both the regulation of body weight by estrogen and in controlling glucose metabolism, and E_2 receptors (ER) are abundantly expressed in the hypothalamic PVN and VMH [48], we hypothesized that the direct, obesity-independent, effects of estrogen on glucose metabolism may be, at least in part, mediated via the hypothalamus and the ANS. To test our hypothesis, we performed a series of experiments that involved the application of reverse microdialysis, selective hepatic autonomic denervations, euglycemic hyperinsulinemic clamps and stable isotope dilution. In order to prevent any effects of increased adiposity on glucose metabolism, all experiments were performed 1 week after OVX, i.e. before any increase in body weight or adiposity occurred.

OVX caused a 17% decrease in plasma glucose. This decrease was completely restored by systemic E_2. On the other hand, infusion of an E_2 antagonist via reverse microdialysis into the PVN or VMH attenuated the restorative effect of systemic E_2 on plasma glucose. In agreement with these results, also the selective administration of E_2 by microdialysis, either in the PVN or in the VMH, restored the decreased in plasma glucose values due to OVX. In subsequent experiments, we showed that E_2 administration in the VMH, but not in the PVN, increased EGP and induced hepatic insulin resistance, whereas E_2 administration in both the PVN and the VMH resulted in peripheral insulin resistance. Finally, the stimulatory effect of E_2 via the VMH on EGP and plasma glucose concentrations was abolished by a sympathetic, but not a parasympathetic, denervation of the liver. On the other hand, autonomic denervation of the liver (either sympathetic or parasympathetic) had no effect on the stimulatory effect of E_2 on plasma glucose concentrations via the PVN [51]. Contrary to the PVN, there is no evidence for a direct neural connection between the VMH and the parasympathetic and sympathetic motoneurons in respectively DMV and IML, although steroidogenic factor-1 (SF1)-containing neurons in the dorsomedial VMH do project to brainstem areas such as the retrotrapezoid nucleus, nucleus of the solitary tract and the rostral ventrolateral medulla [52]. In addition, the VMH has also pronounced projections to the PVN, i.e. the final neuroendocrine and autonomic output nucleus from the hypothalamus. ER-α is expressed in the majority of glutamatergic neurons in the VMH [53] and the PVN is known to receive a strong glutamatergic input from the VMH [52]. Therefore, we propose that the ER-α-containing glutamatergic neurons in the VMH that project to the PVN are activated by local administration of E_2. This may excite sympathetic pre-autonomic neurons in the PVN that in turn stimulate the hepatic sympathetic tone. Indeed, in 2007, Tong et al. [54] elegantly demonstrated that the knockout of glutamate specifically from the SF-1 neurons in the VMH resulted in a significantly impaired counterregulatory response. In order to explain the opposite effect of the VMH on muscle-dedicated and liver-dedicated pre-autonomic neurons we propose that the glutamatergic projection of the VMH to the muscle-dedicated pre-autonomic neurons involves a GABAergic interneuron in the subPVN which contacts and inhibits the muscle-dedicated pre-autonomic neurons directly (fig. 5). Clearly this hypothesis needs to be investigated further in future studies.

The ANS not only affects hepatic glucose production, but also peripheral glucose uptake. Activation of adrenergic receptors was reported to inhibit insulin-stimulated glucose uptake by 2T3-L1 adipocytes and to stimulate glucose uptake in brown adipocytes. It is not possible to perform similar surgical denervations of muscle as we did for the liver, but β-adrenergic antagonists and knockdown of skeletal β-adrenergic receptors attenuated the modulatory effects of VMH signaling on glucose uptake. We observed that both PVN and VMH E_2 signaling decreased insulin-dependent glucose uptake, taking into account the studies mentioned above, this indicates that E_2 signaling in the PVN and VMH may also regulate glucose uptake by changing autonomic nervous activity. The effect of E_2 in the PVN on glucose uptake indicates that the pre-autonomic neurons in the PVN that control the autonomic nervous input to the muscle probably contain ERs, in contrast to the pre-autonomic PVN neurons that control hepatic glucose production (fig. 5).

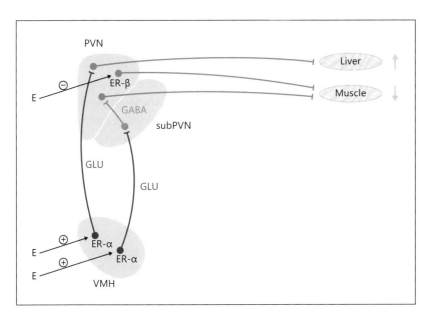

Fig. 5. Graphical representation of the hypothalamic connections that might be involved in the effects of estrogen on glucose metabolism. ER-α-containing glutamatergic (GLU) neurons in the VMH are proposed to project to sympathetic pre-autonomic neurons in the PVN, either directly or indirectly via GABAergic interneurons in the subPVN. Estrogen administration in the VMH will result in a glutamatergic stimulation of the sympathetic input to the liver and thereby increase hepatic glucose production. At the same time, sympathetic pre-autonomic neurons connected to the muscle will be inhibited (due to the GABAergic interneuron) and glucose uptake will be reduced. In addition, we propose that estrogen administration in the PVN can reduce peripheral glucose uptake via pre-autonomic neurons in the PVN that are connected to the muscle and contain the ER-β.

A number of studies have indicated that increased body weight after OVX is not only the result of increased food intake, but also of reduced energy expenditure, as OVX rats need less calories to maintain body weight compared to intact rats. One of the determinants of energy expenditure is adaptive thermogenesis in BAT. Of interest, sympathetic denervation of BAT markedly impairs the estrogen-induced increase in oxygen consumption [55]. This may be explained, at least in part, by effects of estrogen on the expression of UCP in BAT, as UCP expression is downregulated by OVX and upregulated by E_2 supplementation. Selective inhibition of estrogen signaling in the hypothalamus also reduces total energy expenditure, suggesting an important role of the hypothalamus in the effects of estrogen on energy homeostasis [49]. Interestingly, we recently found both β-adrenergic receptor and UCP gene expression in BAT to be increased after hypothalamic E_2 administration, further supporting the idea that indeed hypothalamic E_2 signaling may also play an important role in the modulation of energy metabolism via its effect on the autonomic input into BAT.

E_2 regulates not only energy expenditure but also body fat distribution [49]. This has been documented in humans and in rodent models, but the mechanism is unknown at present. Fat deposition in WAT is mainly regulated by the rate-limiting enzymes involved in lipogenesis and lipolysis, i.e. FAS and lipoprotein lipase (LPL) on the one hand and hormone-sensitive lipase (HSL) on the other. LPL is the rate-limiting enzyme for hydrolysis of the triglyceride component of circulating lipoproteins and thereby is essential for lipogenesis. HSL functions to hydrolyze the first fatty acid from stored triacylglycerol molecules, and is considered the rate-limiting step in lipolysis. Previous studies have shown that systemic E_2 may regulate LPL and FAS gene expression in heart and adipose tissue. In WAT, we found lower HSL and LPL expression after OVX. These observations are in line with other studies showing a lower HSL gene expression in the liver after OVX. Interestingly, higher LPL gene expression was found in subcutaneous WAT after OVX as compared to intact animals. The changes in LPL expression therefore appear to reflect the redistribution of body fat in favor of the abdominal compartment in OVX animals. E_2 administration in either the PVN or VMH acutely reversed the lowered HSL expression in the visceral fat compartments of OVX animals. LPL expression, however, was regulated by hypothalamic estrogen signaling only in gonadal WAT. We did not observe any significant effects of OVX or hypothalamic E_2 signaling on FAS gene expression, suggesting that the hypothalamic E_2 signal affects fat accumulation and distribution primarily by modulating lipolytic genes. We found no effect of hypothalamic E_2 on subcutaneous WAT, again pointing to the concept that the hypothalamic E_2 regulation of fat distribution is primarily effectuated through the accumulation of visceral fat. Previously it was shown that intra-abdominal and subcutaneous fat depots are innervated by separate sets of autonomic neurons [56] and, moreover, that these autonomic neurons in the spinal cord and brainstem are controlled by separate sets of pre-autonomic neurons in higher brain areas [57]. In addition, these neurons were shown to contain estrogen, as well as androgen and glucocorticoid receptors, and subtle neurochemical differences were found between WAT projecting neurons in males and females [58]. Thus, these neural pathways may represent the anatomical substrate for the selectivity of the molecular effects of hypothalamic E_2 as found with the microdialysis studies just described (fig. 6).

Taken together, estrogens also display a nucleus-specific action within the hypothalamus to modulate energy balance, particularly within the ARC, VMH and PVN. VMH-specific delivery of adenoassociated viral vectors silencing ER-α in mice and rats leads to marked obesity, impaired glucose tolerance and reduced energy expenditure [49]. Of note, those animals remain hyperphagic, indicating that estrogens actions in the VMH modulates for energy expenditure but not feeding behavior. In keeping with this, current evidence has also demonstrated that female mice lacking ER-α in hypothalamic SF1 neurons of the VMH exhibit reduced energy expenditure and BAT-mediated thermogenesis, leading to obesity, despite normal feeding. In contrast, deletion of ER-α in POMC of the ARC leads to hyperphagia without changes in energy expenditure. Concomitant deletion of ER-α from both SF1 and POMC neurons recapitulates both phenotypes, causing hypometabolism, hyperphagia, and severe obesity

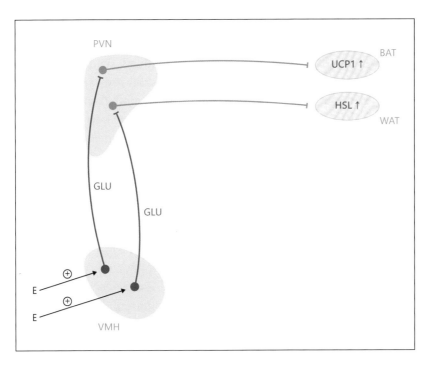

Fig. 6. Graphical representation of the hypothalamic connections that might be involved in the effects of estrogen on lipid metabolism. ER-α-containing glutamatergic (GLU) neurons in the VMH are proposed to project to sympathetic pre-autonomic neurons in the PVN. Estrogen administration in the VMH will result in a glutamatergic stimulation of the sympathetic pre-autonomic neurons and thereby increase UCP1 expression in BAT and HSL expression in WAT.

[50]. In addition, estrogen modulates the activity of the pre-autonomic neurons in the PVN either directly or via its action on other neurons, such as the GABA-containing neurons in the periPVN region, the glutamate-containing neurons in the VMH, and the NPY-containing neurons in the ARC. Future studies are needed to further unravel the neural pathways involved in the different effects of estrogen, as well its local intrahypothalamic interaction with other hormones such as leptin, insulin and thyroid hormone that may use very much similar neural pathways to impose their effect.

Menopause is associated with a shift towards a more masculine body fat distribution, metabolic syndrome and osteoporosis. Although estrogen hormone replacement therapy is one of the most efficient ways to relieve these symptoms, the clinical treatment is challenging since systemic estrogen replacement increases the risk of breast cancer and venous thrombosis. Based on recent studies, indicating central pathways for effects of estrogen that occur independently of estrogen concentrations in the circulation, it may be worthwhile to develop new and more specific ER modulators that primarily target estrogen signaling in the brain [59]. In view of the selectivity of estrogen's central effects, this may be an alternative way to prevent or at least relieve the systemic side effects including increased risk of breast cancer.

Glucocorticoids

Clinical conditions with glucocorticoid excess such as Cushing's syndrome are accompanied by deranged glucose metabolism and hepatic insulin resistance, which is often reversible after treatment. As described above, several hypothalamic nuclei including the ARC and the PVN have recently been shown to mediate hormonal effects on hepatic glucose production and insulin sensitivity. Thus, we wondered whether in addition to their well-known direct peripheral effects, glucocorticoids may also affect glucose metabolism through receptor activation in defined circuits of the central nervous system (CNS).

Glucocorticoid signaling involves two receptor systems, i.e. the mineralocorticoid receptor, which in the CNS is mainly restricted to the septum, hippocampus and amygdala, and the glucocorticoid receptor, which is more widely expressed in different brain regions including the hypothalamus [60]. In the hypothalamus, glucocorticoid receptors are expressed abundantly in the PVN and ARC as demonstrated by immunohistochemistry, in situ hybridization and receptor autoradiography studies. Mineralocorticoid receptors show weak immunoreactivity in the PVN and its mRNA expression is not detectable by in situ hybridization methods. The strong expression of glucocorticoid receptors in the PVN, especially in the parvocellular subdivision, is thought to be mainly involved in the negative feedback of corticosterone on the hypothalamus-pituitary-adrenal (HPA) axis. However, the PVN not only governs neuroendocrine pathways but also represents an important hypothalamic center for the control of the ANS as reflected by the abundance of pre-autonomic neurons. As accumulating evidence suggests that the ANS plays an essential role in the regulation of hepatic glucose metabolism and insulin sensitivity, we hypothesized that glucocorticoid action in the CNS might affect glucose metabolism through activation of receptors on pre-autonomic neurons in the PVN. Interestingly, ICV infusion of dexamethasone (Dex, i.e. a glucocorticoid receptor agonist) stimulates food intake and body weight gain [61], while it decreases peripheral glucose uptake [62]. The specific neuronal targets for these effects of Dex in the CNS have not been clearly identified yet. One obvious possibility is that this phenomenon involves glucocorticoid signaling in the ARC, thereby antagonizing the effects of insulin on NPY-containing ARC neurons. This is supported by the observations that peripheral administration of Dex or corticosterone increases NPY mRNA expression in the ARC [63] (fig. 7).

We investigated whether modulation of hypothalamic glucocorticoid signaling specifically in the ARC or the PVN would influence peripheral glucose metabolism. In all experiments, the retrodialysis technique was used to slowly and exclusively deliver Dex locally into specific hypothalamic nuclei under stress-free experimental conditions. EGP was measured by the stable isotope dilution method and hepatic insulin sensitivity was determined using hyperinsulinemic-euglycemic clamps.

Selective administration of Dex within the PVN and ARC had no effect on either basal plasma glucose concentrations or basal EGP. However, local administration of

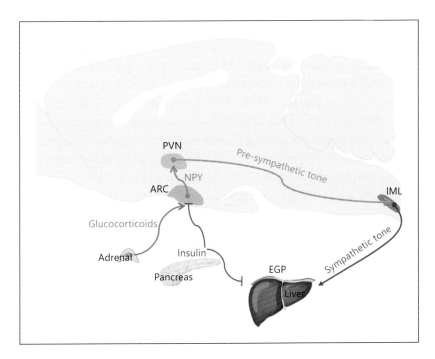

Fig. 7. Mid-sagittal view of the rat brain with a schematic representation of the hypothalamic connections involved in the regulatory effects of circulating glucocorticoids and insulin on hepatic glucose production. Increased plasma insulin concentrations will inhibit hepatic glucose production directly at the level of the liver as well as by inhibiting the activity of the NPY neurons in the ARC. It is well known that increased levels of plasma glucocorticoids will increase hepatic glucose production by increasing gluconeogenesis. We showed that glucocorticoids also counteract the inhibitory effect of insulin at the central level by increasing ARC NPY synthesis and release.

Dex into the ARC, but not into the PVN, during a hyperinsulinemic-euglycemic clamp induced severe hepatic insulin resistance. Dex-ARC-induced hepatic insulin resistance was completely prevented by either ICV co-administration of the NPY1 receptor antagonist BIBP3226 or by hepatic sympathetic denervation [20]. Our data indicate that specific activation of glucocorticoid receptors in the ARC stimulates NPY release, which in turn activates sympathetic pre-autonomic output from hypothalamus to liver [7, 64]. The counteractive effect of Dex on the insulin-induced inhibition of hepatic glucose production thus seems to be mediated by a very specific subset of hypothalamic neurons. On the other hand, the inhibitory effect of Dex on the HPA axis did not differ between ARC and PVN or the area surrounding these two nuclei, as shown by an equal inhibition of the circadian rise in circulating plasma corticosterone levels in all Dex-treated groups [20]. Thus, the feedback action of Dex on the HPA axis seems to be based on a more widespread phenomenon mediated via several hypothalamic circuits. Although all three Dex-treated groups showed a similar inhibitory pattern with regard to the daily rise in plasma corticosterone, the Dex effects on hepatic insulin sensitivity clearly differed between groups. Together, these data indicate that the inhibitory effect of Dex on hepatic insulin sensitivity probably does not involve a change in glucocorticoid signaling within the liver. The clearest evidence for glucocorticoids directly acting on ARC neurons are the changes induced by glucocorticoids in NPY expression and release [63] in conjunction with the presence of glucocorticoid-binding elements in the NPY gene. Together, these data indicate that glucocorticoids capably interact with ARC signaling and that this cross-talk may represent a key mechanism by which ARC neurons control glucose metabolism. Previously, we showed that ICV administration of NPY could prevent the inhibitory effect of systemic hyperinsulinemia on hepatic glucose production. In addition, we showed that the NPY-induced insulin resistance was mediated via sympathetic innervation of the liver [12]. However, owing to the generalized CNS effect inherent to the ICV administration protocols, we were not able to pinpoint the effect of insulin to any specific subpopulation of NPY receptor-containing neurons. In the current study, we uncover a role for the NPY-containing ARC neurons with the help of the more anatomically refined microdialysis technique. The antagonistic effect of the ICV administration of NPY1R receptor antagonist clearly indicates that the main action of Dex in the ARC was to increase NPY activity and release. Our studies suggest that the increased release of NPY by the ARC in turn induces hepatic insulin resistance. Indeed ICV administration of NPY causes an increased EGP [22]. The results of our observations in rodent models with hepatic denervations in our previous study [12] and the current study clearly implicate the sympathetic branch of the ANS in the stimulatory effect of NPY on hepatic glucose production. In view of the ICV administration route of the NPY1R antagonist, however, it is not clear yet which pre-autonomic neurons in the hypothalamus are responsible for the increased sympathetic input to the liver, but recently tyrosine hydroxylase-containing pre-autonomic neurons have been implicated in the stimulatory effect of NPY of BAT activity via the SNS [26]. Chronic ICV infusion of Dex (for 2 days) increases food intake and decreases muscle tissue glucose uptake, and both effects require an intact subdiaphragmatic vagus nerve. Interestingly, some of the metabolic effects of chronic ICV infusion of NPY depend on the presence of circulating corticosterone, since bilateral adrenalectomy prevents the effects on muscle glucose uptake and insulin sensitivity of adipose tissue. Moreover, these effects also depend on an intact subdiaphragmatic vagus nerve [65]. In summary, these data support synergisms in metabolic control on multiple levels between hypothalamic NPY signaling and corticosteroid action in the CNS as well as in the periphery. Intriguingly, some of these earlier experiments implicate the parasympathetic branch of the ANS in the joint metabolic effects of Dex and NPY, whereas in our experiment [20] we did not find any evidence of the involvement of hepatic parasympathetic innervation. Differences in surgical denervation protocols and acute versus chronic study design may account for some of the discordance between studies. Collectively, all available data indicate that depending on the metabolic (im)balance NPY projections orchestrate the balance between sympathetic and parasympathetic pre-autonomic neurons to efficiently adjust hepatic glucose metabolism.

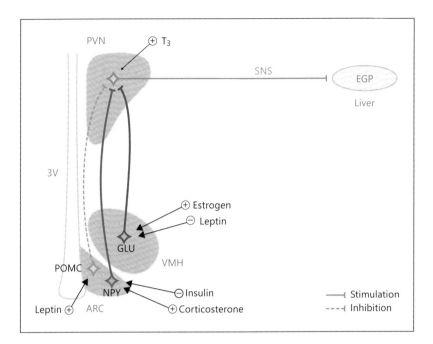

Fig. 8. Graphical representation of the hypothalamic pathways that may be involved in mediating the effects of hormonal feedback on EGP. The most important 'targets' for the hormonal feedback seem to be the NPY-containing neurons in the ARC and glutamatergic (GLU) neurons in the VMH. These neurons can either be stimulated (glucocorticoids, estrogen (E_2)) or inhibited (insulin, leptin) and subsequently increase or decrease the sympathetic (SNS) input to the liver via their connections to the pre-autonomic neurons in the PVN. In addition, thyroid hormone (T_3) may act directly at the level of the pre-autonomic neurons in the PVN, but effects of thyroid hormone via the ARC or VMH have not been excluded.

In conclusion, as the current study used an acute hypercortisolism in specific hypothalamic nuclei to study its effects on hepatic insulin sensitivity, the mechanistic insight reported here only represents a first step towards a better understanding of the metabolic side effects of hypercortisolism. Therefore, whether the currently presented mechanism can fully explain the pathological changes during long-term hypercortisolism (such as Cushing's syndrome) or therapeutic Dex requires further investigation including complex combinations of cell-specific genetic loss- and gain-of-function studies.

Conclusion

As a result of a less complete blood-brain barrier in circumventricular organs, the ARC, next to the median eminence, represents a population of neurons in the brain that is accessible for many blood-borne signals such as insulin, leptin, thyroid hormone, ghrelin, and glucocorticoids. Moreover, the receptors for all of these hormones

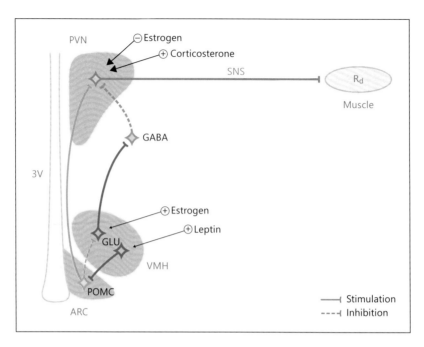

Fig. 9. Graphical representation of the hypothalamic pathways that may be involved in mediating the effects of hormonal feedback on systemic glucose uptake. The most important 'targets' for the hormonal feedback on glucose uptake seem to be the VMH and the PVN. The VMH neurons seem to project to the pre-autonomic neurons in the PVN either via GABAergic neurons in the subPVN or via POMC-containing neurons in the ARC.

are abundantly expressed in this nucleus. The NPY-containing neurons in the ARC represent an important conduit for numerous afferent signals to sense, process, and convey feedback messages to higher brain centers and subsequently back to the periphery. The present overview has provided clear evidence for a mediatory role of the ARC NPY neurons in the effects of insulin and corticosterone on hepatic glucose production and lipid metabolism. These ARC neurons may also contribute to the effects of thyroid hormone, estrogen and leptin on hepatic glucose production (fig. 8). Although at present direct evidence for such a mediatory role is not available, and alternative pathways have been proposed for these hormones, all three have been shown to affect the expression of NPY in the ARC. In addition, the NPY neurons have been assigned a mediatory role in other effects of these hormones, such as the effects of leptin and estrogen on feeding behavior and the effects of thyroid hormone on BAT activity.

As clearly indicated by the reduced heart rate and diastolic blood pressure in the face of severe obesity in MC4R-deficient mice and humans [29], α-MSH also seems to affect the activity of pre-autonomic neurons as well as the ones that are involved in the control glucose metabolism. Indeed, as described above, there are many indications that also the ARC POMC neurons are involved in the control of glucose

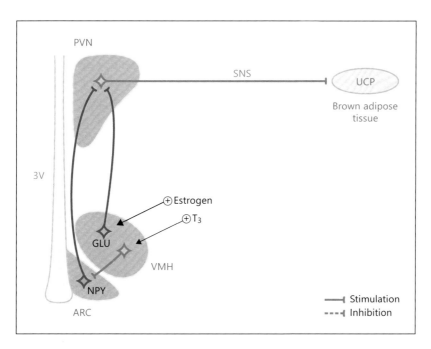

Fig. 10. Graphical representation of the hypothalamic pathways that may be involved in mediating the effects of hormonal feedback on BAT activity. The most important 'targets' for the hormonal feedback on BAT activity seems to be the VMH. The stimulatory effect of thyroid hormone (T_3) seems to involve the projection of NPY-containing neurons in the ARC to the pre-autonomic neurons in the PVN. For estrogen (E_2) it is not clear whether is also involves the NPY-containing neurons in the ARC or direct (glutamatergic) projections from the VM to the pre-autonomic PVN neurons.

metabolism, although it is unclear whether this involves direct projections to the PVN or indirect projections via the VMH. Therefore, at present the exact mechanism remains elusive.

For some hormones the VMH seems to be the primary target as it relates to their effects on glucose metabolism, but still the ARC might be involved in their ultimate effect through the direct projection of many VMH neurons to the ARC [52]. Especially for the effects of leptin via the VMH on glucose uptake, some clear evidence is available for an involvement of the POMC-containing ARC neurons [32] (fig. 9). In a similar way the effect of thyroid hormone in the VMH seems to involve a connection via the NPY-containing neurons in the ARC and their projections to pre-autonomic neurons in the PVN [26] (fig. 10). On the other hand, in the study of Toda et al. [32] it also became clear that leptin influences hepatic glucose production via other, non-ARC, projections of the VMH. Likely this non-ARC connection involves the glutamatergic projections from the VMH to the PVN as proposed in our study investigating the effects of hypothalamic estrogen on glucose metabolism (fig. 6, 8).

The PVN does not seem to be the prime target as it concerns the glucoregulatory effects of many hormones. Inhibition of EGP was seen after GLP-1 administration in the ARC, but GLP-1 had no effect on EGP after injection in the third ventricle or PVN. In contrast, ARC GLP-1 injection had no effect on food intake, but food intake was suppressed after GLP-1 injection in the PVN [66]. On the other hand, we did find that local administration of thyroid hormone increased hepatic glucose production and that local administration of estrogen and Dex decreased and increased glucose uptake, respectively (fig. 9). Although the receptors for all three hormones are present in the PVN, it is not known whether they are present on the pre-autonomic neurons that control the autonomic input to the muscle or whether this involves an indirect effect of these hormones.

It may be clear that although we have come a long way to unravel and understand the hypothalamic control of glucose and lipid metabolism, a more detailed deciphering of the neuroanatomical details is still necessary to come to a full understanding.

References

1 Buijs RM, Kalsbeek A: Hypothalamic integration of central and peripheral clocks. Nat Neurosci Rev 2001;2:521–526

2 Colwell CS: Preventing dehydration during sleep. Nat Neurosci 2010;13:403–404.

3 Kalsbeek A, Yi CX, La Fleur SE, Fliers E: The hypothalamic clock and its control of glucose homeostasis. Trends Endocrinol Metab 2010;21:402–410.

4 Campfield LA, Smith FJ, Guisez Y, Devos R, Burn P: Recombinant mouse OB protein: evidence for a peripheral signal linking adiposity and central neural networks. Science 1995;269:546–549.

5 Obici S, Feng Z, Karkanias G, Baskin DG, Rossetti L: Decreasing hypothalamic insulin receptors causes hyperphagia and insulin resistance in rats. Nat Neurosci 2002;5:566–572.

6 Obici S, Zhang BB, Karkanias G, Rossetti L: Hypothalamic insulin signaling is required for inhibition of glucose production. Nat Med 2002;8:1376–1382.

7 Stanley S, Pinto S, Segal J, et al: Identification of neuronal subpopulations that project from hypothalamus to both liver and adipose tissue polysynaptically. Proc Natl Acad Sci USA 2010;107:7024–7029.

8 La Fleur SE, Kalsbeek A, Wortel J, Buijs RM: Polysynaptic neural pathways between the hypothalamus, including the suprachiasmatic nucleus, and the liver. Brain Res 2000;871:50–56.

9 Buijs RM, la Fleur SE, Wortel J, et al: The suprachiasmatic nucleus balances sympathetic and parasympathetic output to peripheral organs through separate pre-autonomic neurons. J Comp Neurol 2003; 464:36–48.

10 Luiten PGM, Ter Horst GJ, Steffens AB: The hypothalamus, intrinsic connections and outflow pathways to the endocrine system in relation to the control of feeding and metabolism. Prog Neurobiol 1987;28:1–54.

11 Yi CX, la Fleur SE, Fliers E, Kalsbeek A: The role of the autonomic nervous liver innervation in the control of energy metabolism. Biochim Biophys Acta 2010;1802:416–431.

12 Van den Hoek AM, van Heijningen C, Schroder-van der Elst JP, et al: Intracerebroventricular administration of neuropeptide Y induces hepatic insulin resistance via sympathetic innervation. Diabetes 2008;57: 2304–2310.

13 Chee MJ, Colmers WF: Y eat? Nutrition 2008;24: 869–877.

14 Marks JL, Waite K: Intracerebroventricular neuropeptide Y acutely influences glucose metabolism and insulin sensitivity in the rat. J Neuroendocrinol 1997; 9:99–103.

15 Van den Hoek AM, Voshol PJ, Karnekamp BN, et al: Intracerebroventricular neuropeptide Y infusion precludes inhibition of glucose and VLDL production by insulin. Diabetes 2004;53:2529–2534.

16 Van den Top M, Spanswick D: Integration of metabolic stimuli in the hypothalamic arcuate nucleus. Prog Brain Res 2006;153:141–154.

17 Pocai A, Obici S, Schwartz GJ, Rossetti L: A brain-liver circuit regulates glucose homeostasis. Cell Metab 2005;1:3–11.

18 Zarjevski N, Cusin I, Vettor R, Rohner-Jeanrenaud F, Jeanrenaud B: Chronic intracerebroventricular neuropeptide-Y administration to normal rats mimics hormonal and metabolic changes of obesity. Endocrinology 1993;133:1753–1758.

19 Rojas JM, Stafford JM, Saadat S, Printz RL, Beck-Sickinger AG, Niswender KD: Central nervous system neuropeptide Y signaling via the Y1 receptor partially dissociates feeding behavior from lipoprotein metabolism in lean rats. Am J Physiol Endocrinol Metab 2012;303:E1479–E1488.

20 Yi CX, Foppen E, Abplanalp W, et al: Glucocorticoid signaling in the arcuate nucleus modulates hepatic insulin sensitivity. Diabetes 2012;61:339–345.

21 Stafford JM, Yu F, Printz R, Hasty AH, Swift LL, Niswender KD: Central nervous system neuropeptide Y signaling modulates VLDL triglyceride secretion. Diabetes 2008;57:1482–1490.

22 Bruinstroop E, Pei L, Ackermans MT, et al: Hypothalamic neuropeptide Y controls hepatic VLDL-triglyceride secretion in rats via the sympathetic nervous system. Diabetes 2012;61:1043–1050.

23 Scherer T, O'Hare J, Diggs-Andrews K, et al: Brain insulin controls adipose tissue lipolysis and lipogenesis. Cell Metab 2011;13:183–194.

24 Coomans CP, Biermasz NR, Geerling JJ, Guigas B, Rensen PC, Havekes LM, Romijn JA: Stimulatory effect of insulin on glucose uptake by muscle involves the central nervous system in insulin-sensitive mice. Diabetes 2011;60:3132–3140.

25 Tiesjema B, Adan RAH, Luijendijk MC, Kalsbeek A, la Fleur SE: Differential effects of recombinant adeno-associated virus-mediated neuropeptide Y overexpression in the hypothalamic paraventricular nucleus and lateral hypothalamus on feeding behavior. J Neurosci 2007;27:14139–14146.

26 Shi YC, Lau J, Lin Z, et al: Arcuate NPY controls sympathetic output and BAT function via a relay of tyrosine hydroxylase neurons in the PVN. Cell Metab 2013;17:236–248.

27 Farooqi IS: Monogenic human obesity. Front Horm Res 2008;36:1–11.

28 Konner AC, Janoschek R, Plum L, et al: Insulin action in AgRP-expressing neurons is required for suppression of hepatic glucose production. Cell Metab 2007;5:438–449.

29 Farooqi S: Obesity genes – it's all about the parents! Cell Metab 2009;9:487–488.

30 Rossi J, Balthasar N, Olson D, et al: Melanocortin-4 receptors expressed by cholinergic neurons regulate energy balance and glucose homeostasis. Cell Metab 2011;13:195–204.

31 Gutierrez-Juarez R, Obici S, Rossetti L: Melanocortin-independent effects of leptin on hepatic glucose fluxes. J Biol Chem 2004;279:49704–49715.

32 Toda C, Shiuchi T, Lee S, et al: Distinct effects of leptin and a melanocortin receptor agonist injected into medial hypothalamic nuclei on glucose uptake in peripheral tissues. Diabetes 2009;58:2757–2765.

33 German J, Kim F, Schwartz GJ, et al: Hypothalamic leptin signaling regulates hepatic insulin sensitivity via a neurocircuit involving the vagus nerve. Endocrinology 2009;150:4502–4511.

34 Perez-Tilve D, Hofmann SM, Basford J, et al: Melanocortin signaling in the CNS directly regulates circulating cholesterol. Nat Neurosci 2010;13:877–882.

35 Lam TK, Gutierrez-Juarez R, Pocai A, et al: Brain glucose metabolism controls the hepatic secretion of triglyceride-rich lipoproteins. Nat Med 2007;13:171–180.

36 Bruinstroop E, la Fleur SE, Ackermans MT, et al: The autonomic nervous system regulates postprandial hepatic lipid metabolism. Am J Physiol Endocrinol Metab 2013;304:E1089–E1096.

37 Tu T, Nash CW: The influence of prolonged hyper- and hypothyroid states on the noradrenaline content of rat tissues and on the accumulation and efflux rates of tritiated noradrenaline. Can J Physiol Pharmacol 1975;53:74–80.

38 Matsukawa T, Mano T, Gotoh E, Minamisawa K, Ishii M: Altered muscle sympathetic nerve activity in hyperthyroidism and hypothyroidism. J Auton Nerv Syst 1993;42:171–175.

39 Chen JL, Chiu HW, Tseng YJ, Chu WC: Hyperthyroidism is characterized by both increased sympathetic and decreased vagal modulation of heart rate: evidence from spectral analysis of heart rate variability. Clin Endocrinol (Oxf) 2006;64:611–616.

40 Haluzik M, Nedvidkova J, Bartak V, et al: Effects of hypo- and hyperthyroidism on noradrenergic activity and glycerol concentrations in human subcutaneous abdominal adipose tissue assessed with microdialysis. J Clin Endocrinol Metab 2003;88:5605–5608.

41 Silva JE, Bianco SD: Thyroid-adrenergic interactions: physiological and clinical implications. Thyroid 2008;18:157–165.

42 Klieverik LP, Coomans CP, Endert E, et al: Thyroid hormone effects on whole-body energy homeostasis and tissue-specific fatty acid uptake in vivo. Endocrinology 2009;150:5639–5648.

43 Fliers E, Unmehopa UA, Alkemade A: Functional neuroanatomy of thyroid hormone feedback in the human hypothalamus and pituitary gland. Mol Cell Endocrinol 2006;251:1–8.

44 Klieverik LP, Janssen SF, van Riel A, et al: Thyroid hormone modulates glucose production via a sympathetic pathway from the hypothalamic paraventricular nucleus to the liver. Proc Natl Acad Sci USA 2009;106:5966–5971.

45 Sjögren M, Alkemade A, Mittag J, et al: Hypermetabolism in mice caused by the central action of an unliganded thyroid hormone receptor α_1. EMBO J 2007;26:4535–4545.

46 Varela L, Martinez-Sanchez N, Gallego R, et al: Hypothalamic mTOR pathway mediates thyroid hormone-induced hyperphagia in hyperthyroidism. J Pathol 2012;227:209–222.

47 Lopez M, Varela L, Vazquez M, et al: Hypothalamic AMPK and fatty acid metabolism mediate thyroid regulation of energy balance. Nat Med 2010;16: 1001–1009.

48 Shughrue PJ, Lane MV, Merchenthaler I: Comparative distribution of estrogen receptor-α and -β mRNA in the rat central nervous system. J Comp Neurol 1997;388:507–525.

49 Musatov S, Chen W, Pfaff DW, et al: Silencing of estrogen receptor α in the ventromedial nucleus of hypothalamus leads to metabolic syndrome. Proc Natl Acad Sci USA 2007;104:2501–2506.

50 Xu Y, Nedungadi TP, Zhu L, et al: Distinct hypothalamic neurons mediate estrogenic effects on energy homeostasis and reproduction. Cell Metab 2011;14: 453–465.

51 Liu J, Bisschop PH, Eggels L, et al: Intrahypothalamic estradiol regulates glucose metabolism via the sympathetic nervous system in female rats. Diabetes 2012;62:435–443.

52 Lindberg D, Chen P, Li C: Conditional viral tracing reveals that steroidogenic factor 1-positive neurons of the dorsomedial subdivision of the ventromedial hypothalamus project to autonomic centers of the hypothalamus and hindbrain. J Comp Neurol 2013; 521:3167–3190.

53 Pompolo S, Pereira A, Scott CJ, Fujiyma F, Clarke IJ: Evidence for estrogenic regulation of gonadotropin-releasing hormone neurons by glutamatergic neurons in the ewe brain: an immunohistochemical study using an antibody against vesicular glutamate transporter-2. J Comp Neurol 2003;465:136–144.

54 Tong Q, Ye C, McCrimmon RJ, Dhillon H, Choi B, Kramer MD, et al: Synaptic glutamate release by ventromedial hypothalamic neurons is part of the neurocircuitry that prevents hypoglycemia. Cell Metab 2007;5:383–393.

55 Bartness TJ, Wade GN: Effects of interscapular brown adipose tissue denervation on body weight and energy metabolism in ovariectomized and estradiol-treated rats. Behav Neurosci 1984;98:674–685.

56 Youngstrom TG, Bartness TJ: Catecholaminergic innervation of white adipose tissue in Siberian hamsters. Am J Physiol 1995;268:R744–R751.

57 Kreier F, Kap YS, Mettenleiter TC, et al: Tracing from fat tissue, liver, and pancreas: a neuroanatomical framework for the role of the brain in type 2 diabetes. Endocrinology 2006;147:1140–1147.

58 Adler ES, Hollis JH, Clarke IJ, Grattan DR, Oldfield BJ: Neurochemical characterization and sexual dimorphism of projections from the brain to abdominal and subcutaneous white adipose tissue in the rat. J Neurosci 2012;32:15913–15921.

59 Finan B, Yang B, Ottaway N, et al: Targeted estrogen delivery reverses the metabolic syndrome. Nat Med 2012;18:1847–1856.

60 Reul JMHM, De Kloet ER: Two receptor systems for corticosterone in rat brain: microdistribution and differential occupation. Endocrinology 1985;117: 2505–2511.

61 Zakrzewska KE, Cusin I, Stricker-Krongrad A, et al: Induction of obesity and hyperleptinemia by central glucocorticoid infusion in the rat. Diabetes 1999;48: 365–370.

62 Cusin I, Rouru J, Rohner-Jeanrenaud F: Intracerebroventricular glucocorticoid infusion in normal rats: induction of parasympathetic-mediated obesity and insulin resistance. Obes Res 2001;9:401–406.

63 Akabayashi A, Watanabe Y, Wahlestedt C, McEwen BS, Paez X, Leibowitz SF: Hypothalamic neuropeptide Y, its gene expression and receptor activity: relation to circulating corticosterone in adrenalectomized rats. Brain Research 1994;665:201–212.

64 Vinuela MC, Larsen PJ: Identification of NPY-induced c-Fos expression in hypothalamic neurones projecting to the dorsal vagal complex and the lower thoracic spinal cord. J Comp Neurol 2001;438:286–299.

65 Sainsbury A, Rohner-Jeanrenaud F, Cusin I, et al: Chronic central neuropeptide Y infusion in normal rats: status of the hypothalamo-pituitary-adrenal axis, and vagal mediation of hyperinsulinaemia. Diabetologia 1997;40:1269–1277.

66 Sandoval D, Cota D, Seeley RJ: The integrative role of CNS fuel-sensing mechanisms in energy balance and glucose regulation. Annu Rev Physiol 2008;70: 513–535.

A. Kalsbeek, PhD
Department of Endocrinology and Metabolism
Academic Medical Center, University of Amsterdam
Meibergdreef 9, NL–1105 AZ Amsterdam (The Netherlands)
E-Mail a.kalsbeek@amc.uva.nl

Delhanty PJD, van der Lely AJ (eds): How Gut and Brain Control Metabolism.
Front Horm Res. Basel, Karger, 2014, vol 42, pp 29–49 (DOI: 10.1159/000358313)

The Blood-Brain Barrier as a Regulator of the Gut-Brain Axis

Marie Schaeffer[a-c] · David J. Hodson[a-d] · Patrice Mollard[a-c]

[a]Institut de Génomique Fonctionnelle, UMR-5203, CNRS, [b]U661, INSERM, and [c]UMR-5203, Universities of Montpellier 1 & 2, Montpellier, France; [d]Section of Cell Biology, Division of Diabetes, Endocrinology and Metabolism, Department of Medicine, Imperial College London, London, UK

Abstract

The gut-brain axis is involved in metabolic homeostasis through optimization of nutrient absorption and appetite regulation, and encompasses a two-way communication between the gastrointestinal tract and neural circuits in the brain. An important feature of this axis is the secretion of gut-derived peptide hormones which signal energy status to the brain, provoking adaptive behaviors such as food intake or satiation. However, the major integrator of gut signals, the arcuate nucleus of the hypothalamus, is protected by blood-brain barrier, an obstacle to free diffusion of circulating molecules. The aim of this chapter is to therefore review and summarize recent findings regarding the mechanisms underlying entry of gastrointestinal tract hormones into the central nervous system, and identify how these become dysregulated in socioeconomically-costly metabolic diseases such as obesity and type 2 diabetes.

The Gut-Brain Axis

Central effects of gut hormones, previously reviewed thoroughly [1], can be both direct and indirect. Firstly, many gut peptides are able to act directly on the hypothalamus to regulate food intake. Since various neurons in the arcuate nucleus (ARC) of the hypothalamus express receptors for appetite-regulating hormones, the ARC constitutes the primary site of integration for nutrient-related peptides in the central nervous system (CNS) [2, 3]. Circulating factors principally modify the activity of two functionally opposing neuron populations within the ARC: the food intake-activating agouti-related peptide/neuropeptide Y (AgRP/NPY)-expressing neurons, and the food intake-inhibiting proopiomelanocortin and cocaine- and amphetamine-related transcript (POMC/CART)-expressing neurons [1]. From the ARC, signals are relayed to postsynaptic neurons charged with evoking a homeostatic response. Indeed, NPY and POMC neuronal populations send axonal projections into the paraventricular nucleus (PVN), and other areas of the brain [1]. In addition, some gut hormones can directly or indirectly act on nuclei linked with feeding behaviors, such as the PVN, but also the ventromedial nucleus (VMN) or the lateral hypothalamic area (LHA) [1]. Besides homeostatic pathways, hormones such as ghrelin can target mesolimbic circuits linked to reward, which can in turn modify feeding behavior and energy homeostasis by biasing preference towards foods associated with pleasure enhancement [for review, see 4]. Secondly, an indirect effect of gut peptides on the ARC is provided via the activation of distant brainstem areas which house key nuclei [5]. For example, signals generated through binding of gut hormones to gastric vagal afferent neurons are thought to be integrated at the level of the nucleus of the tractus solitarius (NTS) before transmission to the ARC [6].

While efforts have historically focused upon understanding the effects of gut-derived hormones on appetite-regulating neurons and central integration of satiety cues, the mechanisms of molecule entry into the CNS remain largely obscure.

Peripheral Signals Regulating Energy Balance

At the beginning of the last century, the discovery of secretin, a molecule liberated by the intestine and capable of stimulating exocrine pancreas secretion, gave rise to the idea that gut function may be regulated by circulating factors. It was not until the mid-seventies that other major gut hormones started to be identified [7]. The gastroenteropancreatic system is now recognized as a major endocrine system, secreting a plethora of hormones [8]. The primary purpose of gut peptides is to participate in nutrient digestion and absorption, as well as promote efficient energy uptake and utilization. In addition, gastrointestinal hormones play a role in nutrient delivery to different compartments by acting on gastric-emptying and gut motility, and affect appetite through control of satiety, which has long-term effects on body weight regulation. It is this latter role in energy homeostasis, coupled with the burgeoning twin epidemics of obesity and diabetes, that has spurred a renewed interest in gut hormone action during recent years.

Peripheral hormones acting on brain areas implicated in homeostatic control of food intake are generally derived from four major sources: the gastrointestinal tract (GIT), the pancreas, the stomach and adipose tissue [8]. While insulin, and leptin, also termed 'adiposity signals', primarily deliver long-term information to the CNS relating to energy stores, nutrient-related gastrointestinal peptides relay short-term signals to the brain, usually to trigger meal termination [9]. Most gut-derived hormones are therefore classified as anorexigenic [2] and act to reduce food

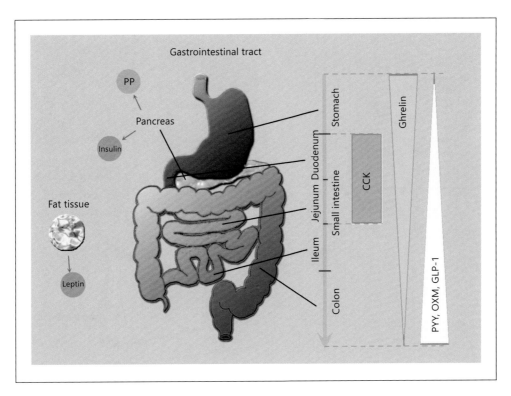

Fig. 1. Peripheral signals modifying food intake and their sites of production. CCK = Cholecystokinin; GLP-1 = glucagon-like peptide 1; OXM = oxyntomodulin; PYY = peptide YY; PP = pancreatic polypeptide.

intake. These satiety signals, secreted principally by the intestine and the pancreas, include cholecystokinin (CCK), peptide YY (PYY), pancreatic polypeptide (PP), oxyntomodulin (OXM), and the incretins gastric inhibitory polypeptide (GIP) and glucagon-like peptide 1 (GLP-1). The only orexigenic hormone is ghrelin, principally produced in conditions of food restriction by the stomach and, to a lower extent, the upper intestine to promote meal initiation [10]. Principal peripheral hormones affecting food intake and their sites of production are summarized in figure 1.

In addition to roles in regulation of immediate food intake, some hormones such as ghrelin and PYY [2, 10] have dual long- and short-term effects on energy homeostasis. Chronic elevation of plasma ghrelin promotes weight gain, and concentrations are inversely correlated with body fat stores [11]. Similarly, levels of the satiety signal PYY are modified by energy store status, being attenuated in obese subjects [3]. As gut hormones and their roles are reviewed in detail elsewhere [8], we will briefly describe the major GIT hormones, with emphasis on their central targets and putative mechanisms of transport into the CNS. An overview of gut hormones and their sites of integration in the brain is provided in figure 2.

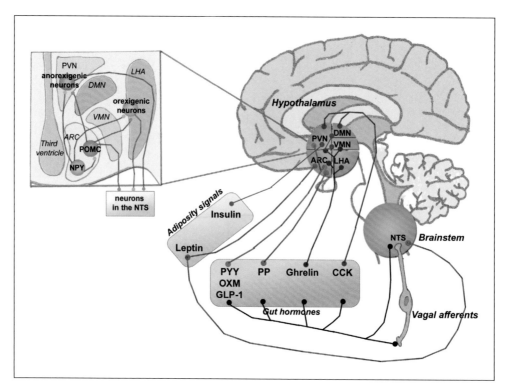

Fig. 2. Central integration of peripheral signals and neuronal circuits regulating appetite. Lines represent direct effects of hormones at target sites. Left insert illustrates neuronal circuits regulating food intake within the hypothalamus. CCK = Cholecystokinin; GLP-1 = glucagon-like peptide 1; OXM = oxyntomodulin; PYY = peptide YY; PP = pancreatic polypeptide; NTS = nucleus of the solitary tract; PVN = paraventricular nucleus; DMN = dorsomedial nucleus; VMN = ventromedial nucleus; LHA = lateral hypothalamic area; ARC = arcuate nucleus; NPY = neuropeptide Y neurons; POMC = proopiomelanocortin neurons.

Gut Hormones

Ghrelin

Ghrelin is an *n*-octanoylated 28-amino-acid peptide (~3 kDa in size), principally secreted preprandially by X/A-like endocrine cells in the gastric fundus [12]. Posttranslational peptide modification is necessary for activity and binding to its specific receptor, the growth hormone secretagogue receptor 1a (GHS-R1a), underlies the majority of ghrelin effects [13]. GHS-R1a expression in the periphery is found in the pituitary gland and reflects the neuroendocrine functions of ghrelin, acting at both pituitary and hypothalamic levels to potentiate growth hormone releasing hormone-stimulated growth hormone (GHRH) release [12]. Ghrelin receptors can also be found in the pancreas, the GIT, immune cells or the heart, and roles for ghrelin in glucose metabolism, intestinal emptying, and immune or cardiac functions have also been described [13].

Schaeffer · Hodson · Mollard

In addition, GHS-R1a is abundantly expressed in the CNS, in particular in hypothalamic neurons of the ARC, as well as other hypothalamic regions involved in food intake control, such as the VMN, the PVN, or the LHA [14], consistent with ghrelin's main role in regulation of energy homeostasis. Although a central production of ghrelin may exist [15], the exact localization of ghrelin-producing cells remains to be clarified [16], the physiological role for central ghrelin has not been elucidated, and it is generally accepted that peripherally-secreted ghrelin plays the major part in generating effects on food intake regulation. In the ARC, GHS-R1a receptors are strongly co-localized with NPY, and ghrelin is able to modulate the electrical activity of both NPY and POMC neurons [15]. Ghrelin respectively stimulates and inhibits NPY and POMC neuron activity through GABAergic inputs originating from NPY axons [15]. In addition, ghrelin is able to bind POMC neurons and similar direct effects have been reported for PVN, VMN, and LHA populations [17]. GHRS-R1a receptors are also expressed in the vagus nerve, and the NTS and area postrema (AP) of the brainstem, from where they may mediate motor responses associated with changes in appetite [13]. Indirect effects of ghrelin on hypothalamic structures may be mediated through: (1) stimulation of brainstem regions; (2) binding to gastric vagal nerve afferents; (3) inhibition of NTS catecholaminergic neurons [18], and (4) actions upon AP neurons [19]. Lastly, GHS-R1a is expressed in areas of the brain involved in emotion, memory and reward-seeking behavior, such as the dentate gyrus, CA2 and CA3 regions of the hippocampus and ventral tegmental area [20], reflecting ghrelin's role in increasing desire for food intake and non-homeostatic feeding behavior. These effects are thought to be mediated through action on GHS-R1a receptor-expressing dopaminergic neurons, inducing dopamine release [4]. In addition, heterodimerization of GHS-R1a with dopamine receptors has been recently described [21], providing a functional role for GHS-R1a in neuronal populations not immediately accessible to peripheral or central ghrelin.

Despite a role for ghrelin in efficiently inducing food intake in both rodents and humans, ghrelin and GHS-R1a knockout mice present normal growth and weight when fed with standard chow [22], perhaps in part due to genomic plasticity induced by embryonic/early postnatal gene deletion. However, chronic ghrelin administration in rodent induces obesity [23], and ghrelin plasma levels are decreased in obese individuals and increased in anorexic patients, presumably to adapt food intake to need [10].

Since peripheral injection of ghrelin can stimulate feeding almost instantly (<10 min) [24], detection of circulating peptide needs to be rapid, and mechanisms of ghrelin transport need to be plastic to adapt to metabolic needs. A recent study investigated the diffusion kinetics of a fully functional fluorescence ghrelin derivative directly in vivo at the level of the median eminence (ME) using a two-photon microscope custom-adapted with long-distance objectives [17], and demonstrated that ghrelin crosses the fenestrated capillaries of the ME by passive diffusion processes, as opposed to a rate-limited active transport. Although a role for receptor-mediated transport cannot be excluded, the kinetics of ghrelin entry into the cerebrospinal fluid (CSF) after intravenous injection (in sheep, rate doubles after 50 min [24]) are not consistent with transport through the choroid plexus to act on appetite-modifying neurons in the ARC, no specific transport mechanism could be identified in the blood-to-brain direction through the blood-brain barrier (BBB), and the rate of transport of ghrelin across the BBB was much lower when studied by brain perfusion than by intravenous injection [25]. Furthermore, fluorescent ghrelin was found to very rapidly (<5 min) label NPY and POMC neurons in the ARC in close proximity to fenestrated capillary loops located in the vmARC projecting from the ME [26]. Similarly, access to brainstem regions could be mediated by passive diffusion of ghrelin through fenestrated vessels of the AP and subsequent delivery to the dorsal vagal complex, known to communicate with hypothalamic centers, although this remains to be investigated.

Cholecystokinin
CCK was one of the first anorexigenic hormones to be described [7]. Levels of this peptide in both the periphery and brain rise rapidly in the immediate postprandial period. In the periphery, CCK is produced by I-cells of the duodenum and the jejunum, while in the brain it is produced by neurons of the PVN and VMH [27]. A number of different bioactive forms result from posttranslational processing events, with the short form, CCK-8, being the major isoform in the CNS [27]. CCK expressed in the CNS acts directly on centers involved in reward-seeking behavior, memory and satiety, while peripheral CCK acts on the vagus [28]. Two different CCK receptors have been identified, CCK-1 and CCK-2, the former being predominantly expressed along the GIT, especially in the vagal nerves pervading the gut, and the latter being localized to the CNS [29]. The main roles of CCK are to inhibit food intake, stimulate gallbladder contraction, and increase secretion of digestive enzymes from the pancreas. Effects of CCK on appetite are mediated both through binding to CCK-1 directly in the CNS, in particular the NTS, the dorsomedial nucleus (DMN) and the AP, and through transmission via vagal afferent fibers from the periphery [27]. CCK-1 receptor knockout rats are obese and hyperphagic [30], which suggests a link between CCK effects on satiety and alterations in food intake. Furthermore, chronic reduction in CCK signaling increases weight gain in rodent models, which supports a role for CCK in long-term energy balance [31].

There is no evidence that CCK is able to translocate across the BBB. However, CCK produced locally in the brain may directly act as a neurotransmitter, as exemplified by its effects on the DMH to suppress NPY levels [30]. In addition, given its small molecular weight (about 1 kDa for CCK-8), peripheral CCK may be able to directly diffuse through fenestrated capillaries of the AP, one of the circumventricular organs (CVOs), and subsequently reach its target neurons in the AP and the NTS, as has been shown for ghrelin [17].

Peptide YY

PYY belongs to the polypeptide-fold (PP) family of proteins, together with NPY and pancreatic PP peptides, which are 36-amino-acid peptides with a C-terminal amidation. The truncated 34-amino-acid long PYY_{3-36} is the major circulating form produced by enteroendocrine L-cells which line the GIT, with increasing expression in the hindgut [32]. PYY is also expressed in the CNS, exclusively in neurons located in the gigantocellular reticular nucleus [33]. In addition to local effects in the digestive tract to suppress secretion, gut motility and gastric emptying, PYY is also a satiety signal, with levels respectively increased and reduced by food ingestion and fasting. Five Y-receptor subtypes mediate the effects of this family of peptides [34]. While uncleaved PYY binds to all five Y-receptor subclasses with similar affinity, PYY_{3-36} promotes satiety and weight loss through specific interaction with Y2 receptors [2]. Y2 receptors are expressed in different tissues, particularly on NPY neurons in the ARC of the hypothalamus [34]. Y1 and Y5 receptors are found in other brain regions involved in food intake, such as the PVN [34]. Centrally produced PYY_{3-36} may exert its orexigenic effects through binding to Y1 receptors since the rodent equivalent of gastric bypass surgery induces a decrease in CNS expression of both PYY and Y1 receptor which is correlated with weight loss [33]. Peripheral PYY_{3-36} inhibits food intake through binding to Y2 receptors on both vagal afferent neurons [35] and NPY neurons in the ARC to reduce NPY expression [2]. This is consistent with peripheral the ability of PYY_{3-36} to enter the brain through CVOs such as the AP and the subfornical organ, and to cross the BBB by transmembrane diffusion [36]. Y2 receptors are also expressed in other regions of the brain, such as the NTS, and additional effects on food inhibition may occur through entry into the AP and subsequent transmission of signals to the ARC [2].

Chronic treatment of rodents with PYY_{3-36} induces a reduction in food intake and weight [2], and PYY secretion in response to food ingestion may be impaired in obese individuals [37], supporting a role for PPY in both rapid food-related signaling of satiety to the CNS and long-term energy homeostasis.

Pancreatic Polypeptide

PP is another member of the PP-fold family. It is secreted postprandially under vagal cholinergic control [38] predominantly in the pancreas by F (or PP) cells located at the islet periphery, although some is also secreted from the distal GIT [39]. To date, there is no evidence for PP expression in the brain [39]. PP effects include inhibition of pancreatic and gallbladder secretions, inhibition of gut motility and signaling of satiety. PP binds preferentially to Y4 receptors, and biological effects on digestion and food intake control involve binding of vagus nerve Y4 receptors [38]. In addition, Y4 receptor-dependent *cfos* induction can be found in regions of the brain involved in depressive behavior, as well as feeding, such as the hypothalamus and the brainstem (NTS and AP) [40]. Knockout mice models of the Y4 receptor present increased feeding behavior and higher levels of PP in the plasma [41]. Mice in which PP is overexpressed conversely present reduced weight gain and food intake [35].

PP is thought to enter the brain through a saturable receptor-mediated transport mechanism at the level of the cerebellum, and entry is highly facilitated in the AP outside the BBB [42]. Again, given PP's small molecular weight (~4 kDa), it may be able to directly diffuse through fenestrated capillaries of CVOs to reach its target neurons. Since effects on reducing anxiety can only be observed following peripheral administration and not following intracerebroventricular injection [43], it is likely that access of PP to the brain is not equivalent in all regions of the CNS, and that this differential access plays a major role in regulating PP effects.

Preproglucagon Cleavage Products (OXM and GLP-1)

OXM is secreted together with GLP-1 and PYY from enteroendocrine intestinal L-cells following food ingestion [44]. OXM is a 37-amino-acid long peptide resulting from cleavage of preproglucagon. Maturation of preproglucagon, also synthesized in pancreatic α-cells and in the CNS (exclusively in NTS neurons projecting into the PVN and the hypothalamus [45]), is tissue-specific. In the brain and the GIT, preproglucagon is mainly cleaved into GLP-1 and OXM, whereas in the pancreas it gives rise to glucagon [46]. OXM actions include inhibition of gastric motility and secretion, stimulation of glycogenolysis, and stimulation of insulin secretion through an incretin-like effect [47]. OXM also acts as a powerful anorectic, inhibiting food intake and energy expenditure, and inducing weight loss [48]. OXM is a full agonist of the GLP-1 receptor (GLP-1R) and the glucagon receptor (GCGR), with reduced affinity compared to GLP-1 and glucagon, respectively [49]. Central anorectic effects of OXM are mediated principally through GLP-1R binding, while effects on glucose metabolism are mainly achieved through GCGR activation [47]. In addition to expression in various peripheral sites such as the pancreas, the heart and the gut, GLP-1R is widely expressed throughout the CNS. It is particularly abundant in a number of areas important in food intake regulation, such as the ARC, the supraoptic nucleus, the NTS and the AP [44]. Although intracerebroventricular injection of exendin-(9–39), a specific GLP-1R antagonist, increases feeding and body weight in rats [50], mice lacking GLP-1R do not present abnormal food intake or obesity [51], suggesting the existence of redundant or compensatory mechanisms permitting satiety signaling to the brain.

GLP-1 corresponds to a C-terminal fragment of preproglucagon, and possesses a non-overlapping sequence with OXM [50]. Release of GLP-1 is stimulated by direct sensing of nutrients by L-cells, bile entry into the intestine and neural pathways [52], and the main circulating bioactive form of the hormone is the N-terminal truncated GLP-1$_{7-36amide}$ [45]. The most studied function of GLP-1 is the incretin effect, whereby insulin secretion is augmented in a glucose-dependent manner [53]. Other functions include promotion of nutrient absorption through inhibition of gastric emptying, motility and secretion [45]. Similarly to OXM, GLP-1 is a potent satiety signal due to binding of GLP-1R in brain areas implicated in energy homeostasis control.

Peripheral and central injections of GLP-1 both induce *cfos* expression in the ARC, the NTS, in particular corticotrophin-releasing neurons, and the AP [54]. GLP-1R have been found on POMC neurons in the ARC [54], although binding of GLP-1 to ARC neurons remains to be demonstrated. Indeed, there is evidence that a large part of GLP-1's anorectic effects are mediated through vagus nerve afferents to the NTS, which then relays the signal to the ARC [45]. Since leptin receptors have been identified on GLP-1-expressing neurons in the NTS projecting to the ARC [55], circulating levels of leptin may play a role in central GLP-1 release and effects on food intake. Furthermore, GLP-1 may be able to enter the brainstem through the BBB-deficient AP [53].

Given that GLP-1R is expressed in regions close to CVOs, peripheral OXM and GLP-1 may enter the brain by passive diffusion through fenestrated vessels to access target neurons involved in food intake control, while CNS-produced OXM and GLP-1 may directly act on neural feeding circuits within the brain. However, mechanisms of entry of OXM and GLP-1 into the brain may differ. Dakin et al. [48] showed that OXM- but not GLP-1-induced satiety signaling could be abolished using an ARC-specific injection of GLP-1 antagonist. This suggests that, unlike GLP-1, OXM can directly act on the ARC, even if the ARC also plays an essential role in mediating the anorexigenic effects of GLP-1. Other results suggest differential access routes and/or signaling pathways between OXM and GLP-1. Indeed, unlike GLP-1, peripheral injection of OXM activates *cfos* in ARC neurons but not the NTS [48]. In addition, different neuronal pathways seem to be activated in the hypothalamus by these two hormones [8].

Adiposity Signals

Insulin and Leptin

While leptin and insulin are not considered to be gut-derived hormones, due to their release from adipocytes and the pancreas, respectively, they nevertheless possess strong effects upon food intake and satiety.

In mammals, circulating insulin is exclusively produced by β-cells within Langerhans' islets of the pancreas. It acts in the periphery as a blood glucose-lowering hormone, by increasing glucose uptake and energy storage [56]. Circulating insulin can also act on the CNS to reduce food intake, and deletion of insulin receptor substrate 2 in neurons is associated with hyperphagia [57]. Indeed, insulin receptors are expressed in various areas of the brain, in particular in regions involved in food intake control such as the hypothalamus (ARC, DMH and PVN) [58].

Insulin enters the brain through a saturable receptor-mediated transport mechanism, which is unidirectional and involves an endocytic process [59]. However, given insulin's molecular size (6 kDa), diffusion through fenestrated capillaries of CVOs, such as those of the ME, may also provide a route by which ARC neurons are targeted;

indeed, recent studies have demonstrated that insulin is capable of reaching BBB-unprotected subfornical organ neurons [60].

Leptin is mainly synthesized by white adipose tissue, and circulating levels are directly correlated to fat mass. Among the three types of existing leptin receptors (long, short, or secreted forms), the Ob-Rb receptor, mainly expressed in the hypothalamus, is involved in the anorectic effects of leptin [61]. Both hypothalamic NPY and POMC neurons express leptin receptors and leptin inhibits NPY neurons, while it activates POMC neurons [1] to reduce food consumption. Moreover, leptin directly depolarizes GLP-1 neurons in the NTS, and this mode of action is postulated to be involved in the anorexic effects of GLP-1 [55]. While leptin deficiency leads to obesity, treatment of obese individuals with exogenous leptin fails to reduce food intake, most likely reflecting leptin resistance due to either modification of receptor signaling [62], or impaired transport across the BBB [63]. However, whereas alterations to leptin receptor signaling account for the physiological hyperphagia observed during pregnancy [64], similar mechanisms are rarely implicated in obesity [65]. An alternate explanation is that leptin is a fat-sparing signal, indicating to the brain when stores are appropriate for energy-expensive processes such as reproduction or pregnancy.

Leptin is transported across the BBB by a saturable transporter system present throughout the CNS, but with highest efficiency at the ARC and the choroid plexus [59]. This transport is most efficient when leptin serum levels are low [66]. A combination of diffusion at the ME through fenestrated capillaries (the molecular weight of leptin is 16 kDa, below the cut-off for vascular pores in physiological conditions), transport across the BBB, and from CSF across the ependymal layer could mediate leptin entry in the ARC. However, the CSF/serum leptin ratio is lower in obese versus lean individuals, supporting a relative predominant role for a saturable transport system [66].

The Blood-Brain Barrier

The main function of the BBB is to prevent the unrestricted entry of circulating molecules into the CNS. Some plasma proteins, such as prothrombin or plasminogen, as well as viral, bacterial and parasitic agents, elicit neuronal activation and apoptosis [67], and must therefore be prevented from entering the CNS. The protein content in the CSF is therefore generally lower than in the plasma. The BBB consists of three main elements: the vascular barrier, the choroid plexus (also referred to as the brain-CSF barrier), and the barriers between CVOs and the rest of the brain, each possessing their own characteristics to prevent leakage into the brain parenchyma (fig. 3).

Since gut peptides are known to interact with feeding behavior, the existence of a gut-brain axis has been long been suspected. It was however thought that effects of

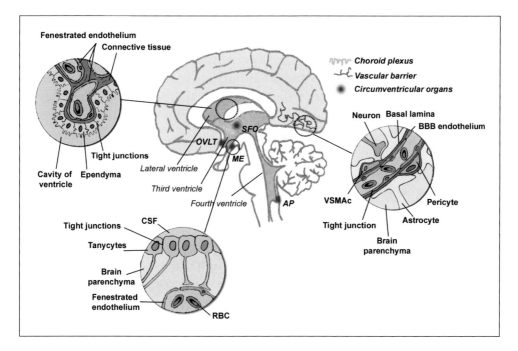

Fig. 3. Structure of the three major blood to brain barriers: the vascular barrier, the choroid plexus and the circumventricular organs. BBB = Blood-brain barrier; ME = median eminence; AP = area postrema; SFO = subfornical organ; OVLT = organum vasculosum laminae terminalis; CSF = cerebrospinal fluid; RBC = red blood cell; VSMAc = vascular smooth muscle actin cell.

peripheral gut hormones on the brain were mainly mediated through vagus nerve afferents due to restriction of molecule entry into the brain by the presence of the BBB at the brain-circulating blood interface. Definite evidence of transport across the BBB was provided with the discovery of an insulin transport mechanism [68]. Now it is not only accepted that gut hormones can be transported through the BBB, but that they also influence the function of brain endothelial cells through modification of transport rates or liberation of signaling molecules [69].

The Vascular Barrier – the BBB

The most studied barrier between the blood and the brain consists in the vascular barrier, commonly referred to as the BBB. It is also the predominant barrier, with ~95% of brain vessels displaying BBB properties. Brain vascular endothelial cells form a very efficient barrier to molecule diffusion, preventing serum proteins in the circulating blood from leaking into the CNS. Several unique features characterize this barrier (fig. 3). Firstly, brain endothelial cells form homotypic interactions through complex tight junctions, composed of different transmembrane proteins [70]. In addition, adherent junctions stabilize these interactions to efficiently disable passage of polar molecules by a paracellular route. Tight junctions are composed of occludins, different claudins, and junctional adhesion molecules, and adherent junctions are composed of scaffold proteins, such as catenins [70]. Secondly, there is an absence of intracellular fenestration and a decreased pinocytotic activity. Lastly, cerebral endothelial cells interact with the surrounding basal lamina, as well as astrocytic end-feet processes, pericytes and neurons [71, 72]. Astrocytes and pericytes are both involved in modulating brain endothelial permeability and in BBB maintenance [71, 72].

Transport Mechanisms across the Vascular Barrier
Transport mechanisms are classified as either saturable or non-saturable processes which depend or not on the existence of molecule transporters. Passive transmembrane diffusion, which does not require transporters, occurs for a wide range of substances and increases with lipid solubility [73]. By contrast, transporters either form pores across the epithelial membrane, or implicate transcytosis and vesicle formation to permit molecules to cross the BBB. An active transport corresponds to an energy-dependent mechanism, whereas energy-independent transporters mediate facilitated diffusion. Facilitated diffusion occurs according to molecule gradient in a bidirectional manner, whereas other transport mechanisms can be uni- or bidirectional due their reliance on ATP as an energy source. A variety of carriers exist at the BBB to mediate diffusion of essential polar nutrients, such as glucose or various amino acids. Existing transport mechanisms are reviewed in detail elsewhere [74].

Since many gut hormones are exclusively produced in the periphery but have defined actions on the CNS where their specific receptors are expressed, it is unsurprising to find that many of these hormones possess specific transporters at the BBB [36, 63]. This transport either occurs through saturable or non-saturable mechanisms. Saturable mechanisms usually involve active receptor-mediated transcytotic transport, whereas the main non-saturable transport mechanism for gut hormones is passive transmembrane diffusion [69]. Incidentally, gastrointestinal signals for which saturable transporters have been identified to date are those for which central expression is not detected (PP, insulin, leptin) [75]. However, transport into the CNS still has to be elucidated for many gut hormones, and other specific transporters at the BBB may still yet be identified.

The Choroid Plexus
The choroid plexus constitutes the blood-CSF barrier and is located in the ventricles of the brain. It is composed of fenestrated capillaries and loose connective tissue separated from the ventricles by tight choroid epithelial cells (fig. 3). Choroid epithelial cells are modified ependymal cells forming a continuous layer linked by tight junctions on the ventricular portion. The choroid epithelium is responsible for CSF production, by filtering fluids across the epithelial layer from the blood into the ventricles [76]. Active transport of molecules also occurs to and from the CSF, in particular of

ions to maintain osmotic balance. In addition, the choroid plexus is thought to play an important role in neuroendocrine signaling, since a variety of hormone receptors have been identified in this structure [76] which may facilitate hormone uptake into the CSF. The main role of the choroid plexus in energy homeostasis is through expression of leptin receptor and leptin transport into the CSF. While the choroid plexus does not have a defined role in gut-brain axis function, this may be uncovered as more details are gleaned about the secreted peptides.

The Circumventricular Organs

CVOs in the brain lack BBB and are composed of fenestrated vessels, which allow facilitated entry of molecules into CNS. The four main CVOs are the ME, the organum vasculosum of the laminae terminalis (OVLT), the AP and the suprafornical organ. While all are sensory organs in that neuronal tissue is in close apposition and can sense peripheral signals, only the ME, located at the base of the hypothalamus, has secretory functions which permit transport of neurohormones to the periphery. With relation to the gut-brain axis, the CVOs are strategically placed, or inversely, are the neuronal circuits involved in feeding behavior. For example, the ME is in close apposition to the ARC region of the hypothalamus, the AP can relay signals from the periphery to the NTS [6], which has strong connections with hypothalamic nuclei involved in feeding behavior, and the suprafornical organ plays important roles in energy homeostasis through direct blood glucose-sensing and neural efferents to the PVN [77]. On a structural basis, CVOs therefore constitute key players in the gut-brain axis, permitting potential free diffusion of peripheral signals to target neurons, precluding the need for active transport across the BBB.

Fenestrated vessels display pores of 50–80 nm diameter closed by a permeable diaphragm 4–6 nm thick composed of radial fibrils interweaving in a central knob [78]. Since passive molecule diffusion may be both size- and charge-limited, following the time course of events at the blood-brain interface in real-time is critical. To characterize the role of the ME in molecule entry into the brain, the in vivo cut-off size of pores on the fenestrated vessels of this structure was recently determined [17]. Using fluorescently-labeled dextran molecules of different molecular sizes and two-photon microscopy to access the ventral side of the brain, the size selectivity of the ME vessels was measured, as well as the molecule diffusion rate from the blood to brain. Molecular size limit for passive diffusion was below 66 kDa (size of albumin), with a stepwise decrease in permeability rate between 20 and 40 kDa. This limit is well above the size of the majority of documented gut hormones, suggesting the diffusion of signals through the ME, and possibly other CVOs, would not be size-limited. As saturable transporters are modulated by physiological events and by pathological conditions [79], it would be of interest to investigate if modification of vessel permeability, for example through modulation of pore radial fibril density, could constitute another level of regulation for molecule diffusion into the metabolic brain.

Entry of Molecules in Feeding-Related Behavior Regions of the Brain
The main integration center of peripheral signals involved in food intake is the ARC of the hypothalamus. In addition, some gut hormones can directly or indirectly act on nuclei linked with feeding control, such as the PVN, but also the VMN and LHA [1]. Several mechanisms of transport of molecules into the ARC have been proposed, and can be divided into three major groups: (1) passive transmembrane diffusion, (2) receptor-mediated transport, and (3) fast feedback route. Firstly and as already discussed, some hormones are able to passively diffuse through the BBB [69]. Secondly, a variety of circulating nutrients and hormones can enter the CNS through a receptor-mediated transport at the BBB and choroid plexus levels [69, 76]. Transport through the choroid plexus permits hormones to enter the CSF and potentially diffuse/be transported into the ARC through the third ventricle. However, a variety of specialized ependymal cells termed tanycytes line the ventricular wall, and tight junctions between these cells form a physical barrier controlling molecule diffusion bidirectionally between the CSF and the brain parenchyma [80]. Incidentally, a recent study has shown the presence of tanycyte-like ependymal cells along the ventricular walls of other CVOs, suggesting that these specialized cells may play an important role in controlling molecule diffusion and regulating barrier properties in all CVOs [81]. Lastly, the ARC is located in close apposition to the ME, one of the CVOs composed of fenestrated capillaries that may provide a direct route of entry for circulating hormones. However, most hypothalamic neurons involved in food intake reside in BBB-protected areas.

Whether molecules from the circulation can diffuse from the ME and enter the ARC has remained controversial. Although tracer diffusion experiments eluded to the existence of a tight barrier between the ME and ARC that could be mediated by tanycyte processes [80], some signals from the circulation were found to diffuse into the ARC [82]. By employing fluorescently-labeled ghrelin to circumvent limitations inherent to dye injections [17], we recently demonstrated that ghrelin diffusion from the circulation to the ME, and subsequently from the ME to the ARC is possible. Indeed, ghrelin-labeled neurons were in close proximity to fenestrated capillary loops located in the vmARC and projecting from the ME [26] (fig. 4). These vessels could therefore permit fast ghrelin entry into the metabolic brain. Given that all gut hormones described to date also have effects on the brainstem, direct access to the dorsal vagal complex could possibly be provided by the BBB-unrestricted AP, although this is still to be demonstrated.

Modulation of BBB Activity
The BBB constitutes a mechanism by which signaling between peripheral tissues and the brain is controlled. Molecule entry into the brain can be altered by two main events. Firstly, transporter properties and rates for many gut hormones can be modulated by different physiological states, and can therefore be adapted to best-fit energetic needs. Secondly, various pathologies have been linked to BBB transporter

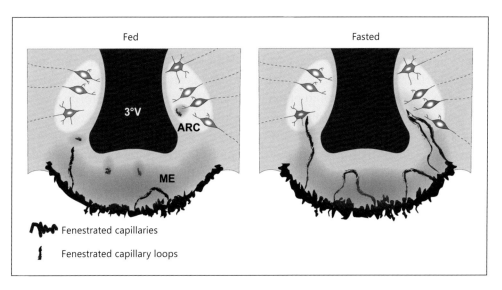

Fig. 4. Schematic of the modulation of ghrelin access to the ARC in fed and fasted states. Pink halo corresponds to peripheral molecule's free diffusion zones. Pink neurons correspond to neurons with direct access to circulating molecules, whereas blue neurons correspond to neurons in BBB-protected areas. Non-permeable BBB-protected capillaries are not represented on the schematic. ME = Median eminence; ARC = arcuates nucleus; 3°V = third ventricle.

dysregulation [79]. Available data exclusively concerns the three main hormones involved in food intake control: leptin, insulin and ghrelin.

In the case of ghrelin, very few reports exist regarding transport through the blood-brain interfaces under different physiological conditions. It has been suggested that obesity, starvation and age may modify the access of ghrelin to the CNS [25]. Indeed, permeation of ghrelin into the CNS decreases with increasing body weight. Peripheral injection of fluorescent bioactive hormone rapidly binds NPY and POMC neurons, and that this can be dynamically regulated by food intake [17]. More ghrelin-labeled neurons were observed following 24 h fasting, and this could be reversed with refeeding. Subsequent studies demonstrated a role for glucose in modulating molecule entry into the brain through a BBB-independent transport mechanism (discussed below), which may explain the facilitated uptake of ghrelin into the brain under conditions of food deprivation [83].

Reports on modulation of insulin transport into the CNS by physiological state, and consequences of insulin transport dysfunction are more extensive. The insulin transporter is saturated by serum levels unable to induce hypoglycemia [59], suggesting a role for central insulin signaling other than reversal of hyperglycemia. Transport of anorectic insulin is dynamically regulated by physiological states such as fasting, aging, and hibernating [84]. In addition, during pregnancy, insulin resistance develops to increase circulating glucose levels and thereby enhance placental glucose transfer to the fetus. However, insulin resistance is also associated with a decrease in insulin transport to the CNS [84]. A decrease in insulin levels in the CSF may reduce the promotion of the baroreflex by insulin, suggesting that the defective baroreceptor responses associated with pregnancy may stem from altered insulin permeation into the CNS [85]. In addition, modification of insulin transport rate is a common sequel to pathologies that provoke glucose intolerance [84]. For instance, transport of insulin across the BBB is decreased during obesity [86], inhibition of insulin transport into the brain by dexamethasone may explain weight gain during glucocorticoid treatment [87], and impaired transport and central effects of insulin are observed in Alzheimer's disease [88]. In the latter, altered insulin signaling likely contributes to the disease, since central delivery of insulin can improve cognition in Alzheimer's patients [88]. By contrast, insulin transport is greatly enhanced by lipopolysaccharide and it has been hypothesized that chronically elevated insulin entry transport into the CNS may underlie the insulin resistance observed during sepsis [84]. However, since the nature of the insulin transporter is not known, exact mechanisms of modulation of insulin transport into the brain remain unclear.

Alterations of leptin transport into the brain are the most studied and the best documented modulations of BBB transport mechanisms. The BBB is thought to play a major role in leptin resistance in obese subjects, displaying increases in plasma leptin not coupled to increases in CSF leptin levels [66], probably due to saturation of leptin transporters [79]. Leptin resistance is likely to be associated with a progressive decrease of transport across the BBB and a default in CNS leptin signaling, although resistance at the BBB level is likely to occur first [86]. Lastly, leptin transport can also be affected by circulating molecules such as triglycerides, insulin, glucose, estrogen, and epinephrine [89].

Modulation of BBB Function
Insulin has been reported to modify BBB function by altering transport of molecules into the brain. However, whether other gastrointestinal hormones are able to directly interact with the BBB to alter transport of molecules, in particular of other gut peptides, is unresolved. The mechanism by which insulin acts on BBB endothelial cells is unclear, but could be mediated through insulin transporters, or insulin receptors [90]. Insulin enhances tyrosine and tryptophan transport across the BBB, which in turn induces an increase in catecholamines and serotonin levels in the CNS, the latter being potentially involved in food intake control through reduction of appetite [91]. Moreover, insulin increases transport of leptin into the brain in non-diabetic states [89], as well as uptake of p-glycoprotein. Decreases in this latter protein have incidentally been linked to amyloid-β protein accumulation, a hallmark of Alzheimer's disease [88]. It is relatively well documented that the BBB can secrete a variety of substances such as cytokines [92] capable of affecting brain functions including food intake regulation. This secretion is polarized, since brain endothelial cells can either secrete substances towards the brain, or the blood compartment. There is some

Schaeffer · Hodson · Mollard

evidence that food-related peptides can modulate cytokine production from brain endothelial cells. For instance, peripheral adiponectin inhibits IL-6 release by the BBB at the brain side [92]. However, whether gastrointestinal hormones can have similar effects is unknown.

Modulation of Other Entry Routes

Plasticity of the mechanisms which dictate BBB-independent hormone uptake into the CNS may also underlie regulation of energy homeostasis. For example, the passive diffusion of ghrelin across fenestrated capillaries of the ME [17] into the ARC is likely to be modified by nutrient intake since the number of labeled NPY neurons can be reversibly modified by fasting. Furthermore, the decrease in glucose levels associated with fasting induces tanycyte VEGF-A expression, increasing the number of fenestrated capillary loops projecting from the ME into the ARC [26] and facilitating molecule entry into the hypothalamus [83] (fig. 4). Whether similar mechanisms play a role in regulating molecule entry at the level of other CVOs, in particular the AP of the brainstem, or in modulating peripheral hormone entry under pathological conditions, remains to be investigated.

Conclusion

The BBB, located at the interface between peripheral circulation-brain compartments, constitutes a critical checkpoint in gut-brain axis function by responding to changes in both molecule concentrations as well as whole-organism requirements. It therefore plays an integral part in feeding behavior regulation, in particular through the regulation and expression of specific hormone transporters. However, most of what we know concerns the adiposity signals leptin and insulin, whereas little is known about mechanisms of GIT hormone entry into the brain. Recent findings, including from our group, have highlighted a role for nutrient levels in molecule access into the metabolic brain, in particular through one of key the CVOs, the ME. Indeed, most gut hormones require access to the ARC and brainstem, and all possess molecular weights consistent with passive diffusion through the fenestrated vessels that infiltrate the CVOs. In addition, the unique vmARC milieu irrigated by fenestrated vessels and in close proximity to the ME may provide a specific niche for a subpopulation of 'scout neurons' that could rapidly sense peripheral signals in a nutrient-dependent manner to coordinate more global responses. This supports a role for both the endothelial cells of the BBB, and more generally, endothelial cells of capillaries in CVOs, in regulating brain function involved in feeding behavior. Future studies will allow a better understanding of how the brain vasculature contributes to energy homeostasis, and how this becomes perturbed during pathologies ranging from obesity to type 2 diabetes.

References

1 Schwartz MW, Woods SC, Porte D Jr, Seeley RJ, Baskin DG: Central nervous system control of food intake. Nature 2000;404:661–671.

2 Batterham RL, Cowley MA, Small CJ, Herzog H, Cohen MA, Dakin CL, Wren AM, Brynes AE, Low MJ, Ghatei MA, Cone RD, Bloom SR: Gut hormone PYY(3–36) physiologically inhibits food intake. Nature 2002;418:650–654.

3 Stanley S, Wynne K, McGowan B, Bloom S: Hormonal regulation of food intake. Physiol Rev 2005; 85:1131–1158.

4 Skibicka KP, Dickson SL: Ghrelin and food reward: The story of potential underlying substrates. Peptides 2011;32:2265–2273.

5 Schwartz GJ: Brainstem integrative function in the central nervous system control of food intake. Forum Nutr 2010;63:141–151.

6 Blouet C, Schwartz GJ: Brainstem nutrient sensing in the nucleus of the solitary tract inhibits feeding. Cell Metabolism 2012;16:579–587.

7 Gibbs J, Young RC, Smith GP: Cholecystokinin decreases food intake in rats. J Comp Physiol Psychol 1973;84:488–495.

8 Chaudhri O, Small C, Bloom S: Gastrointestinal hormones regulating appetite. Philos Trans R Soc Lond B Biol Sci 2006;361:1187–1209.

9 Strader AD, Woods SC: Gastrointestinal hormones and food intake. Gastroenterology 2005;128:175–191.

10 Tschöp M, Smiley DL, Heiman ML: Ghrelin induces adiposity in rodents. Nature 2000;407:908–913.

11 Otto B, Cuntz U, Fruehauf E, Wawarta R, Folwaczny C, Riepl RL, Heiman ML, Lehnert P, Fichter M, Tschöp M: Weight gain decreases elevated plasma ghrelin concentrations of patients with anorexia nervosa. Eur J Endocrinol 2001;145:R5–R9.

12 Kojima M, Hosoda H, Date Y, Nakazato M, Matsuo H, Kangawa K: Ghrelin is a growth-hormone-releasing acylated peptide from stomach. Nature 1999;402: 656–660.

13 Van der Lely AF, Tschöp M, Heiman ML, Ghigo E: Biological, physiological, pathophysiological, and pharmacological aspects of ghrelin. Endocr Rev 2004;25:426–457.

14 Harrold JA, Dovey T, Cai XJ, Halford JCG, Pinkney J: Autoradiographic analysis of ghrelin receptors in the rat hypothalamus. Brain Res 2008;1196:59–64.

15 Cowley MA, Smith RG, Diano S, Tschop M, Pronchuk N, Grove KL, Strasburger CJ, Bidlingmaier M, Esterman M, Heiman ML, Garcia-Segura LM, Nillni EA, Mendez P, Low MJ, Sotonyi P, Friedman JM, Liu H, Pinto S, Colmers WF, Cone RD, Horvath TL: The distribution and mechanism of action of ghrelin in the CNS demonstrates a novel hypothalamic circuit regulating energy homeostasis. Neuron 2003;37:649–661.

16 Sakata I, Nakano Y, Osborne-Lawrence S, Rovinsky SA, Lee CE, Perello M, Anderson JG, Coppari R, Xiao G, Lowell BB, Elmquist JK, Zigman JM: Characterization of a novel ghrelin cell reporter mouse. Regul Pept 2009;155:91–98.

17 Schaeffer M, Langlet F, Lafont C, Molino F, Hodson DJ, Roux T, Lamarque L, Verdie P, Bourrier E, Dehouck B, Baneres JL, Martinez J, Mery PF, Marie J, Trinquet E, Fehrentz JA, Prevot V, Mollard P: Rapid sensing of circulating ghrelin by hypothalamic appetite-modifying neurons. Proc Natl Acad Sci USA 2013;110:1512–1517.

18 Cui RJ, Li XJ, Appleyard SM: Ghrelin inhibits visceral afferent activation of catecholamine neurons in the solitary tract nucleus. J Neurosci 2011;31:3484–3492.

19 Fry M, Ferguson AV: Ghrelin modulates electrical activity of area postrema neurons. Am J Physiol Regul Integr Comp Physiol 2009;296:R485–R492.

20 Zigman JM, Jones JE, Lee CE, Saper CB, Elmquist JK: Expression of ghrelin receptor MRNA in the rat and the mouse brain. J Comp Neurol 2006;494:528–548.

21 Kern A, Albarran-Zeckler R, Walsh HE, Smith RG: Apo-ghrelin receptor forms heteromers with DRD2 in hypothalamic neurons and is essential for anorexigenic effects of DRD2 agonism. Neuron 2012;73: 317–332.

22 Sun YX, Ahmed S, Smith RG: Deletion of ghrelin impairs neither growth nor appetite. Mol Cell Biol 2003;23:7973–7981.

23 Wren AM, Small CJ, Abbott CR, Dhillo WS, Seal LJ, Cohen MA, Batterham RL, Taheri S, Stanley SA, Ghatei MA, Bloom SR: Ghrelin causes hyperphagia and obesity in rats. Diabetes 2001;50:2540–2547.

24 Grouselle D, Chaillou E, Caraty A, Bluet-Pajot MT, Zizzari P, Tillet Y, Epelbaum J: Pulsatile cerebrospinal fluid and plasma ghrelin in relation to growth hormone secretion and food intake in the sheep. J Neuroendocrinol 2008;20:1138–1146.

25 Banks WA, Burney BO, Robinson SM: Effects of triglycerides, obesity, and starvation on ghrelin transport across the blood-brain barrier. Peptides 2008; 29:2061–2065.

26 Ciofi P, Garret M, Lapirot O, Lafon P, Loyens A, Prevot V, Levine JE: Brain-endocrine interactions: a microvascular route in the mediobasal hypothalamus. Endocrinology 2009;150:5509–5519.

27 Rehfeld JF: Cholecystokinin. Best Pract Res Clin Endocrinol Metab 2004;18:569–586.

28 Moran TH, Baldessarini AR, Salorio CF, Lowery T, Schwartz GJ: Vagal afferent and efferent contributions to the inhibition of food intake by cholecystokinin. Am J Physiol Regul Integr Comp Physiol 1997; 272:R1245–R1251.

29 Wank SA: Cholecystokinin receptors. Am J Physiol Gastrointest Liver Physiol 1995;269:G628–G646.

30 Bi S, Ladenheim EE, Schwartz GJ, Moran TH: A role for NPY overexpression in the dorsomedial hypothalamus in hyperphagia and obesity of OLETF rats. Am J Physiol Regul Integr Comp Physiol 2001;281:R254–R260.

31 Meereis-Schwanke K, Klonowski-Stumpe H, Herberg L, Niederau C: Long-term effects of CCK-agonist and -antagonist on food intake and body weight in Zucker lean and obese rats. Peptides 1998;19:291–299.

32 Adrian TE, Long RG, Fuessl HS, Bloom SR: Plasma peptide YY (PYY) in dumping syndrome. Dig Dis Sci 1985;30:1145–1148.

33 Gelegen C, Chandarana K, Choudhury AI, Al-Qassab H, Evans IM, Irvine EE, Hyde CB, Claret M, Andreelli F, Sloan SE, Leiter AB, Withers DJ, Batterham RL: Regulation of hindbrain PYY expression by acute food deprivation, prolonged caloric restriction, and weight loss surgery in mice. Am J Physiol Endocrinol Metab 2012;303:E659–E668.

34 Karra E, Chandarana K, Batterham RL: The role of peptide YY in appetite regulation and obesity. J Physiol 2009;587:19–25.

35 Ueno H, Yamaguchi H, Mizuta M, Nakazato M: The role of PYY in feeding regulation. Regul Pept 2008;145:12–16.

36 Nonaka N, Shioda S, Niehoff ML, Banks WA: Characterization of blood-brain barrier permeability to PYY3–36 in the mouse. J Pharmacol Exp Ther 2003;306:948–953.

37 Batterham RL, Heffron H, Kapoor S, Chivers JE, Chandarana K, Herzog H, Le Roux CW, Thomas EL, Bell JD, Withers DJ: Critical role for peptide YY in protein-mediated satiation and body-weight regulation. Cell Metab 2006;4:223–233.

38 Field BCT, Chaudhri OB, Bloom SR: Bowels control brain: gut hormones and obesity. Nat Rev Endocrinol 2010;6:444–453.

39 Ekblad E, Sundler F: Distribution of pancreatic polypeptide and peptide YY. Peptides 2002;23:251–261.

40 Tasan RO, Lin S, Hetzenauer A, Singewald N, Herzog H, Sperk G: Increased novelty-induced motor activity and reduced depression-like behavior in neuropeptide Y (NPY)-Y4 receptor knockout mice. Neuroscience 2009;158:1717–1730.

41 Edelsbrunner ME, Painsipp E, Herzog H, Holzer P: Evidence from knockout mice for distinct implications of neuropeptide-Y Y2 and Y4 receptors in the circadian control of locomotion, exploration, water and food intake. Neuropeptides 2009;43:491–497.

42 Banks WA, Kastin AJ, Jaspan JB: Regional variation in transport of pancreatic-polypeptide across the blood-brain barrier of mice. Pharmacol Biochem Behav 1995;51:139–147.

43 Asakawa A, Inui A, Yuzuriha H, Ueno N, Katsuura G, Fujimiya M, Fujino MA, Niijima A, Meguid MM, Kasuga M: Characterization of the effects of pancreatic polypeptide in the regulation of energy balance. Gastroenterology 2003;124:1325–1336.

44 Kieffer TJ, Habener JL: The glucagon-like peptides. Endocr Rev 1999;20:876–913.

45 Holst JJ: The physiology of glucagon-like peptide 1. Physiol Rev 2007;87:1409–1439.

46 Habib AM, Richards P, Cairns LS, Rogers GJ, Bannon CAM, Parker HE, Morley TCE, Yeo GSH, Reimann F, Gribble FM: Overlap of endocrine hormone expression in the mouse intestine revealed by transcriptional profiling and flow cytometry. Endocrinology 2012;153:3054–3065.

47 Du XB, Kosinski JR, Lao JL, Shen XL, Petrov A, Chicchi GG, Eiermann GJ, Pocai A: Differential effects of oxyntomodulin and GLP-1 on glucose metabolism. Am J Physiol Endocrinol Metab 2012;303:E265–E271.

48 Dakin CL, Small CJ, Batterham RL, Neary NM, Cohen MA, Patterson M, Ghatei MA, Bloom SR: Peripheral oxyntomodulin reduces food intake and body weight gain in rats. Endocrinology 2004;145:2687–2695.

49 Pocai A, Carrington PE, Adams JR, Wright M, Eiermann G, Zhu L, Du XB, Petrov A, Lassman ME, Jiang GQ, Liu F, Miller C, Tota LM, Zhou GC, Zhang XP, Sountis MM, Santoprete A, Capito E, Chicchi GG, Thornberry N, Bianchi E, Pessi A, Marsh DJ, SinhaRoy R: Glucagon-like peptide 1/glucagon receptor dual agonism reverses obesity in mice. Diabetes 2009;58:2258–2266.

50 Meeran K, O'Shea D, Edwards CMB, Turton MD, Heath MM, Gunn I, Abusnana S, Rossi M, Small CJ, Goldstone AP, Taylor GM, Sunter D, Steere J, Choi SJ, Ghatei MA, Bloom SR: Repeated intracerebroventricular administration of glucagon-like peptide-1(7–36) amide or exendin(9–39) alters body weight in the rat. Endocrinology 1999;140:244–250.

51 Scrocchi LA, Brown TJ, MacLusky N, Brubaker PL, Auerbach AB, Joyner AL, Drucker DJ: Glucose intolerance but normal satiety in mice with a null mutation in the glucagon-like peptide 1 receptor gene. Nat Med 1996;2:1254–1258.

52 Parker HE, Wallis K, le Roux CW, Wong KY, Reimann F, Gribble FM: Molecular mechanisms underlying bile acid-stimulated glucagon-like peptide-1 secretion. Brh J Pharmacol 2012;165:414–423.

53 Drucker DJ, Nauck MA: The incretin system: glucagon-like peptide-1 receptor agonists and dipeptidyl peptidase-4 inhibitors in type 2 diabetes. Lancet 2006;368:1696–1705.

54 Sandoval DA, Bagnol D, Woods SC, D'Alessio DA, Seeley RJ: Arcuate glucagon-like peptide 1 receptors regulate glucose homeostasis but not food intake. Diabetes 2008;57:2046–2054.

55 Hisadome K, Reimann F, Gribble FM, Trapp S: Leptin directly depolarizes preproglucagon neurons in the nucleus tractus solitarius electrical properties of glucagon-like peptide-1 neurons. Diabetes 2010; 59:1890–1898.

56 Tang-Christensen M, Vrang N, Larsen PJ: Glucagon-like peptide 1(7–36) amide's central inhibition of feeding and peripheral inhibition of drinking are abolished by neonatal monosodium glutamate treatment. Diabetes 1998;47:530–537.

57 Choudhury AI, Heffron H, Smith MA, Al-Qassab H, Xu AW, Selman C, Simmgen M, Clements M, Claret M, MacColl G, Bedford DC, Hisadome K, Diakonov I, Moosajee V, Bell JD, Speakman JR, Batterham RL, Barsh GS, Ashford MLJ, Withers DJ: The role of insulin receptor substrate 2 in hypothalamic and β-cell function. J Clin Invest 2005;115:940–950.

58 Corp ES, Woods SC, Porte D, Dorsa DM, Figlewicz DP, Baskin DG: Localization of I-125 insulin binding sites in the rat hypothalamus by quantitative autoradiography. Neurosci Lett 1986;70:17–22.

59 Zlokovic BV, Jovanovic S, Miao W, Samara S, Verma S, Farrell CL: Differential regulation of leptin transport by the choroid plexus and blood-brain barrier and high affinity transport systems for entry into hypothalamus and across the blood-cerebrospinal fluid barrier. Endocrinology 2000;141:1434–1441.

60 Lakhi S, Snow W, Fry M: Insulin modulates the electrical activity of subfornical organ neurons. Neuroreport 2013;24:329–334.

61 Tartaglia LA: The leptin receptor. J Biol Chem 1997; 272:6093–6096.

62 Munzberg H: Leptin-signaling pathways and leptin resistance. Forum Nutr 2010;63:123–132.

63 Banks WA: Leptin transport across the blood-brain barrier: Implications for the cause and treatment of obesity. Curr Pharm Des 2001;7:125–133.

64 Ladyman SR, Grattan DR: Region-specific reduction in leptin-induced phosphorylation of signal transducer and activator of transcription-3 (STAT3) in the rat hypothalamus is associated with leptin resistance during pregnancy. Endocrinology 2004;145: 3704–3711.

65 Farooqi IS, O'Rahilly S: Genetics of obesity in humans. Endocr Rev 2006;27:710–718.

66 Caro JF, Kolaczynski JW, Nyce MR, Ohannesian JP, Opentanova I, Goldman WH, Lynn RB, Zhang PL, Sinha MK, Considine RV: Decreased cerebrospinal-fluid/serum leptin ratio in obesity: a possible mechanism for leptin resistance. Lancet 1996;348:159–161.

67 Abbatecola AM, Ferrucci L, Grella R, Bandinelli S, Bonafe M, Barbieri M, Corsi AM, Lauretani F, Franceschi C, Paolisso G: Diverse effect of inflammatory markers on insulin resistance and insulin-resistance syndrome in the elderly. J Am Geriatr Soc 2004;52: 399–404.

68 King GL, Johnson SM: Receptor-mediated transport of insulin across endothelial cells. Science 1985;227: 1583–1586.

69 Banks WA: The blood-brain barrier as a regulatory interface in the gut-brain axes. Physiol Behav 2006; 89:472–476.

70 Wolburg H, Lippoldt A: Tight junctions of the blood-brain barrier: development, composition and regulation. Vascul Pharmacol 2002;38:323–337.

71 Abbott NJ, Ronnback L, Hansson E: Astrocyte-endothelial interactions at the blood-brain barrier. Nat Rev Neurosci 2006;7:41–53.

72 Armulik A, Genove G, Mae M, Nisancioglu MH, Wallgard E, Niaudet C, He LQ, Norlin J, Lindblom P, Strittmatter K, Johansson BR, Betsholtz C: Pericytes regulate the blood-brain barrier. Nature 2010; 468:557–561.

73 Banks WA, Kastin AJ: Peptides and the blood-brain barrier – lipophilicity as a predictor of permeability. Brain Res Bull 1985;15:287–292.

74 Abbott NJ, Patabendige AAK, Dolman DEM, Yusof SR, Begley DJ: Structure and function of the blood-brain barrier. Neurobiol Dis 2010;37:13–25.

75 Banks WA: Blood-brain barrier and energy balance. Obesity (Silver Spring) 2006;14(suppl 5):234S–237S.

76 Skipor J, Thiery JC: The choroid plexus – cerebrospinal fluid system: undervaluated pathway of neuroendocrine signaling into the brain. Acta Neurobiol Exp 2008;68:414–428.

77 Medeiros N, Dai L, Ferguson AV: Glucose-responsive neurons in the subfornical organ of the rat – a novel site for direct CNS monitoring of circulating glucose. Neuroscience 2012;201:157–165.

78 Bearer EL, Orci L: Endothelial fenestral diaphragms: a quick-freeze, deep-etch study. J Cell Biol 1985;100: 418–428.

79 Burguera B, Couce ME, Curran GL, Jensen MD, Lloyd RV, Cleary MP, Poduslo JF: Obesity is associated with a decreased leptin transport across the blood-brain barrier in rats. Diabetes 2000;49:1219–1223.

80 Mullier A, Bouret SG, Prevot V, Dehouck B: Differential distribution of tight junction proteins suggests a role for tanycytes in blood-hypothalamus barrier regulation in the adult mouse brain. J Comp Neurol 2010;518:943–962.

81 Langlet F, Mullier A, Bouret SG, Prevot V, Dehouck B: Tanycyte-like cells form a blood-cerebrospinal fluid barrier in the circumventricular organs of the mouse brain. J Comp Neurol 2013;521:3389–3405.

82 Cheunsuang O, Stewart AL, Morris R: Differential uptake of molecules from the circulation and CSF reveals regional and cellular specialisation in CNS detection of homeostatic signals. Cell Tissue Res 2006;325:397–402.

83 Langlet F, Levin BE, Luquet S, Mazzone M, Messina A, Dunn-Meynell AA, Balland E, Lacombe A, Mazur D, Carmeliet P, Bouret SG, Prevot V, Dehouck B: Tanycytic VEGF-A boosts blood-hypothalamus barrier plasticity and access of metabolic signals to the arcuate nucleus in response to fasting. Cell Metab 2013;17:607–617.

84 Banks WA, Coon AB, Robinson SM, Moinuddin A, Shultz JM, Nakaoke R, Morley JE: Triglycerides induce leptin resistance at the blood-brain barrier. Diabetes 2004;53:1253–1260.

85 Daubert DL, Chung MY, Brooks VL: Insulin resistance and impaired baroreflex gain during pregnancy. Am J Physiol Regul Integr Comp Physiol 2007; 292:R2188–R2195.

86 Halaas JL, Boozer C, Blair-West J, Fidahusein N, Denton DA, Friedman JM: Physiological response to long-term peripheral and central leptin infusion in lean and obese mice. Proc Natl Acad Sci USA 1997; 94:8878–8883.

87 Baura GD, Foster DM, Kaiyala K, Porte D, Kahn SE, Schwartz MW: Insulin transport from plasma into the central nervous system is inhibited by dexamethasone in dogs. Diabetes 1996;45:86–90.

88 Reger MA, Watson GS, Green PS, Wilkinson CW, Baker LD, Cholerton B, Fishel MA, Plymate SR, Breitner JCS, DeGroodt W, Mehta P, Craft S: Intranasal insulin improves cognition and modulates β-amyloid in early ad. Neurology 2008;70:440–448.

89 Kastin AJ, Akerstrom V: Glucose and insulin increase the transport of leptin through the blood-brain barrier in normal mice but not in streptozotocin-diabetic mice. Neuroendocrinology 2001;73: 237–242.

90 Pardridge WM, Eisenberg J, Yang J: Human blood-brain barrier insulin-receptor. J Neurochem 1985; 44:1771–1778.

91 Bello NT, Liang NC: The use of serotonergic drugs to treat obesity – is there any hope? Drug Des Devel Ther 2011;5:95–109.

92 Spranger J, Verma S, Gohring I, Bobbert T, Seifert J, Sindler AL, Pfeiffer A, Hileman SM, Tschöp M, Banks WA: Adiponectin does not cross the blood-brain barrier but modifies cytokine expression of brain endothelial cells. Diabetes 2006;55:141–147.

Dr. Patrice Mollard & Dr. Marie Schaeffer
Department of Endocrinology
Institute of Functional Genomics
141, rue de la Cardonille
FR–34094 Montpellier (France)
E-Mail Patrice.Mollard@igf.cnrs.fr & Marie.Schaeffer@igf.cnrs.fr

Delhanty PJD, van der Lely AJ (eds): How Gut and Brain Control Metabolism.
Front Horm Res. Basel, Karger, 2014, vol 42, pp 50–58 (DOI: 10.1159/000358314)

The Brain Modulates Insulin Sensitivity in Multiple Tissues

Edwin T. Parlevliet[a–c] · Claudia P. Coomans[d] · Patrick C.N. Rensen[b, c] · Johannes A. Romijn[a]

[a]Department of Medicine, Academic Medical Center, University of Amsterdam, Amsterdam, [b]Department of Endocrinology and Metabolic Diseases, [c]Einthoven Laboratory for Experimental Vascular Medicine, and [d]Department of Molecular Cell Biology, Leiden University Medical Center, Leiden, The Netherlands

Abstract

Insulin sensitivity is determined by direct effects of circulating insulin on metabolically active tissues in combination with indirect effects of circulating insulin, i.e. via the central nervous system. The dose-response effects of insulin differ between the various physiological effects of insulin. At lower insulin concentrations, circulating insulin inhibits endogenous glucose production through a combination of direct and indirect effects. At higher insulin concentrations, circulating insulin also stimulates glucose uptake and fatty acid uptake in adipose tissue, again through direct and indirect effects. High-fat diet induces insulin resistance in the central nervous system, which contributes considerably to overall insulin resistance of liver and peripheral tissues. Central insulin resistance is amendable to therapeutic intervention, reflected in the central effects of topiramate and glucagon-like peptide-1 on hepatic and peripheral insulin resistance in insulin resistant mice.

© 2014 S. Karger AG, Basel

Insulin is the best studied hormone with more than 300,000 citations in PubMed. Insulin was the first protein of which the complete amino acid sequence was determined by Sanger and the insulin receptor was one of the first hormone receptors to be detailed. These discoveries, paved with various Nobel Prizes, indicate that insulin is a prismatic hormone for endocrinology.

Insulin is a very strong anabolic hormone with pleiotropic effects in multiple tissues. In contrast to many other hormones, the in vivo effects of insulin can be readily measured by assessing glucose metabolism and, to a lesser extent, plasma lipid metabolism. This has enabled characterization of the tissue-specific effects of insulin on glucose and lipid metabolism. These effects are of major importance in physiological conditions. This is illustrated by type 1 diabetes mellitus: absence of insulin

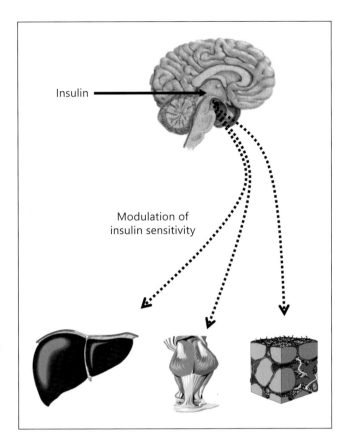

Fig. 1. Circulating insulin acts in the CNS to modulate insulin sensitivity in peripheral organs, possibly through mechanisms that involve alterations in the autonomous nervous system.

results in extreme catabolism, ultimately resulting in ketoacidotic coma and death in the absence of insulin substitution. Excessive autonomous insulin secretion, exemplified by insulinomas, results in severe hypoglycemia. Insulin and insulin sensitivity are crucial factors in the pathophysiology of obesity and type 2 diabetes mellitus. These conditions are associated with a combination of decreased β-cell function and insulin resistance in multiple tissues, in the case of type 2 diabetes mellitus resulting in hyperglycemia.

In general, the implicit notion was until recently that insulin acts from the blood only on peripheral tissues directly. However, the central nervous system (CNS) also actively participates in the orchestration of tissue-specific insulin sensitivity. The brain is an insulin-sensitive organ and insulin receptors are widely distributed throughout the brain [1]. Insulin crosses the blood-brain barrier through insulin receptor-mediated active transport [2]. The origin of insulin in the brain is mostly peripheral and only a modest amount is synthesized locally [3]. In this review, we focus on the indirect effects of circulating insulin on peripheral tissues, i.e. the effects of circulating insulin via the CNS (fig. 1). The pathways of insulin-mediated signaling within the CNS are beyond the scope of the current review.

Insulin in the Brain Modulates Insulin Sensitivity of Plasma Glucose Metabolism

Physiology
The CNS is involved in the physiological regulation of whole-body glucose metabolism. There are multiple lines of evidence supporting this notion. These studies have been done in experimental models, since there are restraints in the experimental approaches in humans for obvious reasons. Nonetheless, these rodent models serve to provide proof of concept.

Central Effects of Circulating Insulin on Endogenous Glucose Production
Insulin inhibits endogenous glucose production by the liver by three major mechanisms: (a) direct effects on the liver [4] (mostly leading to rapid inhibition of glycogenolysis); (b) indirect effects mediated via peripheral actions of insulin [5] (mostly on lipolysis), and (c) indirect effects mediated via activation of central insulin signaling [6–8]. Here, we focus on these indirect hepatic effects of circulating insulin mediated through the brain.

Central administration of insulin, resulting in activation of insulin signaling in the brain without elevating plasma insulin levels, decreases plasma glucose levels by inhibiting endogenous glucose production [6, 8]. Insulin activates ATP-sensitive potassium channels (K_{ATP} channels) in neurons of the hypothalamus, including POMC/CART- and AgRP/NPY-expressing neurons [9, 10]. Inhibition of these neuronal K_{ATP} channels by intracerebroventricular (ICV) administration of sulfonylurea (either tolbutamide or glibenclamide) impairs the inhibitory effect of circulating insulin on endogenous glucose production [6, 11]. Inhibition of K_{ATP} channels in the dorsal vagal complex appears to abolish the inhibiting effect on glucose production as well, although the insulin signaling pathway differs from that in the hypothalamus [8]. Conversely, activation of hypothalamic or dorsal vagal complex K_{ATP} channels enhances insulin-mediated inhibition of endogenous glucose production [8, 12]. Finally, restoration of hepatic insulin signaling in insulin receptor knockout mice fails to normalize the in vivo inhibitory response of hepatic glucose production to insulin, proving that hepatic insulin signaling per se is insufficient for the full hepatic effect of circulating insulin [7]. Therefore, these studies by various groups employing different methodological approaches consistently point towards the notion that central effects of circulating insulin are required for the full inhibitory effect on hepatic glucose production.

Central Effects of Circulating Insulin on Peripheral Glucose Uptake
Insulin signaling in the brain not only substantially contributes to the inhibitory effect of circulating insulin on glucose production, but also to the insulin-stimulated glucose uptake by muscle. ICV administration of tolbutamide decreased insulin-stimulated muscle glucose uptake in chow-fed mice, not by decreasing insulin signaling in skeletal muscle as phosphorylation of PKB and PRAS40 were unaffected by ICV tolbutamide, but, through other, indirect, effects of insulin exerted via the CNS [8].

A number of studies focusing on the role of central K_{ATP} channels in glucose metabolism do not show an effect on glucose disposal [6, 8, 12]. Consequently, the notion might appear that the central effects of circulating insulin are required only for the hepatic effects of insulin, but not for the peripheral effects of insulin on glucose uptake. However, there are some important methodological differences between the different studies, including animal models, insulin levels and duration of fasting. In initial experiments, we carefully characterized insulin dose-response characteristics on endogenous glucose production versus glucose disposal in mice [13]. These data indicate that increased insulin levels up to three times the basal levels inhibit endogenous glucose production, but do not stimulate glucose disposal. Therefore, in a follow-up study aimed at studying the indirect effects of circulating insulin on glucose disposal [11], we even increased insulin levels up to fivefold during the clamp as compared to the basal levels, compared to lower levels in previous studies [6, 8]. Using these insulin levels, we were not only capable of reproducing the central effects of circulating insulin on endogenous glucose production as reported by others [6, 8], but, in addition, to document central effects of insulin on muscle glucose uptake. We speculate that the discrepancy in the effects of central K_{ATP} channel modulation on insulin-mediated glucose uptake during hyperinsulinemia between our study and other studies is explained by the higher insulin levels in our study. Furthermore, the observation that ICV administration of K_{ATP} channel inhibitors did not impact on glucose disposal rate, were performed in rats fasted for 6 h or after food restriction [6, 8], which is in contrast to our observations in overnight fasted mice. Differences between the duration of fasting may be involved to explain the differential effects of ICV K_{ATP} channel inhibitors on insulin-stimulated glucose uptake between these studies. Therefore, it is important to consider the details in study designs between the different experimental approaches in order to reach balanced conclusions.

Pathophysiology: Insulin Resistance

The above-mentioned physiological observations indicate that hepatic and muscle insulin sensitivity is determined by two components: direct effects of insulin on liver and muscle and indirect effects, through the CNS, on liver and muscle. Interestingly, high-fat feeding induces insulin resistance, which includes impaired indirect insulin effects through the CNS.

High-Fat Feeding Inhibits the Central Effects of Circulating Insulin on Endogenous Glucose Production

Dedicated studies in rodents have assessed the effects of high-fat feeding on the ability of insulin to inhibit endogenous glucose production [8, 11, 14]. Our mouse model was designed to develop obesity in combination with partial, rather than complete, insulin resistance, and, as a result, effects of central insulin antagonism in these diet-induced obese mice could still be obtained. Indeed, the high-fat diet caused partial insulin resistance, since insulin was still able, although to a lesser extent, to inhibit glucose production. The high-fat diet abolished the inhibitory effect of ICV tolbutamide on insulin-mediated inhibition of endogenous glucose production. High-fat feeding in rats blunted central insulin signaling pathways, and, as a consequence, infusion of insulin both into the mediobasal hypothalamic nuclei and dorsal vagal complex, failed to suppress glucose production [8, 14]. Collectively, these studies indicate that central insulin resistance contributes to hepatic insulin resistance induced by high-fat feeding in rodents.

High-Fat Feeding Inhibits the Central Effects of Circulating Insulin on Peripheral Glucose Uptake

We assessed the effects of high-fat feeding on the insulin sensitivity of glucose disposal. High-fat feeding strongly reduced insulin-mediated glucose disposal. Remarkably, the inhibitory effects of ICV administration of tolbutamide on insulin-stimulated glucose uptake by skeletal muscle were abolished after high-fat feeding [8]. Interestingly, in quantitative terms, insulin-stimulated muscle glucose uptake in chow-fed conditions during ICV tolbutamide infusion was not different from muscle glucose uptake during high-fat conditions. This remarkable observation indicates that muscle-specific insulin resistance was present for the centrally mediated effects of insulin, rather than for the direct effects of insulin on muscle, at least within the constraints of our high-fat diet mouse model. These observations indicate that central insulin resistance is a major contributor to insulin resistance in muscle induced by high-fat feeding in mice.

Our in vivo observations in diet-induced obese mice extend the in vitro observations by Spanswick et al. [10], showing that physiological levels of insulin activate K_{ATP} channels in glucose responsive neurons of lean, but not of obese rats, suggesting that K_{ATP} channels are already inhibited in the insulin-resistant state. Moreover, stimulation of K_{ATP} channels by administration of diazoxide, ICV or into the dorsal vagal complex, during peripheral insulin infusion did not improve muscle glucose uptake in diet-induced obese insulin-resistant mice or whole-body glucose uptake in rats respectively [8, 11]. The absence of effects of ICV tolbutamide in diet-induced obese mice might also involve reduced insulin transport across the blood-brain barrier [15]. Although the precise mechanisms remain to be elucidated, these studies indicate that high-fat diet decreases the central effects of insulin on both endogenous glucose production and muscle glucose uptake, which contributes to the pathophysiology of diet-induced insulin resistance.

Therapeutic Implications

The question arises to which extent central insulin resistance might be amenable to therapeutic interventions, which might be used to treat insulin resistance. Interestingly, several lines of evidence indicate that there are therapeutic options.

Topiramate Reduces Central Insulin Resistance
Topiramate is used as an antiepileptic drug. In obese, diabetic rats, topiramate reduced plasma glucose levels and improved insulin sensitivity independently of weight loss [16]. We have demonstrated that topiramate improved insulin sensitivity by increasing glucose uptake by skeletal and cardiac muscle and by adipose tissue in insulin-resistant, high-fat-fed mice [17]. In addition, inhibition of the central action of circulating insulin by ICV administration of tolbutamide prevented this insulin-sensitizing effect of topiramate. Topiramate had no direct effect on muscle insulin signaling and glucose uptake in vivo and in vitro. Collectively, these data indicate that topiramate improves peripheral insulin sensitivity indirectly via the brain, rather than by directly targeting peripheral organs. Therefore, this proof of concept indicates that central insulin resistance is potentially amendable to therapeutic intervention.

Glucagon-Like Peptide-1 Reduces Central Insulin Resistance
Glucagon-like peptide-1 (GLP-1) improves insulin sensitivity in humans and rodents. We studied the impact of central GLP-1 receptor antagonism on the metabolic effects of peripheral GLP-1 administration in mice. High-fat-fed insulin-resistant mice were treated with continuous subcutaneous infusion of GLP-1 with or without concomitant ICV infusion of the GLP-1 receptor antagonist exendin-9 [18]. Interestingly, high-fat feeding induced central insulin resistance (see above). Peripheral administration of GLP-1 decreased hepatic and peripheral insulin resistance in high-fat-fed mice, involving central effects of GLP-1. Therefore, GLP-1 may be another approach to improve central insulin resistance, at least in high-fat-induced insulin-resistant mice.

Insulin in the Brain Modulates Triglyceride Metabolism

Insulin has many pleiotropic effects, which also holds true for triglyceride (TG) metabolism. In accordance with the major central effects of insulin on glucose metabolism, insulin also has major central effects on TG metabolism [19–21].

White adipose tissue (WAT) releases TG-derived non-esterified fatty acids (FA) into the circulation to serve as energy substrates, predominantly for muscle. Excessive release of FA may result in ectopic deposition of TG in non-adipose tissues like liver and muscle, associated with insulin resistance and steatosis. Conversely, WAT is also an important metabolic storage facility for TG, clearing and storing circulating FA and very low density lipoprotein (VLDL)-TG, thereby protecting other organs from ectopic lipid accumulation. The central effects of insulin have profound effects on the functions of WAT.

Physiology: Effects of Insulin in the Brain on White Adipose Tissue Metabolism
Neuronal and in particular hypothalamic insulin action is a critical regulator of WAT metabolism. Brain insulin action restrains lipolysis by reducing sympathetic outflow to WAT and controls de novo lipogenesis in adipose tissue. Impaired hypothalamic

insulin signaling increases lipolytic flux and decreases de novo lipogenesis [20]. Apparently, brain insulin action has an important anabolic function in WAT maintenance, which complements direct effects of insulin on adipocytes. Accordingly, the presence of the brain insulin receptor is critically important to prevent lipodystrophy in mice [19].

The stimulatory effects of brain insulin on WAT lipogenesis plus the finding that the absence of the neuronal insulin receptor impairs the lipogenic capacity of WAT suggest that the dysregulation of WAT lipogenesis in obesity is at least in part a function of brain insulin resistance [20].

Insulin also stimulates uptake of VLDL-TG-derived FA and albumin-bound FA in WAT from the blood [22]. Centrally administered insulin stimulated retention of both FA sources in a similar manner but without activating insulin signaling in WAT. Tolbutamide decreased this insulin-stimulated FA partitioning to WAT during peripheral insulin infusion, and it even abolished this effect during ICV co-administration with insulin [22]. Taken together, we showed that the central effects of circulating insulin contribute on average ~30% to TG-derived FA uptake in WAT and ~66% to albumin-derived FA uptake in WAT of the total effects of circulating insulin during hyperinsulinemic clamp conditions. These observations indicate that the effects of circulating insulin on FA uptake in WAT from plasma are for a considerable extent dependent on the central effects of insulin (fig. 1).

Pathophysiology: High-Fat Feeding Impairs the Effects of Insulin in the Brain on White Adipose Tissue Metabolism

The group of Buettner [20] tested whether diet-induced insulin resistance impairs the ability of hypothalamic insulin to regulate WAT lipolysis. Three days of high-fat diet in rats abolished the ability of mediobasal hypothalamic insulin to suppress WAT lipolysis as assessed by glycerol flux, but did not impair insulin signaling in WAT. Therefore, overfeeding impairs hypothalamic insulin action, which may contribute to unrestrained lipolysis seen in human obesity and type 2 diabetes.

Moreover, in diet-induced obese mice, centrally administered insulin was unable to stimulate FA retention in WAT. Furthermore, inhibition of central action of ICV administered insulin or circulating insulin by tolbutamide did not affect FA retention in WAT [22]. Therefore, overfeeding induces central insulin resistance to multiple effects of insulin on adipose tissue. These effects of overfeeding may contribute to the pathophysiology of obesity and type 2 diabetes.

Therapeutic Implications

At present, the studies targeting central insulin resistance have focused mainly on glucose metabolism. It is challenging to speculate that the effects of topiramate and GLP-1 via improvement of central insulin resistance with respect to glucose metabolism may also exert effects on lipid metabolism. Central infusion of GLP-1 beneficially impacts on lipid metabolism in WAT [23]. However, this effect is lost in diet-induced obese animals, implicating that overfeeding leads to central GLP-1 resistance. This contradicts findings on glucose metabolism and might imply that GLP-1 treatment of central insulin resistance of WAT metabolism is not a straight-forward approach, in contrast to the beneficial effects of GLP-1 on central insulin resistance of glucose metabolism.

Conclusion

Insulin acts on peripheral tissues both directly and indirectly, through the CNS. Insulin sensitivity is not a fixed entity, but is modulated dependent on (patho)physiological conditions. Likewise, the central effects of insulin are not fixed. Studies employing overfeeding have clearly demonstrated that central insulin resistance contributes considerably to an overall decrease in insulin effects on glucose and fat metabolism. There are indications that central insulin resistance is amenable to therapeutic interventions, at least with respect to glucose metabolism.

Acknowledgment

P.C.N.R. is an Established Investigator of the Dutch Heart Foundation (2009T038).

References

1 Havrankova J, Roth J, Brownstein M: Insulin receptors are widely distributed in the central nervous system of the rat. Nature 1978;272:827–829.

2 Gerozissis K: Brain insulin: regulation, mechanisms of action and functions. Cell Mol Neurobiol 2003;23:1–25.

3 Banks WA: The source of cerebral insulin. Eur J Pharmacol 2004;490:5–12.

4 Sindelar DK, et al: Basal hepatic glucose production is regulated by the portal vein insulin concentration. Diabetes 1998;47:523–529.

5 Rebrin K, Steil GM, Mittelman SD, Bergman RN: Causal linkage between insulin suppression of lipolysis and suppression of liver glucose output in dogs. J Clin Invest 1996;98:741–749.

6 Obici S, Zhang BB, Karkanias G, Rossetti L: Hypothalamic insulin signaling is required for inhibition of glucose production. Nat Med 2002;8:1376–1382.

7 Okamoto H, Obici S, Accili D, Rossetti L: Restoration of liver insulin signaling in Insr knockout mice fails to normalize hepatic insulin action. J Clin Invest 2005;115:1314–1322.

8 Filippi BM, Yang CS, Tang C, Lam TK: Insulin activates Erk1/2 signaling in the dorsal vagal complex to inhibit glucose production. Cell Metab 2012;16:500–510.

9 Karschin C, Ecke C, Ashcroft FM, Karschin A: Overlapping distribution of K_{ATP} channel forming Kir6.2 subunit and the sulfonylurea receptor SUR1 in rodent brain. FEBS Lett 1997;401:59–64.

10 Spanswick D, Smith MA, Mirshamsi S, Routh VH, Ashford ML: Insulin activates ATP-sensitive K^+ channels in hypothalamic neurons of lean, but not obese rats. Nat Neurosci 2000;3:757–758.

11 Coomans CP, Biermasz NR, Geerling JJ, Guigas B, Rensen PC, Havekes LM, Romijn JA: Stimulatory effect of insulin on glucose uptake by muscle involves the central nervous system in insulin-sensitive mice. Diabetes 2011;60:3132–3140.

12 Pocai A, Lam TK, Gutierrez-Juarez R, Obici S, Schwartz GJ, Bryan J, Guilar-Bryan L, Rossetti L: Hypothalamic K_{ATP} channels control hepatic glucose production. Nature 2005;434:1026–1031.

13 Den Boer MA, Voshol PJ, Kuipers F, Romijn JA, Havekes LM: Hepatic glucose production is more sensitive to insulin-mediated inhibition than hepatic VLDL-triglyceride production. Am J Physiol Endocrinol Metab 2006;291:E1360–E1364.

14 Ono H, Pocai A, Wang Y, Sakoda H, Asano T, Backer JM, Schwartz GJ, Rossetti L: Activation of hypothalamic S6 kinase mediates diet-induced hepatic insulin resistance in rats. J Clin Invest 2008;118: 2959–2968.

15 Kaiyala KJ, Prigeon RL, Kahn SE, Woods SC, Schwartz MW: Obesity induced by a high-fat diet is associated with reduced brain insulin transport in dogs. Diabetes 2000;49:1525–1533.

16 Wilkes JJ, Nelson E, Osborne M, Demarest KT, Olefsky JM: Topiramate is an insulin-sensitizing compound in vivo with direct effects on adipocytes in female ZDF rats. Am J Physiol Endocrinol Metab 2005;288:E617–E624.

17 Coomans CP, Geerling JJ, van den Berg SAA, van Diepen HC, Garcia-Tardón H, Thomas A, Schröder-van der Elst JP, Ouwens DM, Pijl H, Rensen PCN, Havekes LM, Guigas B, Romijn JA: The insulin-sensitizing effect of topiramate involves K_{ATP} channel activation in the central nervous system. Br J Pharmacol 2013;170:908–918.

18 Parlevliet ET, de Leeuw van Weenen JE, Romijn JA, Pijl H: GLP-1 treatment reduces endogenous insulin resistance via activation of central GLP-1 receptors in mice fed a high-fat diet. Am J Physiol Endocrinol Metab 2010;299:E318–E324.

19 Koch L, Wunderlich FT, Seibler J, Könner AC, Hampel B, Irlenbusch S, Brabant G, Kahn CR, Schwenk F, Bruning JC: Central insulin action regulates peripheral glucose and fat metabolism in mice. J Clin Invest 2008;118:2132–2147.

20 Scherer T, O'Hare J, Diggs-Andrews K, Schweiger M, Cheng B, Lindtner C, Zielinski E, Vempati P, Su K, Dighe S, Milsom T, Puchowicz M, Scheja L, Zechner R, Fisher SJ, Previs SF, Buettner C: Brain insulin controls adipose tissue lipolysis and lipogenesis. Cell Metab 2011;13:183–194.

21 Scherer T, Lindtner C, Zielinski E, O'Hare J, Filatova N, Buettner C: Short-term voluntary overfeeding disrupts brain insulin control of adipose tissue lipolysis. J Biol Chem 2012;287:33061–33069.

22 Coomans CP, Geerling JJ, Guigas B, van den Hoek AM, Parlevliet ET, Ouwens DM, Pijl H, Voshol PJ, Rensen PC, Havekes LM, Romijn JA: Circulating insulin stimulates fatty acid retention in white adipose tissue via K_{ATP} channel activation in the central nervous system only in insulin-sensitive mice. J Lipid Res 2011;52:1712–1722.

23 Nogueiras R, Pérez-Tilve D, Veyrat-Durebex C, Morgan DA, Varela L, Haynes WG, Patterson JT, Disse E, Pfluger PT, López M, Woods SC, DiMarchi R, Diéguez C, Rahmouni K, Rohner-Jeanrenaud F, Tschöp MH: Direct control of peripheral lipid deposition by CNS GLP-1 receptor signaling is mediated by the sympathetic nervous system and blunted in diet-induced obesity. J Neurosci 2009;29:5916–5925.

Johannes A. Romijn, MD, PhD
Department of Medicine, Academic Medical Center
University of Amsterdam, PO Box 22660
NL–1100 DD Amsterdam (The Netherlands)
E-Mail j.a.romijn@amc.uva.nl

Delhanty PJD, van der Lely AJ (eds): How Gut and Brain Control Metabolism.
Front Horm Res. Basel, Karger, 2014, vol 42, pp 59–72 (DOI: 10.1159/000358858)

The Important Role of Sleep in Metabolism

Georges Copinschi[a] · Rachel Leproult[b] · Karine Spiegel[c]

[a]Laboratory of Physiology, Université Libre de Bruxelles (ULB) and [b]Neuropsychology and Functional Neuroimaging Research Unit, Center for Research in Cognition and Neurosciences and ULB Neuroscience Institute, ULB, Brussels, Belgium; [c]Integrated Physiology and Physiology of Brain Arousal Systems, Lyon Neuroscience Research Center, INSERM U1028 – UMR 5292, Faculty of Medicine Lyon Est, Université Claude Bernard Lyon 1, Lyon, France

Abstract

Both reduction in total sleep duration with slow-wave sleep (SWS) largely preserved and alterations of sleep quality (especially marked reduction of SWS) with preservation of total sleep duration are associated with insulin resistance without compensatory increase in insulin secretion, resulting in impaired glucose tolerance and increased risk of type 2 diabetes. When performed under rigorously controlled conditions of energy intake and physical activity, sleep restriction is also associated with a decrease in circulating levels of leptin (an anorexigenic hormone) and an increase in circulating levels of ghrelin (an orexigenic hormone), hunger and appetite. Furthermore, sleep restriction is also associated with a stimulation of brain regions sensitive to food stimuli, indicating that sleep loss may lead to obesity through the selection of high-calorie food. There is also evidence that sleep restriction could provide a permissive environment for the activation of genes that promote obesity. Indeed, the heritability of body mass index is increased in short sleepers. Thus, chronic sleep curtailment, which is on the rise in modern society, including in children, is likely to contribute to the current epidemics of type 2 diabetes and obesity.

Sleep involves two states of distinct brain activity that are each generated in specific brain regions: rapid eye movement (REM) or paradoxical sleep, and non-REM sleep. Physiological sleep is initiated by light non-REM stages (stages 1 and 2), followed by a deeper non-REM stage (stage 3, or slow-wave sleep, SWS), then by REM sleep and possibly by transient awakenings. In healthy young subjects, this pattern lasts approximately 90 min and is usually repeated 4–6 times per night. As the night progresses, the number and duration of awakenings increase, non-REM sleep becomes shallower and the duration of REM episodes becomes longer. Aging is characterized by marked alterations in sleep architecture [1]. After 35 years of age, the duration of SWS is already dramatically reduced. Thereafter, the duration of REM sleep progressively declines, in mirror image of an equivalent increase in the proportion of time spent awake.

With a few exceptions, virtually all endocrine-metabolic systems are, at least partially, regulated by the sleep-wake homeostasis. For instance, it is now clearly established that sleep is a major determinant of growth hormone (GH) secretion, and that SWS is associated with GH secretory episodes [2]. The 24-hour rhythm of cortisol, while primarily driven by the circadian clock, is also regulated by the sleep-wake cycle [3]: at sleep onset, SWS is consistently associated with a drop in circulating cortisol levels. Conversely, cortisol secretion is triggered by awakenings, whether transient or final. During aging, the progressive increase in evening cortisol levels occurs as a mirror image of the decline in REM sleep [1].

Although it had already been observed in 1959 that glucose levels remain stable during nocturnal sleep despite prolonged fasting [4], no attempt was made for years to investigate possible relationships between sleep and metabolic function. Over the last 15 years however, a growing number of studies emphasized the importance of the sleep-wake homeostasis in the regulation of energy metabolism. Sleep curtailment was shown to be associated with major disruptions of energy metabolism.

The mechanisms of the physiological regulation by the sleep-wake cycle of appetite, energy intake and expenditure, and glucose metabolism, and the disruptions induced by sleep restrictions, are reviewed in the following sections.

Glucose Regulation and Insulin Secretion

Relationship between Sleep and Glucose Regulation
Brain mass represents only 2% of the body mass, but the blood flow destined to the brain represents about 10% of cardiac output. Indeed, brain energy requirements are extraordinarily high, since its oxygen and glucose utilization account for at least 20% of total body requirements [5]. Not surprisingly, any modification in glucose utilization by the brain may profoundly affect glucose tolerance. Cerebral glucose utilization is lower during SWS than during either REM sleep or wake [6, 7]. Using PET scans, a strong correlation was evidenced between slow-wave activity, an index of the intensity of SWS, and regional blood flow in the prefrontal brain [6, 7]. Furthermore, experimental studies, involving continuous enteral nutrition or intravenous glucose infusion while allowing for normal nocturnal sleep, have shown that glucose tolerance is minimal during the first half of the sleep period, i.e. when SWS is the dominant sleep stage. These findings confirm the existence of a robust link between SWS and glucose tolerance. In addition, studies performed in normal subjects under constant glucose infusion indicate that sleep-associated elevations in

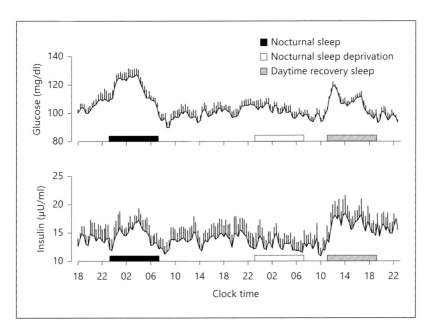

Fig. 1. Mean (+SEM) 24-hour profiles of plasma glucose and insulin in 8 normal young men (20–27 years old) during a 53-hour period that included 8 h of nocturnal sleep, 8 h of nocturnal sleep deprivation and 8 h of daytime sleep recovery. Blood samples were obtained at 20-min intervals [adapted from 35].

circulating glucose levels correlate positively with the amount of concomitant secretion of GH, a counter-regulatory hormone of insulin. Thus, decreased glucose tolerance appears to result from decreased glucose utilization both by the brain and by peripheral tissues [7, 8]. These effects subside during the second part of the night, when sleep becomes shallower and fragmented, and GH is no longer secreted. Under prolonged fasting condition, circulating glucose levels remain stable or decline only minimally during nocturnal sleep, contrasting with the clear decrease observed during daytime fasting.

Investigations involving a 12-hour delay of the sleep period have shown that decreased glucose tolerance is also observed during daytime sleep, but not during nocturnal sleep deprivation, attesting that glucose regulation is modulated by sleep per se, rather than by circadian rhythmicity (fig. 1).

Effects of Sleep Deprivation on Glucose Regulation

Recurrent sleep loss has consistently been found to be associated with marked alterations of glucose tolerance. In a *princeps* study published in 1999 [9], young healthy normal-weight men were successively submitted to three baseline nights with 8 h in bed (from 23:00 to 07:00 h), six nights of sleep curtailment (4 h in bed, from 01:00 h to 05:00 h) and six nights of sleep extension (12 h in bed, from 21:00 to 09:00 h), under strictly controlled conditions of physical activity and caloric intake. In all three conditions, time in bed was centered around 03:00 h in order to avoid circadian disruption. Total sleep time per night averaged (±SEM) 7 h 14 ± 5 min during baseline, 3 h 49 ± 2 min during the sleep restriction period, and 9 h 03 ± 15 min during the sleep extension period. Sleep restriction involved important decreases in durations of stages 1 and 2, of REM sleep, and of awakenings, while SWS was largely preserved. Sleep curtailment was associated with marked alterations of glucose metabolism compared with the fully rested condition. The overall glucose response to a standardized breakfast was increased despite similar insulin secretory response, indicating a decrease in insulin sensitivity, as assessed by an elevation of the HOMA (homeostatic model assessment, an index of insulin resistance) [10]. Following intravenous glucose infusion, acute insulin response, insulin sensitivity, glucose tolerance and glucose effectiveness (an index of insulin-independent glucose disposal) were all markedly reduced [9, 11] (fig. 2). Glucose tolerance fell to values reported in 61- to 80-year-old subjects with impaired glucose tolerance and the disposition index (product of acute insulin response to glucose and insulin sensitivity), a marker of diabetes risk, was reduced by more than 30%.

Subsequently, deleterious effects on glucose metabolism of sleep curtailment to 4–5.5 h per night for 5–14 nights were also found in a number of well-controlled experimental investigations performed in healthy young subjects, using intravenous glucose tolerance test or euglycemic-hyperinsulinic clamp: insulin sensitivity was reduced by 18–24%, without compensatory increase in insulin levels, resulting in impaired glucose tolerance [12]. A few studies, which also included assessments following sleep recovery, found that metabolic disturbances associated with sleep curtailment were, at least partially, reversible [12].

Though a progressive adaptation to prolonged sleep curtailment cannot be excluded, this bulk of data strongly suggests that, voluntary or not, recurrent partial sleep deprivation may increase the risk of diabetes. Moreover, those findings are supported by the results of multiple large cross-sectional and prospective population studies, with 5–17 years duration. A meta-analysis including a total of 107,756 individuals concluded that the relative risk of developing type 2 diabetes was 1.28 for self-reported short sleepers (≤5–6 h per night) after adjusting for possible confounders [12]. Of course, a major limitation of these population studies is the absence of objective determination of sleep duration.

Interestingly, reduced sleep quality with preservation of sleep duration also results in marked alterations of glucose tolerance. In a very elegant study, healthy young subjects were each investigated in a randomized crossover protocol under two experimental conditions: after two consecutive nights of undisturbed baseline sleep, and after three consecutive nights of all-night selective suppression of SWS, obtained by delivering appropriate acoustic stimuli [13] (fig. 2). The resulting 90% reduction in SWS was compensated by increased durations of lighter non-REM sleep (stage 2), while total sleep time, REM sleep, and the duration of wake after sleep onset were not affected. Despite preserved total sleep duration, SWS reduc-

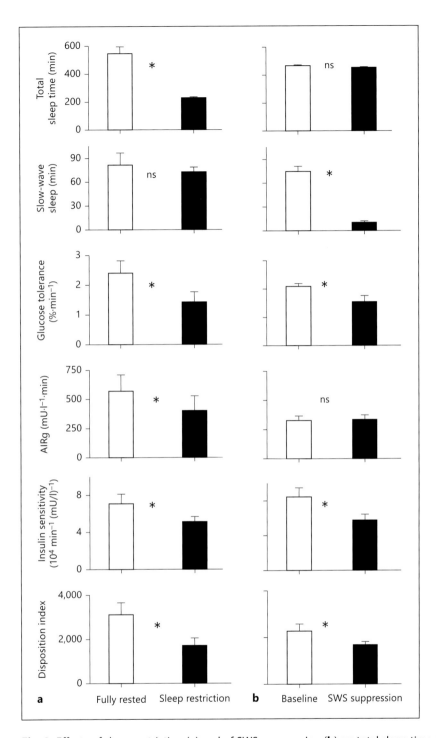

Fig. 2. Effects of sleep restriction (**a**) and of SWS suppression (**b**) on total sleep time, SWS, glucose tolerance, acute insulin response to glucose (AIRg), insulin sensitivity and disposition index in normal young subjects. Values shown are means + SEM. Asterisks denote statistically significant differences (p < 0.05) [adapted from 9, 11, 13].

tion was associated with a nearly 25% decrease in insulin sensitivity, not compensated by an appropriate increase in insulin release, resulting in a lower disposition index and a reduction of glucose tolerance to the range found in the elderly with impaired glucose tolerance. A strong correlation was evidenced between the magnitude of SWS reduction and the magnitude of the decrease in insulin sensitivity. In another study, random sleep fragmentation across all sleep stages, obtained by auditory and mechanical stimuli in healthy volunteers, induced a marked reduction in SWS and a less important but significant reduction in REM sleep, with a compensatory increase in stage 1 sleep, without any change in total sleep time and in stage 2 sleep. These alterations resulted in decreased insulin sensitivity and glucose effectiveness [14]. Thus, both reduced sleep duration with preservation of SWS, and alterations of sleep quality (especially reduction of SWS) with preservation of total sleep duration, have clear negative impacts on glucose metabolism and enhance the risk of type 2 diabetes. In addition, a few studies indicate that glycemic control in type 2 diabetes might be affected by sleep duration [12].

Obstructive Sleep Apnea and Glucose Regulation
Obstructive sleep apnea (OSA), the most common type of sleep apnea, caused by obstruction of the upper airway, is characterized by repetitive 20- to 40-second pauses in breathing during sleep. It results in intermittent hypoxia, shallow and fragmented sleep, lower amounts of SWS and reduced total sleep time. The severity of apnea and hypopnea episodes is greater during REM sleep than during non-REM sleep, possibly because of a reduction in pharyngeal muscle activity during REM sleep. OSA is particularly frequent in obese individuals, especially in men [12]. The impact of hypoxia on glucose metabolism was investigated in healthy volunteers, submitted while awake to 5 h/day of intermittent hypoxia, resulting in desaturation episodes equivalent to moderate OSA [15]. Glucose effectiveness and insulin sensitivity were significantly reduced, without concomitant increase in insulin secretion. In another study comparing healthy lean young men with OSA to healthy control subjects, glucose levels during an oral glucose tolerance test were similar in both groups, but at the cost of an increase in insulin release, indicating that OSA was associated with insulin resistance [16]. These results suggest that OSA-related hypoxia could increase diabetes risk. They are consistent with the findings of numerous large population-based studies, which found strong associations between OSA and insulin resistance, resulting in glucose intolerance in non-diabetic subjects after adjusting for possible confounders, including body mass index (BMI) [12]. In addition, in several population studies, individual degrees of insulin resistance and glucose intolerance appeared to be correlated to the severity of OSA [12]. Furthermore, several – but not all – prospective cohort studies found, after adjusting for possible confounders, that severe OSA predicted incident diabetes at the end of a follow-up period [12].

Hormonal Appetite Regulation: Leptin and Ghrelin

Relationship between Sleep and Leptin Regulation

Leptin is an anorexigenic hormone, mainly released by adipocytes, which provides information about energy status to hypothalamic centers. Leptin levels reflect cumulative energy balance: they increase in response to overfeeding, together with a decrease in hunger, and they decrease in response to underfeeding, together with an increase in hunger [17, 18]. In normal subjects, 24-hour circulating leptin profiles show important diurnal variations with minimum values during daytime and maximum values during early to mid-nocturnal sleep period [19, 20]. Diurnal variations are markedly dependent on the timing of meals: eating and fasting are associated with increased and decreased leptin levels, respectively [21]. However, diurnal variations were found to persist, albeit with reduced amplitude, in subjects receiving continuous enteral nutrition [22] and in subjects submitted to continuous wakefulness during 88 consecutive hours [23, 24]. Following an abrupt shift of the sleep period, a nocturnal rise was observed despite sleep deprivation, and the onset of daytime recovery sleep was associated with another leptin peak [22]. Thus, the 24-hour leptin profiles result from the interaction of the food intake schedule, the circadian pacemaker and the sleep-wake homeostasis.

Relationship between Sleep and Ghrelin Regulation

The acylated form of ghrelin (which also stimulates GH secretion) is an orexigenic hormone [25]. In healthy subjects, daytime profiles are primarily dependent on the timing of meals. In a rigorous experimental study performed in healthy young lean men under controlled conditions of sleep-wake cycles, dark-light cycles, energy intake and activity levels, total and acylated ghrelin levels, measured at frequent intervals during 24 h, were found to rapidly decline after each meal, irrespective of time of day, to reach minimum levels 90–120 min after meal presentation, followed by a rebound until the next meal. Following evening dinner, this rebound persisted during the first part of the sleep period, then ghrelin levels progressively declined until morning awakening, despite prolonged fasting. Moreover, during sleep, the ratio of acylated to total ghrelin was lower than during wake [25]. Altogether, these findings are consistent with a sleep-associated inhibition of the orexigenic signal. In another experimental study involving 3 days of fasting, ghrelin profiles showed diurnal variations, in mirror image of cortisol variations, with minimum levels in early morning, peak levels in the afternoon and a progressive nocturnal decrease [26] (but possible effects of the sleep-wake cycle were not explored). Altogether, available data suggest that the 24-hour ghrelin profiles also result from the interaction of the food intake schedule, the circadian pacemaker and the sleep-wake homeostasis.

Effects of Sleep Deprivation on Leptin, Ghrelin and Hunger Regulation

In a pioneering study published in 2004, healthy normal-weight young men were included in a randomized crossover investigation, performed under strictly controlled conditions of physical activity and caloric intake [27]. All volunteers participated in two sessions that were spaced at least 6 weeks apart. One session involved two consecutive nights of sleep restriction (4 h in bed, from 01:00 to 05:00 h; mean total sleep time 3 h 53 min). The other session involved two consecutive nights of sleep extension (10 h in bed, from 22:00 to 08:00 h; mean total sleep time 9 h 8 min). In both conditions, time in bed was centered around 03:00 h in order to avoid circadian disruption. Weight was similar in both sleep conditions. The day after the two consecutive nights of sleep restriction/extension, participants rated every hour their hunger and appetite for various food categories on validated visual analog scales, and blood samples were obtained at frequent intervals from 08:00 to 21:00 h for the measurement of leptin and ghrelin, while caloric intake was limited to an intravenous glucose infusion at a constant rate. Leptin levels were consistently lower and ghrelin levels consistently higher after sleep restriction than after sleep extension, so that the ghrelin-to-leptin ratio increased by 71% with 4 h in bed compared with 10 h in bed (fig. 3a). Simultaneously, hunger and appetite ratings were 23–24% higher after sleep restriction than after sleep extension, especially for calorie-dense foods (fig. 3a). The increase in hunger was proportional to the increase in ghrelin-to-leptin ratio [27] (fig. 3b). An increase in ghrelin levels under sleep restriction has been observed in most subsequent studies. Discrepant results were reported in studies with ad libitum access to food [12].

Evidence for a dose-response relationship between sleep length and the 24-hour temporal evolution of circulating leptin has been provided in a separate study [10]. Figure 3c shows the 24-hour leptin profiles observed after six days of 12, 8, and 4 h in bed in healthy lean young men studied at bed rest and under identical caloric consumption. Weight was similar in the three sleep conditions. The 24-hour mean, the acrophase and the amplitude of the 24-hour leptin variations gradually decreased from the 12-hour in bed to the 4-hour in bed condition. Of note, the reduction in the acrophase of the leptin profile (26%) between the 12- and the 4-hour in bed condition was similar to the changes reported in healthy subjects fed only 70% of their energy requirements during 3 consecutive days under normal sleep conditions. A decrease in leptin levels under sleep restriction was observed in subsequent studies performed in healthy normal-weight men, when similarly performed under well-controlled conditions of caloric intake, using multiple rather than single blood samplings. Inconsistent findings were observed in leptin-resistant obese subjects and in studies performed under ad libitum access to food.

The effects of sleep restriction in an environment that promoted inactivity and increased food intake were examined in a study that included middle-aged overweight sedentary subjects in a crossover study with ad libitum access to food [28]. Subjects were submitted in random order, at least 3 months apart, to 14 consecutive nights of

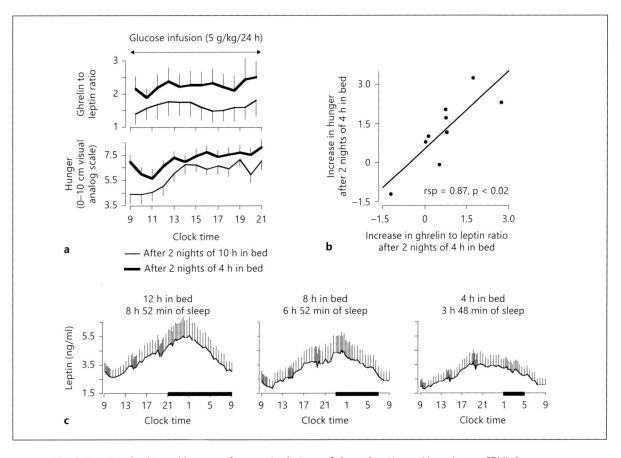

Fig. 3. Leptin, ghrelin and hunger after manipulations of sleep duration. **a** Mean (+ or − SEM) day-time profiles of ghrelin-to-leptin ratio and ratings of hunger obtained in 9 young healthy men studied at bed rest and under glucose infusion after two nights of 4 h in bed and after two nights of 10 h in bed. **b** Association between the increase in ghrelin-to-leptin ratio and the increase in hunger ratings when time in bed was restricted to 4 h as compared to extended to 10 h. **c** Mean (+SEM) 24-hour leptin profiles obtained after 6 days of 12, 8, and 4 h in bed in 9 healthy lean men studied at bed rest and under identical caloric intake. The subjects slept an average of 8 h 52 min at the end of the 12-hour in bed condition, 6 h 52 min at the end of the 8-hour in bed condition, and 3 h 48 min at the end of the 4-hour in bed condition. Note that all the characteristics of the 24-hour leptin profile (overall mean, nocturnal maximum, amplitude) gradually decreased from the 12-hour to the 4-hour in bed condition. The black bars represent the sleep periods [adapted from 10, 27].

sleep restriction (5.5 h in bed without circadian disruption; mean total sleep time 5 h 11 min) and to 14 nights of normal sleep duration (8.5 h in bed; mean total sleep time 7 h 13 min). Sleep restriction was associated with increased intake of calories from snacks, while regular meal intake was not affected, confirming that recurrent sleep curtailment in an obesity-promoting environment may induce excessive consumption of calorie-dense foods.

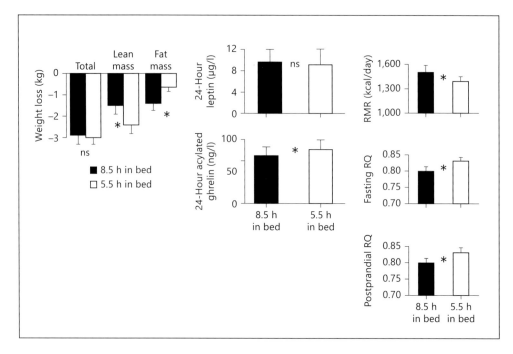

Fig. 4. Effects of sleep restriction on weight loss, 24-h levels of leptin and acylated ghrelin, resting metabolic rate (RMR), fasting and postprandial respiratory quotients (RQ) in middle-aged over-weight subjects submitted to identical moderate caloric restriction during 14 consecutive nights of normal sleep and during 14 consecutive nights of sleep restriction, in a randomized crossover study. Values shown are means + SEM. Asterisks denote statistically significant differences ($p < 0.05$) [adapted from 29].

A similar protocol involving 14 consecutive nights of sleep restriction (5.5 h in bed) versus 14 nights of normal sleep duration (8.5 h in bed) was conducted in middle-aged overweight subjects, with identical moderate caloric restriction in both conditions [29]. Total weight loss (approx. 3 kg) was quite similar in both conditions, but sleep restriction, compared with normal sleep, resulted in a 55% reduction in fat loss and a 60% increase in lean mass loss, suggesting the existence of mechanistic relationships between sleep and energy metabolism (fig. 4). Indeed, despite similar energy consumption, sleep restriction was associated with higher 24-hour levels of acylated ghrelin, an orexigenic hormone known to reduce energy expenditure, promote fat retention and increase hepatic production of glucose. Consistent with a reduced oxidation of fat, fasting and postprandial respiratory quotient values were increased and resting metabolic rate was decreased in the sleep restriction condition.

The effects of sleep restriction on energy expenditure and energy intake were investigated in healthy young normal-weight subjects, in a crossover study involving five consecutive nights of sleep restriction without circadian disruption (5 h in bed, mean total sleep time ~4 h 40 min) and five consecutive nights of normal sleep duration (9 h in bed, mean total sleep time ~7 h 40 min), with ad libitum access to food [30]. Both sessions were counterbalanced. As expected, sleep restriction induced an increase (~5%) in total daily energy expenditure. However, food intake (especially at night after dinner) was found to increase beyond what was needed to maintain energy balance, resulting in a weight gain averaging ~0.8 kg in 5 days.

The impact of sleep restriction on central brain mechanisms regulating the appetitive food desire was explored in two recent experimental studies. In a first crossover study, healthy middle-aged normal-weight volunteers were randomly assigned, 4 weeks apart, to either six consecutive nights of habitual sleep (9 h per night in bed, mean total sleep time ~7 h 38 min) or restricted sleep (4 h per night in bed, mean total sleep time ~3 h 46 min) [31]. During the first 4 days of each phase, they were given a controlled diet. Beginning on day 5, they had ad libitum access to food. Brain functional magnetic resonance, performed on the morning of day 6 after an overnight fast, showed that sleep restriction was associated with increased activation of brain regions sensitive to food stimuli. Consistent results were obtained in another study, where healthy young normal-weight volunteers completed two experimental sessions placed at least 7 days apart and counterbalanced in order across participants: one night of normal sleep and one night of total sleep deprivation [32]. The morning following sleep deprivation, the desire for high-calorie food was higher than following the normal night, and brain functional magnetic resonance showed that during food desirability choices, sleep deprivation was associated with a decrease in activity in appetitive evaluation cortical regions (leading to improper food choice selection), together with an amplification of activity within the amygdala (leading to stimulate desire for high-calorie food) (fig. 5). Furthermore, following sleep deprivation, the desire for high-calorie food correlated positively with subjective sleepiness. Most recently it was also reported that on the morning following one night of total sleep deprivation, healthy normal-weight men, given a fixed budget to get food at their best convenience, purchased more calories and grams than after one night of normal sleep [33].

Lastly, a large population study, involving more than 1,000 pairs of twins, has shown, as expected, that longer sleep duration was associated with decreased BMI [34]. Most importantly, it was also evidenced that the heritability of BMI when sleep duration was less than 7 h per night was more than twice as large than the heritability when sleep duration was more than 9 h per night. Thus, sleep restriction could provide a permissive environment for the expression of genes that promote obesity.

Conclusions and Perspectives

Though a progressive adaptation to chronic partial sleep deprivation cannot be excluded, this bulk of laboratory studies provides consistent evidence that recurrent sleep curtailment may increase the risk of obesity and diabetes, accelerate the senes-

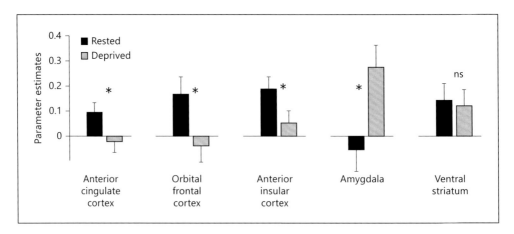

Fig. 5. Effects of sleep deprivation on reactivity to food desirability in five cortical and subcortical regions. Note the reduction in activity after sleep deprivation in the regions (anterior cingulate cortex, orbital frontal cortex and anterior insular cortex) necessary for optimal choice of food stimuli, and the amplification of activity after sleep deprivation within the amygdala, resulting in increased desire for high-calorie food. Values shown are means + or – SEM. Asterisks denote statistically significant differences (p < 0.05) [adapted from 32; data kindly provided by M.S. Greer].

cence of endocrine-metabolic function and compromise the efficacy of dietary energy-restriction strategies in obese patients. Moreover, these findings are corroborated by several cross-sectional and prospective studies, which consistently indicate that chronic short sleep is associated with obesity and/or type 2 diabetes.

Large interventional field studies incorporating objective determinations of sleep duration are now needed to determine if strategies aiming to optimize sleep duration and quality have preventive or therapeutic effects in obesity and diabetes. Considering the rapidly increasing morbidity and mortality of the current epidemics of diabetes and obesity, the identification of potentially modifiable risk factors, such as sleep curtailment, is particularly important.

Acknowledgments

Some of the research described in this article was supported by US National Institute of Health grants P01 AG-11412, R01 HL-075079, P60 DK-20595, R01 DK-0716960, R01 HL-075025, and M01 RR000055, by US Department of Defense award W81XWH-07-2-0071, by Belgian 'Fonds de la Recherche Scientifique Médicale' (FRSM-3.4583.02) and 'Fonds National de la Recherche Scientifique' (FNRS), and by the Integrated Physiology and Physiology of Brain Arousal Systems team, Lyon Neuroscience Research Center, INSERM U1028-CNRS UMR 5292, Claude Bernard University, Lyon, France. Dr. Leproult is currently a recipient of a grant 'Brains Back to Brussels' from the Brussels Institute for Research and Innovation (Belgium).

References

1 Van Cauter E, Leproult R, Plat L: Age-related changes in slow-wave sleep and REM sleep and relationship with growth hormone and cortisol levels in healthy men. JAMA 2000;284:861–868.

2 Van Cauter E, Kerkhofs M, Caufriez A, Van Onderbergen A, Thorner MO, Copinschi G: A quantitative estimation of GH secretion in normal man: reproducibility and relation to sleep and time of day. J Clin Endocrinol Metab 1992;74:1441–1450.

3 Van Cauter E, Blackman JD, Roland D, Spire JP, Refetoff S, Polonsky KS: Modulation of glucose regulation and insulin secretion by circadian rhythmicity and sleep. J Clin Invest 1991;88:934–942.

4 Robin ED, Travis DM, Julian DG, Boshell BR: Metabolic patterns during physiologic sleep. I. Blood glucose regulation during sleep in normal and diabetic subjects. J Clin Invest 1959;38:2229–2233.

5 Magistretti PJ: Neuron-glia metabolic coupling and plasticity. J Exp Biol 2006;209:2304–2311.

6 Maquet P: Positron emission tomography studies of sleep and sleep disorders. J Neurol 1997;244:S23–S28.

7 Maquet P: Functional neuroimaging of normal human sleep by positron emission tomography. J Sleep Res 2000;9:207–231.

8 Scheen AJ, Byrne MM, Plat L, Van Cauter E: Relationships between sleep quality and glucose regulation in normal humans. Am J Physiol 1996;271:E261–E270.

9 Spiegel K, Leproult R, Van Cauter E: Impact of sleep debt on metabolic and endocrine function. Lancet 1999;354:1435–1439.

10 Spiegel K, Leproult R, L'Hermite-Baleriaux M, Copinschi G, Penev PD, Van Cauter E: Leptin levels are dependent on sleep duration: relationships with sympathovagal balance, carbohydrate regulation, cortisol, and thyrotropin. J Clin Endocrinol Metab 2004;89:5762–5771.

11 Leproult R, Van Cauter E: Role of sleep and sleep loss in hormonal release and metabolism. Endocr Dev 2010;17:11–21.

12 Reutrakul S, Van Cauter E: Interactions between sleep, circadian function and glucose metabolism: implications for risk and severity of diabetes. Ann NY Acad Sci, in press.

13 Tasali E, Leproult R, Ehrmann DA, Van Cauter E: Slow-wave sleep and the risk of type 2 diabetes in humans. Proc Natl Acad Sci USA 2008;105:1044–1049.

14 Stamatakis KA, Punjabi NM: Effects of sleep fragmentation on glucose metabolism in normal subjects. Chest 2010;137:95–101.

15 Louis M, Punjabi NM: Effects of acute intermittent hypoxia on glucose metabolism in awake healthy volunteers. J Appl Physiol (1985) 2009;106:1538–1544.

16 Pamidi S, Wroblewski K, Broussard J, Day A, Hanlon EC, Abraham V, Tasali E: Obstructive sleep apnea in young lean men: impact on insulin sensitivity and secretion. Diabetes Care 2012;35:2384–2389.

17 Kershaw EE, Flier JS: Adipose tissue as an endocrine organ. J Clin Endocrinol Metab 2004;89:2548–2556.

18 Flier JS: Obesity wars: molecular progress confronts an expanding epidemic. Cell 2004;116:337–350.

19 Sinha MK, Ohannesian JP, Heiman ML, Kriauciunas A, Stephens TW, Magosin S, Marco C, Caro JF: Nocturnal rise of leptin in lean, obese and non-insulin-dependent diabetes mellitus subjects. J Clin Invest 1996;97:1344–1347.

20 Saad MF, Riad-Gabriel MG, Khan A, Sharma A, Michael R, Jinagouda SD, Boyadjian R, Steil GM: Diurnal and ultradian rhythmicity of plasma leptin: effects of gender and adiposity. J Clin Endocrinol Metab 1998;83:453–459.

21 Schoeller DA, Cella LK, Sinha MK, Caro JF: Entrainment of the diurnal rhythm of plasma leptin to meal timing. J Clin Invest 1997;100:1882–1887.

22 Simon C, Gronfier C, Schlienger JL, Brandenberger G: Circadian and ultradian variations of leptin in normal man under continuous enteral nutrition: relationship to sleep and body temperature. J Clin Endocrinol Metab 1998;83:1893–1899.

23 Shea SA, Hilton MF, Orlova C, Ayers RT, Mantzoros CS: Independent circadian and sleep/wake regulation of adipokines and glucose in humans. J Clin Endocrinol Metab 2005;90:2537–2544.

24 Mullington JM, Chan JL, Van Dongen HP, Szuba MP, Samaras J, Price NJ, Meier-Ewert HK, Dinges DF, Mantzoros CS: Sleep loss reduces diurnal rhythm amplitude of leptin in healthy men. J Neuroendocrinol 2003;15:851–854.

25 Spiegel K, Tasali E, Leproult R, Scherberg N, Van Cauter E: Twenty-four-hour profiles of acylated and total ghrelin: relationship with glucose levels and impact of time of day and sleep. J Clin Endocrinol Metab 2011;96:486–493.

26 Espelund U, Hansen TK, Hojlund K, Beck-Nielsen H, Clausen JT, Hansen BS, Orskov H, Jorgensen JO, Frystyk J: Fasting unmasks a strong inverse association between ghrelin and cortisol in serum: studies in obese and normal-weight subjects. J Clin Endocrinol Metab 2005;90:741–746.

27 Spiegel K, Tasali E, Penev P, Van Cauter E: Brief communication: Sleep curtailment in healthy young men is associated with decreased leptin levels, elevated ghrelin levels, and increased hunger and appetite. Ann Intern Med 2004;141:846–850.

28 Nedeltcheva AV, Kilkus JM, Imperial J, Kasza K, Schoeller DA, Penev PD: Sleep curtailment is accompanied by increased intake of calories from snacks. Am J Clin Nutr 2009;89:126–133.

29 Nedeltcheva AV, Kilkus JM, Imperial J, Schoeller DA, Penev PD: Insufficient sleep undermines dietary efforts to reduce adiposity. Ann Intern Med 2010; 153:435–441.

30 Markwald RR, Melanson EL, Smith MR, Higgins J, Perreault L, Eckel RH, Wright KP Jr: Impact of insufficient sleep on total daily energy expenditure, food intake, and weight gain. Proc Natl Acad Sci USA 2013;110:5695–5700.

31 St-Onge MP, McReynolds A, Trivedi ZB, Roberts AL, Sy M, Hirsch J: Sleep restriction leads to increased activation of brain regions sensitive to food stimuli. Am J Clin Nutr 2012;95:818–824.

32 Greer SM, Goldstein AN, Walker MP: The impact of sleep deprivation on food desire in the human brain. Nat Commun 2013;4:2259.

33 Chapman CD, Nilsson EK, Nilsson VC, Cedernaes J, Rangtell FH, Vogel H, Dickson SL, Broman JE, Hogenkamp PS, Schioth HB, Benedict C: Acute sleep deprivation increases food purchasing in men. Obesity (Silver Spring) 2013;21:E555–E560.

34 Watson NF, Harden KP, Buchwald D, Vitiello MV, Pack AI, Weigle DS, Goldberg J: Sleep duration and body mass index in twins: a gene-environment interaction. Sleep 2011;35:597–603.

35 Van Cauter E, Spiegel K: Circadian and sleep control of endocrine secretions; in Turek FW, Zee PC (eds): Circadian and Sleep Control of Endocrine Secretions. New York, Dekker, 1999, vol 13, pp 43–61.

Karine Spiegel, PhD
Physiologie Intégrée du Système d'Éveil
Centre de Recherche en Neurosciences de Lyon
INSERM U1028 – UMR 5292, Faculté de Médecine Lyon Est
Université Claude Bernard Lyon 1
8, avenue Rockefeller, FR–69373 Lyon Cedex 08 (France)
E-Mail karine.spiegel@univ-lyon1.fr

Delhanty PJD, van der Lely AJ (eds): How Gut and Brain Control Metabolism.
Front Horm Res. Basel, Karger, 2014, vol 42, pp 73–82 (DOI: 10.1159/000358315)

Metabolic Interplay between Gut Bacteria and Their Host

Frank Duca[a–c] · Philippe Gérard[a, b] · Mihai Covasa[a, b, d, e] · Patricia Lepage[a, b]

[a]UMR1319, Micalis, INRA and [b]Micalis, AgroParisTech, Jouy-en-Josas, France; [c]Toronto General Research Institute, University Health Network, Toronto, Ont., Canada; [d]Department of Basic Medical Sciences, College of Osteopathic Medicine, Western University of Health Sciences, Pomona, Calif., USA; [e]Department of Human and Health Development, University of Suceava, Suceava, Romania

Abstract

Shifts in the bacterial composition of the human gut microbiota (i.e. dysbiosis) have been associated with digestive tract dysfunctions such as inflammatory bowel diseases. More strikingly, strong evidence, from both human studies and germ-free animal models, links intestinal microbiota dysbiosis with metabolic disorders, such as obesity and liver diseases. This chapter focuses on the changes and impact of the gut microbiota during these diseased states, and describes the possible direct and indirect mechanisms that an aberrant gut microbiota can promote metabolic dysregulations. The possible involvement of the 'microbiota-gut-brain' axis in the development of obesity is further discussed, as is the perspective of meta-omic technologies that give insight into the functions and potential effect of the non-cultured intestinal bacteria on the host health. Understanding how modifications in this finely tuned ecosystem lead to these pathological processes is crucial for the development of new therapeutic approaches to treat and hopefully ameliorate these metabolic diseases.

© 2014 S. Karger AG, Basel

The Human Gut Bacterial Consortium: A Huge Reservoir of Yet Undescribed Functions

The human gastrointestinal tract hosts more than 100 trillion bacteria and *Archaea*, constituting the gut microbiota. The amount of bacteria in the gut outnumbers human cells by a factor of 10, and regulated mechanisms allow these microorganisms to colonize and survive within the host in a commensalism relationship. The restricted number of phyla (mainly Firmicutes, Bacteroidetes, Actinobacteria and Proteobacteria) as compared to other ecosystems strongly suggests a co-evolution between the intestinal microbiota and its host along ages, leading to physiological intestinal homeostasis. The human host provides a nutrient-rich environment to the microbiota, which, in turn, provides indispensable functions that humans cannot exert themselves. These functions are metabolic (colonic fermentation and short-chain fatty acid-associated production), protective (strengthening resistance to colonization by exogenous or opportunistic pathogens, antimicrobial peptides secretion), but also structural (maturation of the intestinal epithelium and immune system).

Chaotic in the early stages of life, the assembly of the human gut microbiota is established by the age of 2 and remains globally stable over time in healthy conditions in the absence of perturbation, such as antibiotic treatments or infections. The sequential bacterial colonization of the neonatal gut appears to be an important period for the development of a diverse, robust, resilient and functionally efficient microbiota [1]. Once stabilized, the average total number of bacterial species is estimated to be close to 400–500 per individual. Each human being harbors its own gut microbial composition. However, Tap et al. [2] described a phylogenetic core of bacteria containing 66 bacterial species (phylotypes or molecular species) that are shared by at least 50% of their studied populations of healthy humans.

Remarkably, shifts in the bacterial makeup of the human gut microbiota have been associated with digestive tract dysfunctions, such as inflammatory bowel disease (IBD) or inflammatory bowel syndrome. More strikingly, links between intestinal microbiota dysbiosis and distant organs have also been described in obesity, metabolic diseases, liver pathologies, allergy, etc. More than 10 years ago, the concept of 'dysbiosis', i.e. an unbalanced composition of the intestinal microbiota, was introduced in the IBD research field as a causal or aggravating agent [3]. Yet, this dysbiosis cannot be solely described as a bacterial compositional shift but also encompasses a functional shift and a disruption of bacterial diversity and ecosystem structure.

However, intestinal bacteria evolve in a highly specific ecological niche, in an anaerobic atmosphere, in close contact with a numerous pool of immune cells but also with food particles and other microorganisms such as parasites, fungi and viruses. Due to these particular conditions, most of the bacteria to date are not cultivable, their genome has not yet been sequenced and their functions are mostly undescribed.

The use of culture-independent approaches, mostly based on the analysis of 16S rRNA gene marker, has revealed a complex intestinal microbial community, with 70% of non-cultivable bacteria in average. Yet these techniques do not allow inferring encoded/expressed functions in the ecosystem.

Meta-omics approaches have hence recently been developed to answer crucial questions such as 'What is the genetic potential of the non-cultured bacterial fraction of the gut microbiota?' and 'What are these microbes really doing?'. Metagenomic, i.e. the analysis of the collective genomes from all the microorganisms present in an ecosystem, allowed the description of a yet unexpected reservoir of functions in the human gut. The human gut microbiome contains 3.3 million non-redundant genes, i.e. 150 times the size of the human genome [4]. A core microbiome of bacterial functions composed of 75 bacterial species highly prevalent in the population has been described.

Defined as our other genome, the gut microbiome complements the human genome by synthesizing health-related molecules. Recently, the notion of 'enterotypes' to describe general population groups based on their microbiome has been introduced [5]. Enterotypes are mainly explained by the abundance of three prevalent bacterial genera: *Bacteroides*, *Ruminococcus* and *Prevotella*. Originally, enterotypes had not been linked to host health status or human habits but a recent study identified a positive correlation between enterotypes and long-term dietary habits [6].

In the field of microbial ecology, the development of high-throughput sequencing technologies is currently leading to a constantly improved understanding of complex ecosystems.

Human Gut Microbiota and Metabolic Disorders

Microbiota and Obesity
Obesity rates have doubled since 1980, and over 10% of the world's population is obese. Obesity is a complex disease, involving a multitude of factors, including genetic, physiological, neural, metabolic, social, and environmental. More recently, it has been established that the gut microbiota strongly contributes to host physiology and metabolism, demonstrating a potential role for changes in gut microbiota in the development of obesity.

By utilizing germ-free (GF) animals, landmark studies led by the group of Gordon [7, 8] demonstrated that mice lacking intestinal microbiota exhibit less adiposity than normal mice, and are resistant to diet-induced obesity when fed a high-fat (HF) diet, which is reversed upon conventionalization. GF mice exhibited an increased expression of intestinal angiopoietin-related protein 4 (Angptl4), a protein that inhibits lipoprotein lipase and which mediates fatty acid uptake into adipocytes. Consequently, while reduced adiposity in GF mice was associated with increased Angptl4, GF Angptl4 KO animals exhibit similar adiposity as normal wild-type mice, furthering the role for intestinal Angptl4 in adiposity [7]. However, not all groups have replicated the reduction in adiposity of GF animals, despite GF status being associated with intestinal, but not plasma, protein levels of Angptl4 [9]. Therefore, while the microbiota affects fat accretion, it is likely not through changes in Angptl4.

Microbiota Changes during Obesity and Weight Loss
Gut microbiota is significantly altered during obesity, with a reduction in total bacterial diversity, as well as overall compositional shifts. Obese rodents and humans exhibit reduced Bacteroidetes abundance, and a proportional increase in the Firmicutes phylum [8, 10]. These observations have led to the hypothesis that the increased abundance of microbiota responsible for bacterial fermentation of indigestible carbohydrates into short-chain fatty acids (SCFAs) promotes adiposity through

increased energy harvesting. Indeed, GF mice have reduced intestinal SCFAs, and increased calories in urine and feces. On the other hand, genetically obese *ob/ob* mice have increased intestinal SCFAs and reduced fecal excretion of calories [10]. However, despite an enrichment in gene functions related to energy harvesting in the microbiome of obese mice and humans [10], the relationship between gut microbiota composition and energy harvest efficiency is more complex, suggesting that other host-microbe interactions contribute to the development of obesity during HF feeding [11].

Interestingly, obese patients receiving gastric bypass displayed, presurgically, a microbiota depleted in bacteria from the *Bacteroides/Prevotella/Porphyromonas* group (Bacteroidetes phylum), and this was correlated with increased corpulence and caloric intake. An increased level of *Escherichia coli* 3 months postsurgery was inversely correlated to fat mass and leptin levels, while reduced proportions of lactic acid bacteria including *Lactobacillus/Leuconostoc/Pediococcus* group and *Bifidobacterium* have been observed [12]. Similarly, a more recent study emphasized that gastric bypass surgery in a mouse model of obesity was associated with rapid and sustained abundance of Gammaproteobacteria *(Escherichia)* and Verrucomicrobia *(Akkermansia)* while transfer of this gut microbiota to GF animals resulted in decreased body weight and adiposity compared to GF mice inoculated with microbiota from sham operated mice [13].

Role of the Diet in Obesity-Associated Changes in Microbiota

Increased consumption of highly palatable, energy-dense foods, especially rich in fats, represents a major cause of excess caloric intake. As such, HF feeding, profoundly alters the profile of the gut microbiota [8, 11, 14, 15]. Interestingly, gnotobiotic mice inoculated with human microbiota exhibit rapid (~1 day) shifts in gut microbial profile and metabolic pathways in the microbiome after HF feeding, changes that precede adiposity increases [15], while genetically lean mice, display decreased Bacteroidetes, and increased Firmicutes during HF feeding [14]. This suggests that diet, independent of phenotype, is the main contributor to changes in the gut microbiota composition [14]. On the other hand, fat- or carbohydrate-restricted diets in humans and rodents produce similar microbiota shifts, suggesting that changes in energy intake or adiposity can also drive changes in gut microbiota profile [8]. Therefore, although the diet can undoubtedly influence the gut microbiota composition, obesity is associated with an aberrant microbial population that is not solely due to obesogenic feeding.

Gut Microbiota and Liver Diseases

Non-alcoholic fatty liver disease (NAFLD) is considered the hepatic manifestation of metabolic syndrome [16]. NAFLD affects 20–30% of populations in Western countries and more than 80% of obese people, with an increasing prevalence in parallel with the epidemic of obesity. It refers to a spectrum of liver damages ranging from simple steatosis (accumulation of triglycerides in the hepatocytes) to non-alcoholic steatohepatitis (NASH), advanced fibrosis, cirrhosis or even hepatocellular carcinoma. The 'two-hit' model is an accepted theory of the pathogenesis of NAFLD, where the first hit consists in the development of hepatic steatosis due to obesity and insulin resistance, and the second hit implies oxidative stress and dysregulated cytokine production leading to NASH. The liver possesses critical immunologic, metabolic and detoxifying functions. It receives 70% of its blood supply from the gut through the portal vein whose flow in humans exceeds 1 l/min. Therefore it constantly confronts gut-derived microbial components and metabolites. Alterations of the gut microbiota in patients with chronic liver diseases was first identified almost one century ago but only recently this microbiota has been regarded as a new environmental factor contributing to liver disease (including NAFLD) development.

It was first demonstrated that an antibiotic treatment reduces hepatic steatosis in humans after intestinal bypass [17]. Later on, chronic exposure to low-dose LPS has been shown to induce NASH in mice, whereas TLR4 knockout mice were protected [18]. Moreover, gut microbiota transplant in GF mice induces obesity development and a twofold increase in triglycerides content in the liver [7]. Recent results provide evidence for a link between inflammasomes, the gut microbiota and NAFLD [19]. Mice genetically deficient in inflammasome components developed more hepatic inflammation than control wild-type mice. Co-housing these immunocompromised mice with wild-type animals conferred the observed predisposition to NAFLD indicating that inflammasome-mediated dysbiosis, as a result of altered interactions between gut microbiota and host, regulates progression of NAFLD. Another study nicely demonstrated that gut microbiota determines development of NAFLD in mice [20]. First, conventional mice were fed a high-fat diet for 16 weeks and two of them were selected based on their opposite response to HF diet. Although both mice were the same weight, one displayed low fasting glycemia and weak steatosis (Non-Responder). The other one displayed insulin resistance and marked steatosis (Responder). Two groups of GF mice were transplanted with the gut microbiota of the two selected mice. After being fed a HF diet, only the mice associated with the Responder microbiota developed fasting hyperglycemia and hyperinsulinemia as well as hepatic macrovesicular steatosis and showed an increased expression of genes involved in lipogenesis. Lachnospiraceae and Barnesiella were found overrepresented in the gut microbiota of these mice, while the group of mice which did not develop NAFLD features had higher population of *Bacteroides vulgatus*. Therefore, an increasing amount of studies showed a link between gut microbiota and NAFLD development and several different mechanisms have been proposed including altered choline metabolism, small intestinal bacterial overgrowth (SIBO), gut leakiness, or ethanol production. Choline is an essential nutrient of the vitamin B complex and choline-deficient diets are known to promote NAFLD. Indeed, free choline is required to form lipoproteins in the liver in order to export free fatty acids. Members of the gut microbiota are able to metabolize choline leading to production of trimethylamine.

Dumas et al. [21] demonstrated that increased choline metabolism by the gut microbiota lead to reduced choline bioavailability to the host and therefore to NAFLD development. NAFLD and NASH have been associated with SIBO and gut leakiness. Moreover, both gut permeability and SIBO correlated with the severity of steatosis [22]. These observations have led to the hypothesis that the decreased intestinal motility associated with liver disease induces colonization of the small intestine by colonic bacteria and then SIBO. Then, increased gut permeability allows translocation of bacteria and endotoxins into the portal flow, promoting TNF-α hepatic release from Kupffer cells and exacerbation of liver damages. Recently, production of ethanol by intestinal bacteria also arose as a possible cause of NAFLD progression. Indeed, it was observed that the blood concentration of ethanol in obese patients with NASH is higher than the one of obese patients without NASH. Moreover, the gut microbiota of obese patients with NASH is enriched with alcohol-producing bacteria (mainly *Escherichia*) [23]. Therefore, these bacteria could deliver a constant supply of ethanol to the liver leading to the generation of reactive oxygen species and, consequently, liver inflammation. Finally, the gut microbiota could also modulate host lipid metabolism and NAFLD development through metabolism of bile acids, by changing their emulsification and absorption properties, which can affect fatty acids storage in the liver.

Interaction of Microbiota and Gut-Brain Axis in Energy Homeostasis

There is a burgeoning appreciation that the gut microbiota can affect host health by impacting the central nervous system (CNS) through neural, endocrine, and immune pathways. The 'gut-brain axis' represents the bidirectional signalling between the brain and gastrointestinal (GI) tract responsible for maintaining homeostasis of the host through both neural and hormonal mechanisms.

Gut Microbiota Alters the CNS Function and Host Behavior
Accumulating evidence demonstrates that the gut microbiota can influence CNS functions, hence the term 'microbiota-gut-brain axis'. First, clinical studies demonstrate that patients with GI diseases, such as IBDs, exhibit an aberrant gut microbiota, which is sometimes associated with psychiatric disorders. Secondly, GF mice exhibit differences in anxiety behavior, motor control, and memory, which is associated with changes in brain chemistry. Likewise, mice strains with differences in exploratory behavior show alterations in gut microbiota. Finally, probiotic treatment normalizes host behavior such as anxiety as well as brain chemistry. This overwhelming evidence for a microbiota-gut-brain axis that has a strong influence on CNS function and overall host behavior provides credence to the idea that the gut microbiota can similarly alter CNS control of energy homeostasis by influencing intestinal nutrient signalling pathways.

Duca · Gérard · Covasa · Lepage

Gut-Brain Signalling in Control of Food Intake and Energy Regulation

Gut-brain signalling is important in the control of food intake and maintenance of normal glycemic levels. As such, the gut senses intestinal nutrients triggering a variety of signals, such as GI peptides, to provide feedback to the brain about both their quality and quantity. Short-term (or episodic) signals, which are released in response to eating, determine the size of the meal (e.g. CCK), and/or control the amount of time between meals (i.e. GLP-1, PYY), also termed satiation and satiety, respectively. These peptides can then act on local sensory nerves innervating the GI tract to relay messages to the hindbrain, or they can act in an endocrine fashion, directly activating receptors in the brain. Although known for their short-term role in energy intake, recent evidence, including rapid increases in GI peptide levels, now indicates a potential long-term role in the maintenance of body weight and development of obesity [see 24 for more].

Germ-Free Studies Contribution

Recent studies with GF animals provide evidence that the gut microbiota can influence the gut-brain axis to alter metabolism. For example, GF mice exhibit upregulated lingual CD36, and reduced intestinal protein expression of GPR40, GPR41, GPR43, and GPR120 [25]. These proteins are involved in sensing of nutrients, and partly mediate gut peptide release from enteroendocrine cells. As such, intestinal protein expression of gut peptides CCK, PYY, and GLP-1 are decreased in GF animals. All of these changes are associated with an increased acceptance of intralipid and sucrose solutions, indicating that reduced intestinal sensing in GF mice promotes energy intake [25, 26]. Furthermore, central neuropeptides responsible for energy homeostasis are altered in GF animals, emphasizing the broad role of the gut microbiota in energy-regulating pathways, both in the periphery and centrally.

Gut Microbiota and Gut-Brain Axis

Changes in peripheral and central peptides observed in GF animals may be secondary to other consequences resultant from a lack of microbiota, such as a depleted energy state from reduced energy harvest. Indeed, extraction of calories from otherwise nondigestible carbohydrates is accomplished through bacterial fermentation in the colon, producing SCFA end-products. However, in addition to energy, SCFAs have been shown to induce peptide release and lower food intake via activation of GPRs. As such, microbial by-products can affect functional expression of intestinal nutrient-responsive GPRs and GI hormones, suggesting a role for gut microbiota and its metabolic by-products in modulating satiation. Specifically, SCFA production is associated with increased GLP-1 and PYY production, possibly mediated through GPR41. Gut microbiota can also exert a direct effect on gut peptides. Indeed, prebiotic-induced changes in gut microbiota are associated with increased L-cell number, and specific bacterial species, such as *Akkermansia muciniphila* were positively correlated with L-cell numbers [27]. Additionally, certain bacterial species were shown to upregulate GPR120 gene expression and downregulate GLP-1 expression in Caco-2 cells

[28]. Together, these studies demonstrate that lack of, or changes in, gut microbiota results in vast alterations in intestinal nutrient-sensing elements that can alter subsequent energy intake.

Microbiota Modulates Gut-Brain Axis in Obesity

Few studies have examined the role of the gut microbiota in altering intestinal nutrient-sensing pathways that may ultimately promote the development of obesity. Interestingly, HF feeding and obesity is associated with reductions in circulating gut peptides, GLP-1, CCK and PYY. Furthermore, HF feeding also results in rapid changes in gut microbiota composition, therefore it is plausible that an aberrant gut microbiota during HF feeding drives changes in intestinal signalling to promote overeating and weight gain. Indeed prebiotic treatment (non-digestible carbohydrates, i.e. oligofructose) has been associated with an increase in the potency of anorexigenic peptides (GLP, PYY) and a corresponding decrease in orexigenic peptides such as ghrelin. Furthermore, prebiotics increases postprandial release of both GLP-1 and PYY, and is associated with reduced food intake. How gut microbiota modulates endocrine functions is still under investigation, however an increase in intestinal L-cell differentiation by SCFA such as acetate and propionate have been reported. Likewise, gut microbiota modulates the activity of proteins involved in gut barrier functions such as glucagon-like peptide-2 (GLP-2) which is co-secreted with GLP-1 by the L-cells. In this regard, prebiotic treatment increases *Bifidobacterium*, and subsequently decreases gut permeability, inflammatory markers, and metabolic endotoxemia possibly through GLP-2 and endocannabinoid-dependent mechanisms [29]. Together, these studies demonstrate the capacity of the gut microbiota to influence both central and peripheral energy-regulating signalling pathways, contributing to the increased energy intake and weight gain.

Conclusion and Perspectives

The knowledge of the capability of the gut microbiota to influence host health and homeostasis is ever expanding. Recent data indicate that the microbes present in the gut may be capable of directly and/or indirectly influencing the gut-brain axis involved in energy homeostasis. Future work deciphering the exact players and roles in this interaction could provide potential therapeutic strategies aimed at reducing energy intake and decreasing the prevalence of obesity. These recent discoveries are now paving the way toward new therapeutic options to modulate the intestinal microbiota, such as fecal transplantation. Applied for decades to treat patients with recurrent and antibiotic-refractory *Clostridium difficile* infections, fecal matter transplantation proved to have some efficacy, at least over a 6-week period, to treat metabolic disease in obese patients [30]. These pioneer results launched the application of fecal transplantation to other pathologies such as IBD. A better understanding of the intestinal ecosystem is still mandatory to comprehend the exact role of human gut microbiota in human health. Access to bacterial functions will surely soon allow us to accurately modulate the microbiome by restoring specific defective functions in individuals evolving in their own environment. Understanding microbes-microbes and microbes-host interactions at the human organism scale constitutes a major step toward the development of personalized medicine, not only in the pathogenesis of chronic gut diseases, but also in host function and homeostasis beyond the gut.

References

1 Mackie RI, Sghir A, Gaskins HR: Developmental microbial ecology of the neonatal gastrointestinal tract. Am J Clin Nutr 1999;69:1035S–1045S.

2 Tap J, Mondot S, Levenez F, Pelletier E, Caron C, Furet JP, Ugarte E, Munoz-Tamayo R, Paslier DL, Nalin R, Dore J, Leclerc M: Towards the human intestinal microbiota phylogenetic core. Environ Microbiol 2009;11:2574–2584.

3 Tamboli CP, Neut C, Desreumaux P, Colombel JF: Dysbiosis in inflammatory bowel disease. Gut 2004; 53:1–4.

4 Qin J, Li R, Raes J, Arumugam M, Burgdorf KS, Manichanh C, Nielsen T, Pons N, Levenez F, Yamada T, Mende DR, Li J, Xu J, Li S, Li D, Cao J, Wang B, Liang H, Zheng H, Xie Y, Tap J, Lepage P, Bertalan M, Batto JM, Hansen T, Le Paslier D, Linneberg A, Nielsen HB, Pelletier E, Renault P, Sicheritz-Ponten T, Turner K, Zhu H, Yu C, Jian M, Zhou Y, Li Y, Zhang X, Qin N, Yang H, Wang J, Brunak S, Dore J, Guarner F, Kristiansen K, Pedersen O, Parkhill J, Weissenbach J, Bork P, Ehrlich SD: A human gut microbial gene catalogue established by metagenomic sequencing. Nature 2010;464:59–65.

5 Arumugam M, Raes J, Pelletier E, Le Paslier D, Yamada T, Mende DR, Fernandes GR, Tap J, Bruls T, Batto JM, Bertalan M, Borruel N, Casellas F, Fernandez L, Gautier L, Hansen T, Hattori M, Hayashi T, Kleerebezem M, Kurokawa K, Leclerc M, Levenez F, Manichanh C, Nielsen HB, Nielsen T, Pons N, Poulain J, Qin J, Sicheritz-Ponten T, Tims S, Torrents D, Ugarte E, Zoetendal EG, Wang J, Guarner F, Pedersen O, de Vos WM, Brunak S, Dore J, Antolin M, Artiguenave F, Blottiere HM, Almeida M, Brechot C, Cara C, Chervaux C, Cultrone A, Delorme C, Denariaz G, Dervyn R, Foerstner KU, Friss C, van de Guchte M, Guedon E, Haimet F, Huber W, van Hylckama-Vlieg J, Jamet A, Juste C, Kaci G, Knol J, Lakhdari O, Layec S, Le Roux K, Maguin E, Merieux A, Melo Minardi R, M'Rini C, Muller J, Oozeer R, Parkhill J, Renault P, Rescigno M, Sanchez N, Sunagawa S, Torrejon A, Turner K, Vandemeulebrouck G, Varela E, Winogradsky Y, Zeller G, Weissenbach J, Ehrlich SD, Bork P: Enterotypes of the human gut microbiome. Nature 2011;473:174–180.

6 Wu GD, Chen J, Hoffmann C, Bittinger K, Chen YY, Keilbaugh SA, Bewtra M, Knights D, Walters WA, Knight R, Sinha R, Gilroy E, Gupta K, Baldassano R, Nessel L, Li H, Bushman FD, Lewis JD: Linking long-term dietary patterns with gut microbial enterotypes. Science 2011;334:105–108.

7 Backhed F, Ding H, Wang T, Hooper LV, Koh GY, Nagy A, Semenkovich CF, Gordon JI: The gut microbiota as an environmental factor that regulates fat storage. Proc Natl Acad Sci USA 2004;101:15718–15723.

8 Turnbaugh PJ, Backhed F, Fulton L, Gordon JI: Diet-induced obesity is linked to marked but reversible alterations in the mouse distal gut microbiome. Cell Host Microbe 2008;3:213–223.

9 Swartz TD, Sakar Y, Duca FA, Covasa M: Preserved adiposity in the Fischer 344 rat devoid of gut microbiota. FASEB J 2013;27:1701–1710.

10 Turnbaugh PJ, Ley RE, Mahowald MA, Magrini V, Mardis ER, Gordon JI: An obesity-associated gut microbiome with increased capacity for energy harvest. Nature 2006;444:1027–1031.

11 Murphy EF, Cotter PD, Healy S, Marques TM, O'Sullivan O, Fouhy F, Clarke SF, O'Toole PW, Quigley EM, Stanton C, Ross PR, O'Doherty RM, Shanahan F: Composition and energy harvesting capacity of the gut microbiota: relationship to diet, obesity and time in mouse models. Gut 2010;59: 1635–1642.

12 Furet JP, Kong LC, Tap J, Poitou C, Basdevant A, Bouillot JL, Mariat D, Corthier G, Dore J, Henegar C, Rizkalla S, Clement K: Differential adaptation of human gut microbiota to bariatric surgery-induced weight loss: links with metabolic and low-grade inflammation markers. Diabetes 2010;59:3049–3057.

13 Liou AP, Paziuk M, Luevano JM Jr, Machineni S, Turnbaugh PJ, Kaplan LM: Conserved shifts in the gut microbiota due to gastric bypass reduce host weight and adiposity. Sci Transl Med 2013;5: 178ra41.

14 Hildebrandt MA, Hoffmann C, Sherrill-Mix SA, Keilbaugh SA, Hamady M, Chen YY, Knight R, Ahima RS, Bushman F, Wu GD: High-fat diet determines the composition of the murine gut microbiome independently of obesity. Gastroenterology 2009;137:1716–1724.e1–e2.

15 Turnbaugh PJ, Ridaura VK, Faith JJ, Rey FE, Knight R, Gordon JI: The effect of diet on the human gut microbiome: a metagenomic analysis in humanized gnotobiotic mice. Sci Transl Med 2009;1:6ra14.

16 Fabbrini E, Sullivan S, Klein S: Obesity and nonalcoholic fatty liver disease: biochemical, metabolic, and clinical implications. Hepatology 2010;51:679–689.

17 Drenick EJ, Fisler J, Johnson D: Hepatic steatosis after intestinal bypass – prevention and reversal by metronidazole, irrespective of protein-calorie malnutrition. Gastroenterology 1982;82:535–548.

18 Rivera CA, Adegboyega P, van Rooijen N, Tagalicud A, Allman M, Wallace M: Toll-like receptor-4 signaling and Kupffer cells play pivotal roles in the pathogenesis of non-alcoholic steatohepatitis. J Hepatol 2007;47:571–579.

19 Henao-Mejia J, Elinav E, Jin C, Hao L, Mehal WZ, Strowig T, Thaiss CA, Kau AL, Eisenbarth SC, Jurczak MJ, Camporez JP, Shulman GI, Gordon JI, Hoffman HM, Flavell RA: Inflammasome-mediated dysbiosis regulates progression of NAFLD and obesity. Nature 2012;482:179–185.

20 Le Roy T, Llopis M, Lepage P, Bruneau A, Rabot S, Bevilacqua C, Martin P, Philippe C, Walker F, Bado A, Perlemuter G, Cassard-Doulcier AM, Gerard P: Intestinal microbiota determines development of non-alcoholic fatty liver disease in mice. Gut 2012; 62:1787–1794.

21 Dumas ME, Barton RH, Toye A, Cloarec O, Blancher C, Rothwell A, Fearnside J, Tatoud R, Blanc V, Lindon JC, Mitchell SC, Holmes E, McCarthy MI, Scott J, Gauguier D, Nicholson JK: Metabolic profiling reveals a contribution of gut microbiota to fatty liver phenotype in insulin-resistant mice. Proc Natl Acad Sci USA 2006;103:12511–12516.

22 Miele L, Valenza V, La Torre G, Montalto M, Cammarota G, Ricci R, Masciana R, Forgione A, Gabrieli ML, Perotti G, Vecchio FM, Rapaccini G, Gasbarrini G, Day CP, Grieco A: Increased intestinal permeability and tight junction alterations in nonalcoholic fatty liver disease. Hepatology 2009;49:1877–1887.

23 Zhu L, Baker SS, Gill C, Liu W, Alkhouri R, Baker RD, Gill SR: Characterization of gut microbiomes in nonalcoholic steatohepatitis (NASH) patients: a connection between endogenous alcohol and NASH. Hepatology 2013;57:601–609.

24 Duca FA, Covasa M: Current and emerging concepts on the role of peripheral signals in the control of food intake and development of obesity. Br J Nutr 2012; 108:778–793.

25 Duca FA, Swartz TD, Sakar Y, Covasa M: Increased oral detection, but decreased intestinal signaling for fats in mice lacking gut microbiota. PLoS One 2012; 7:e39748.

26 Swartz TD, Duca FA, de Wouters T, Sakar Y, Covasa M: Up-regulation of intestinal type 1 taste receptor 3 and sodium glucose luminal transporter-1 expression and increased sucrose intake in mice lacking gut microbiota. Br J Nutr 2011;107:621–630.

27 Everard A, Lazarevic V, Derrien M, Girard M, Muccioli GM, Neyrinck AM, Possemiers S, Van Holle A, Francois P, de Vos WM, Delzenne NM, Schrenzel J, Cani PD: Responses of gut microbiota and glucose and lipid metabolism to prebiotics in genetic obese and diet-induced leptin-resistant mice. Diabetes 2011;60:2775–2786.

28 Fredborg M, Theil PK, Jensen BB, Purup S: G protein-coupled receptor 120 (GPR120) transcription in intestinal epithelial cells is significantly affected by bacteria belonging to the Bacteroides, Proteobacteria, and Firmicutes phyla. J Anim Sci 2012;90(suppl 4): 10–12.

29 Cani PD, Possemiers S, Van de Wiele T, Guiot Y, Everard A, Rottier O, Geurts L, Naslain D, Neyrinck A, Lambert DM, Muccioli GG, Delzenne NM: Changes in gut microbiota control inflammation in obese mice through a mechanism involving GLP-2-driven improvement of gut permeability. Gut 2009;58:1091–1103.

30 Vrieze A, Van Nood E, Holleman F, Salojarvi J, Kootte RS, Bartelsman JF, Dallinga-Thie GM, Ackermans MT, Serlie MJ, Oozeer R, Derrien M, Druesne A, Van Hylckama Vlieg JE, Bloks VW, Groen AK, Heilig HG, Zoetendal EG, Stroes ES, de Vos WM, Hoekstra JB, Nieuwdorp M: Transfer of intestinal microbiota from lean donors increases insulin sensitivity in individuals with metabolic syndrome. Gastroenterology 2012;143:913–916.e7.

Frank Duca, PhD
Toronto General Research Institute, University Health Network
MaRS Centre, TMDT 10th Floor, Room 10-701G
101 College Street, Toronto, ON M5G 1L7 (Canada)
E-Mail fduca@uhnresearch.ca

Delhanty PJD, van der Lely AJ (eds): How Gut and Brain Control Metabolism.
Front Horm Res. Basel, Karger, 2014, vol 42, pp 83–92 (DOI: 10.1159/000358316)

The Brain-Stomach Connection

C. Folgueira[a, c] · L.M. Seoane[a, c] · F.F. Casanueva[b, c]

[a]Grupo Fisiopatologia Endocrina, Instituto de Investigación Sanitaria de Santiago de Compostela (IDIS), Complexo Hospitalario Universitario de Santiago (CHUS/SERGAS), [b]Laboratorio de Endocrinologia Molecular y Celular, IDIS, CHUS/SERGAS, and [c]CIBER Fisiopatologia Obesidad y Nutricion (CB06/03), Instituto de Salud Carlos III, Santiago de Compostela, Spain

Abstract

The stomach-brain connection has been revealed to be one of the most promising targets in treating obesity. The stomach plays a key role in the homeostatic mechanism implicating stomach-brain communication regulated under neural and hormonal control. The present review explores specific topics related to gut-brain interactions focus on the stomach-brain connection through the different known systems implied in energy balance control as ghrelin, and nesfatin. Moreover, novel mechanisms for energy balance regulation involving gastric-brain communication are described including the role of the gastric intracellular mTOR/S6K1 pathway mediating the interaction among ghrelin, nesfatin and endocannabinoid gastric systems to modulate metabolism.

© 2014 S. Karger AG, Basel

The Brain-Stomach Connection

Obesity constitutes a major public health problem in the developed countries. However, currently employed therapies are not successful with the exception of gastric surgery, which, at present, is the most effective treatment for this pathology. This finding suggests that the signals from the gastrointestinal tract are crucial for the regulation of energy balance. Recent progress in the fight against obesity has involved investigating the increasing number of peripheral hunger and satiety signals that require central integration. In this context, the stomach-brain communication has been revealed to be one of the most promising targets in treating obesity.

Immediately after ingestion, nutrients interact with different areas of the gastrointestinal tract, which respond by secreting various hunger and satiety signals that require central integration to allow efficient energy homeostasis. These neurohormonal signals communicate nutritional status to the brain centers.

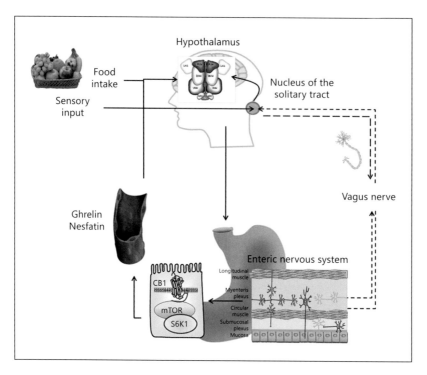

Fig. 1. Neural control of the brain-stomach connection (see text for details).

In this scenario, the stomach plays a key role in the homeostatic mechanism, implicating stomach-brain communication, which is regulated under neural and hormonal control and is responsible for maintaining body weight.

Neural Control of the Brain-Stomach Connection

The stomach is not only a reservoir of food but is also a complex, highly regulated organ with a neural mechanism that connects with higher brain areas, which are associated with central functions, such as reward and appetite [1]. In this context, the neural control of this regulatory system is managed by the nervous system and affects the gastrointestinal tract (fig. 1). The neural control of the gastrointestinal tract is exerted by the autonomic nervous system innervating the stomach, which can be further divided into the sympathetic (excitatory innervations) and the parasympathetic (inhibitory innervations) divisions of the nervous system [1]. The parasympathetic division is composed of the vagal and pelvic nerves, and the sympathetic division includes the splanchnic nerves.

The vagus nerve has recently been shown to regulate energy homeostasis as a mediator of the interaction between stomach and brain [2]. Food-related stimuli activate

Folgueira · Seoane · Casanueva

the sensors of the afferent fibers in the stomach modulating gastrointestinal tract functions and food intake [3]. The afferent fibers of the vagus reach the dorsal brainstem, primarily the nucleus of the solitary tract, and from here to different brain centers as the hypothalamus, to modulate orexigenic and anorexigenic signals in charge of regulate energy (fig. 1) [1].

The enteric nervous system is composed by a complex network of nervous cells located in the gastrointestinal tract. This system is required for major gastrointestinal functions as gut motility, secretion and blood flow [4]. The neurons from the enteric nervous system innervate the stomach and are localized in the myenteric and the submucous plexus. The submucous plexus is primarily involved in responding to nutrient signaling, whereas the myenteric plexus is primarily involved in the coordination of motility patterns [3]. It was recently demonstrated that the myenteric plexus is endowed with a medium-term memory, suggesting that enteric neurons have an intermediate-term memory [5].

Hormonal Control of the Brain-Stomach Connection

The gastrointestinal tract has been revealed as the largest endocrine organ in the body. More than 30 different gastric-derived peptides are secreted from enteroendocrine cells in response to ingested food regulating, in addition to digestive functions, energy balance [6]. These functions are, in part, mediated by the action of the gastric-derived peptides at a central level and, especially, in the hypothalamus, the main center regulator of appetite. At the hypothalamic level, the arcuate NPY/AgRP neurons are in charge of sensing and responding to a wide variety of hormones and nutrient-derived signals in the blood that are relevant to both the short- and long-term aspects of energy homeostasis (fig. 1) [7].

In this context, the gastrointestinal-derived peptides involved in the control of energy homeostasis have recently garnered a notable degree of attention. Among these peptides, ghrelin is considered the most relevant, as demonstrated by the considerable volume of works published about this hormone and its actions [8]. In addition, nesfatin-1, a stomach-derived peptide involved in food intake regulation, which was recently discovered, is receiving increasing interest as a regulator of energy homeostasis [9].

Ghrelin

Ghrelin was isolated from the stomach in 1999 by Kojima et al. [10] as an endogenous ligand for the growth hormone secretagogues orphan receptor. Thirty percent of the circulating levels of this 28-amino-acid peptide present acylation by an *n*-octanoic acid in the Ser3 residue. The remaining 70% circulates as unacylated ghrelin. The acyltransferase that catalyzes ghrelin octanoylation has recently been identified as ghrelin O-acyltransferase and appears to be a key factor in ghrelin function [11].

In humans and rodents, ghrelin-circulating levels were decreased by 65% after gastrectomy, suggesting that the stomach is the main source of ghrelin in the organism. In particular, the main ghrelin-producing cells in the stomach are X/A-like cells, although ghrelin expression throughout the entire gastrointestinal tract has also been described [11]. In addition, ghrelin expression has also been detected in other tissues, such as the hypothalamus, pituitary, ovary, testis, heart and placenta [11].

The diversity of ghrelin physiological actions underlines the key role of the stomach in energy balance regulation. Following exogenous administration of ghrelin, its neuroendocrine functions and effects on GH secretion, as well the corticotroph axis and prolactin secretion were shown [12]. The effects of ghrelin on the digestive tract include an increase of gastric acid secretion and gastric motility. In addition to these functions, this peptide is involved in vasodilatation and cellular proliferation [12].

Ghrelin constitutes the main gastric-derived peptide regulating energy balance as a connection between the stomach and brain. In fact, it has been reported that AgRP/NPY neurons are the primary targets of ghrelin orexigenic actions in the hypothalamus (fig. 1) [7].

Gastric Ghrelin Regulation

Regulation of endogenous ghrelin levels are influence by chronic or acute nutritional status changes in animals and humans. Thus, in food deprivation conditions ghrelin levels are elevated in plasma, while low levels of this peptide are seen after feeding [5]. Until recently, the mechanism that directly regulates ghrelin production in the stomach remained unclear, leading to the assumption that any changes in plasma ghrelin reflect changes in gastric ghrelin release.

In 2007, a novel organ culture model was developed assessing gastric ghrelin secretion directly from gastric tissue explants [5]. Using this new system, it was demonstrated that food-mediated changes in plasma ghrelin levels are due to variations in ghrelin release by the stomach [5]. In addition, it was further demonstrated that the effect of food intake on circulating ghrelin levels involves a more complex mechanism of action than previously thought. In the mentioned article, it became clear that the ghrelin secretion directly from the stomach is not only due to direct mechanical contact with the gastric wall, digestion or absorption of nutrients. The exposure to food-related sensory stimuli, without real intake, is able to modify gastric ghrelin secretion and its circulating levels, in the same way as true feeding [5]. This fact indicates that a relevant factors involved in this process are the central nervous system sensorial stimuli, including ghrelin as a neural-mediated integrative factor that constitutes a link between the sensory qualities of food, neural activation and nutrient metabolism. Furthermore, the regulation of ghrelin production by sensory stimulus is blocked after surgical vagotomy in rats implying the mediation of vagus nerve in ghrelin action [5].

In addition to the implication of the vagus nerve in the gastric control of ghrelin production, it has been demonstrated that the neuronal network of the myenteric plexus is endowed with medium-term memory. Seoane et al. [5] reported that gastric tissue excised from the organism that maintained the previous secretor status for a period of 3 h after excision, suggesting that the neurons from the enteric system of the gastric tissue have medium-term memory. These data were supported by previous studies demonstrating that synaptic activity memory exists in the enteric nervous system.

In addition to food intake-related factors, other metabolic stimuli, such as the classical components of the somatotrope axis pathways, are implicated in gastric ghrelin regulation. These factors comprise somatostatin (SS), growth hormone-releasing hormone (GHRH), insulin-like growth factor 1 (IGF-1) and growth hormone (GH) [13]. It has been demonstrated that SS and GH in vitro inhibits gastric ghrelin secretion though specific receptors for both hormones in the stomach [13].

Nesfatin-1

Nesfatin-1 is an 82-amino-acid peptide identified in 2006 by Oh-I et al. [14] that is derived from a 396-amino-acid precursor, nucleobinding protein 2 (NUCB2), which, after processing, produces three different subtypes: nesfatin-1, nesfatin-2 and nesfatin-3. Currently, only nesfatin-1 has been demonstrated to have an effect on metabolism regulation.

The expression of NUCB2 was initially found in the hypothalamic nucleus involved in food intake control and co-expressed with other appetite-regulator peptides (MCH, CART, α-MSH and NPY). However, recently, it was demonstrated also to be expressed in other brain areas together with other hypothalamic peptides involved in pituitary hormonal secretion, such as CRF, TRH, GHRH and SS and stress response (neurotensin, CRF, serotonin) [15]. At the peripheral level, nesfatin-1 expression has been described in different organs, such as the stomach, heart, pancreas, testis, pituitary and adipose tissue. Co-expression of nesfatin-1 with ghrelin in the stomach and pancreas has been described [16].

The first physiological function described for nesfatin-1 was the reduction of food intake in the dark phase after central injection in rats. In addition, a reduction in weight gain and fat depots most likely related to the anorexigenic action was also observed [14]. In this context, all of the evidence suggests a physiological role for nesfatin-1 as a negative regulator of food intake [16].

With respect to nesfatin-1 production regulation, higher levels of expression in the brain have been found in the hypothalamic nucleus, which suggests a potential role in food intake and metabolism regulation. Moreover, this peptide's hypothalamic levels vary with energy status modifications, being inhibited in fasting or under food deprivation and increased after refeeding. However, contradictory effects have been described with regard to the effect of nesfatin-1 central injection. In male rats, anti-NUCB2 antibody injection in the third ventricle of the brain increases food intake [14]. In contrast, a study demonstrated that inactivation of hypothalamic NUCB2 in female rats does not affect appetite or body weight [9]. In addition, the central administration of nesfatin-1 has been demonstrated to be involved in different digestive processes, including producing a delaying in gastric emptying and suppression of gastric motility [15]. These findings suggest a regulatory role for nesfatin on gastric motor activity as the mediator of its anorexigenic actions.

In the stomach, X/A gastric cells that produce ghrelin have been demonstrated to express nesfatin-1 at a tenfold higher level than in the brain. In addition, peripherally administered nesfatin-1 has been demonstrated to be able to cross the blood-brain barrier. The implication of the vagus nerve in the anorexigenic effect of nesfatin was demonstrated by the lack of effect of this hormone when peripherally administered in mice subject to vagal communication blockade from capsaicin administration [16].

Taken together, these findings suggest that as with ghrelin, the main source in the organism for nesfatin is the stomach. Furthermore, considering the opposite effects of ghrelin and nesfatin on body weight, adiposity and food intake, it has been recently proposed that nesfatin-1 counteracts ghrelin to regulate energy homeostasis.

The Endocannabinoid System

A wide variety of therapeutic actions of *Cannabis sativa* have been described [17]. The characterization of the specific receptors for cannabinoids CB1 and CB2 and the isolation of cannabinoids in organisms indicate the existence of an endocannabinoid system. This system has been assumed to have effects on food intake and energy metabolism regulation through various poorly characterized mechanisms.

The endocannabinoid system, at the peripheral level, plays a role in glucose homeostasis, lipogenesis and insulin sensitivity regulation [18]. Among the different factors activating this regulatory system, hunger, fasting and stress are the most relevant. Functional evidence indicates the possible influence of the CB1 receptors in appetite control in rat and humans at the gastric and intestinal levels. The upregulation of CB1 receptors selectively located in vagal terminals has been demonstrated to be a consequence of the fasting state [18]. In addition, CB1 presents a relatively high constitutive activity at this level, and it modulates vagal nerve function even in the absence of endogenous cannabinoid ligand [19]. It was recently demonstrated that CB1 receptors are localized in the stomach in the neuroendocrine gastric cells producing ghrelin [20]. All of the recent studies regarding the involvement of gastric cannabinoid system suggest that any regulator mechanism at this level can be implicated in gastric-brain communication and the mediation of energy balance control.

Novel Mechanisms for Energy Balance Regulation Involving Gastric-Brain Communication

mTOR/S6K1 Intracellular Pathway

The mTOR (mammalian target of rapamycin) is a highly conserved serine-threonine kinase component of at least two multiprotein complexes: mTOR complex 1 (mTORC1) and mTOR complex 2 (mTORC2). mTORC1 phosphorylates and modulates the activity of the serine/threonine ribosomal protein S6 kinase 1 (S6K1). In turn, S6K1 phosphorylates and activates S6, a ribosomal protein involved in translation [21]. The intracellular pathway mTOR/S6K1 has become a subject of considerable interest in studies focusing on metabolic control. This route has been proposed as an intracellular ATP sensor because it is altered by changes in energy status, such as fasting and obesity. Studies on insulin-resistant obese rats under high-fat diets have demonstrated the activation of mTOR signaling in several peripheral tissues, such as liver and skeletal muscle [22]. At the central level, it was found that mTOR signaling in hypothalamic neurons is involved in the neuronal sensing of nutrient availability and regulates food intake and energy balance.

Ghrelin/mTOR/Cannabinoid Gastric System

Recent studies have examined the gastric mTOR pathway and its role in mediating both hormonal and neural control of gastric regulation of energy balance. Expression of the active form of mTOR (phospho-mTOR) has been described in the endocrine cells producing ghrelin in the stomach [23]. Furthermore, the mTOR signaling pathway in gastric endocrine cells has been demonstrated to function as a peripheral fuel sensor that is able to modulate the expression of various gastric-derived peptides, primarily ghrelin and nesfatin (fig. 1) [23, 24]. The intracellular pathway indirectly participates in the brain-stomach connection regulation of energy balance through the action of gastric peptides on hypothalamic neurons, which regulates food intake (fig. 1). In addition, nutritional status, such as fasting and refeeding, modulates mTOR phosphorylation in gastric tissue. Moreover, a reciprocal relationship exists between gastric mTOR signaling and the expression and secretion of ghrelin during changes in energy status. Therefore, the inhibition of gastric mTOR signaling leads to increased expression of ghrelin mRNA, ghrelin O-acyltransferase mRNA, tissue preproghrelin content, and circulating ghrelin, but the activation of gastric mTOR signaling suppresses the expression and secretion of ghrelin [23].

Recently, a study performed in rats described the existence of a gastric mechanism that consists of the interaction between the endogenous cannabinoid system (CB1) and ghrelin through the intracellular mTOR pathway, which results in the central regulation of food intake under the neural control of the vagus nerve (fig. 1). The study emerged as the result of research into the physiological mechanism involved in the anorexigenic effect of a CB1 receptor antagonist. This antagonist, rimonabant, was proposed several years ago as one of the promising pharmacological therapies against obesity. However, shortly after being placed on market, rimonabant was withdrawn because of non-desired central-level effects. Knowledge of the peripheral effects of rimonabant would be notably helpful in the development of future anti-obesity therapies to aid in avoiding non-desired effects. Traditionally, the regulation of appetite has been attributed to the CB1 cannabinoid receptors located in the brain [17]. However, the expression of CB1 in the gastric mucosa and concretely in the fundus of the stomach, where ghrelin is synthesized and secreted, suggests a possible functional interaction at the gastric level between these two systems. In addition, it was demonstrated that rimonabant does not have anorexigenic effects when it is directly injected into the brain in food-deprived animals [25]. On the contrary, it was demonstrated that rimonabant, when peripherally injected, has a potent food intake-reducing effect, both basal and in response to central ghrelin administration. Moreover, an intact vagus connection is required for the cannabinoid system effects on appetite. Accordingly, using gastric explants from rats in vivo treated with rimonabant, it was demonstrated that the local effect of rimonabant in the stomach reduces the elevated ghrelin secretion characteristic of fasting and reduces ghrelin-circulating levels [20]. However, this inhibitory effect disappears in animals under surgical vagotomy, which indicates that the vagus nerve connection is mandatory for the local interaction between the ghrelinergic and cannabinoid systems in the stomach and the consequent anorexigenic effect. The intracellular pathway in charge of modulating this gastric system is the mTOR/S6K1 pathway, as the blockade of peripheral CB1 receptors by both rimonabant and AM281 (another antagonist for CB1) activates the intracellular pathway (as indicated by the increase in the phosphorylation of mTOR and S6K1), which coincides with a decrease in ghrelin secretion and circulating levels [20]. In addition, in animals with in vivo blockade of mTOR/S6K1 pathway via rapamycin treatment, rimonabant injection is not effective in reducing ghrelin. In summary, this newly discovered gastric mechanism demonstrates that the pharmacological blockade of the cannabinoid receptor is sensed by the hungry gastric cells as a satiety signal comparable to food intake, and as a consequence, the gastric tissue responds by decreasing the increased ghrelin secretion characteristic of fasting states, which, consequently, decreases food intake via inhibition of the orexigenic message vagally communicated to the brain (fig. 1). This mechanism is most likely the clearest current example of the stomach-brain connection-based system physiologically involved in energy balance regulation.

mTOR-Nesfatin-1
There is currently little information concerning the involvement of nesfatin-1 in this new gastric mechanism of energy balance regulation. Previously, it was demonstrated that the mTOR signaling molecule pS6K co-localizes with nesfatin-1/NUCB2-expressing cells in the gastric oxyntic mucosa and that alteration in mTOR activity is linked to nesfatin-1/NUCB2 production [24]. The relation between the mTOR pathway and nesfatin-1 is opposed to those found with ghrelin as a parallel relationship

between gastric mTOR activity and the expression of nesfatin-1/NUCB2 during changes in energy status, such as during fasting and obesity. Future research should seek to demonstrate if the cannabinoid system in the stomach is involved in this interaction between nesfatin-1 and the mTOR pathway and if this interaction has any final effect on food intake regulation at the central level via the vagal connection between the stomach and brain.

Conclusions

In conclusion, the stomach-brain communication has been revealed to be one of the most promising targets in treating obesity. Among the novel gastric systems requiring central integration that directly or indirectly participates in the regulation of energy balance by the brain-stomach connection, the endocannabinoid, ghrelin and nesfatin systems together with the intracellular mTOR/S6K1 pathway have become key factors.

References

1 Al-Massadi O, Pardo M, Casanueva FF, Seoane LM: The stomach as an energy homeostasis regulating center. An approach for obesity. Recent Pat Endocr Metab Immune Drug Discov 2010;4:75–84.

2 Sawchenko PE: Central connections of the sensory and motor nuclei of the vagus nerve. J Auton Nerv Syst 1983;9:13–26.

3 Berthoud HR: The vagus nerve, food intake and obesity. Regul Pept 2008;149:15–25.

4 Konturek SJ, Brzozowski T, Konturek PC, Schubert ML, Pawlik WW, Padol S, Bayner J: Brain-gut and appetite regulating hormones in the control of gastric secretion and mucosal protection. J Physiol Pharmacol 2008;59(suppl 2):7–31.

5 Seoane LM, Al-Massadi O, Caminos JE, Tovar SA, Dieguez C, Casanueva FF: Sensory stimuli directly acting at the central nervous system regulate gastric ghrelin secretion. An ex vivo organ culture study. Endocrinology 2007;148:3998–4006.

6 Rehfeld JF: Accurate measurement of cholecystokinin in plasma. Clin Chem 1998;44:991–1001.

7 Seoane LM, Lopez M, Tovar S, Casanueva FF, Senaris R, Dieguez C: Agouti-related peptide, neuropeptide Y, and somatostatin-producing neurons are targets for ghrelin actions in the rat hypothalamus. Endocrinology 2003;144:544–551.

8 Komarowska H, Jaskula M, Stangierski A, Wasko R, Sowinski J, Ruchala M: Influence of ghrelin on energy balance and endocrine physiology. Neuro Endocrinol Lett 2012;33:749–756.

9 Garcia-Galiano D, Tena-Sempere M: Emerging roles of NUCB2/nesfatin-1 in the metabolic control of reproduction. Curr Pharm Des 2013;19:6966–6972.

10 Kojima M, Hosoda H, Date Y, Nakazato M, Matsuo H, Kangawa K: Ghrelin is a growth-hormone-releasing acylated peptide from stomach. Nature 1999;402:656–660.

11 Al Massadi O, Tschop MH, Tong J: Ghrelin acylation and metabolic control. Peptides 2011;32:2301–2308.

12 Wren AM, Bloom SR: Gut hormones and appetite control. Gastroenterology 2007;132:2116–2130.

13 Seoane LM, Al-Massadi O, Barreiro F, Dieguez C, Casanueva FF: Growth hormone and somatostatin directly inhibit gastric ghrelin secretion. An in vitro organ culture system. J Endocrinol Invest 2007;30:RC22–RC25.

14 Oh-I S, Shimizu H, Satoh T, Okada S, Adachi S, Inoue K, Eguchi H, Yamamoto M, Imaki T, Hashimoto K, Tsuchiya T, Monden T, Horiguchi K, Yamada M, Mori M: Identification of nesfatin-1 as a satiety molecule in the hypothalamus. Nature 2006;443:709–712.

15 Goebel-Stengel M, Wang L: Central and peripheral expression and distribution of NUBC2/nesfatin-1. Curr Pharm Des 2014, Epub ahead of print.

16 Stengel A, Goebel M, Tache Y: Nesfatin-1: a novel inhibitory regulator of food intake and body weight. Obes Rev 2011;12:261–271.

17 Kirkham TC, Williams CM: Endogenous cannabinoids and appetite. Nutr Res Rev 2001;14:65–86.

18 Di Marzo V, Petrosino S: Endocannabinoids and the regulation of their levels in health and disease. Curr Opin Lipidol 2007;18:129–140.

19 Burdyga G, Lal S, Varro A, Dimaline R, Thompson DG, Dockray GJ: Expression of cannabinoid CB1 receptors by vagal afferent neurons is inhibited by cholecystokinin. J Neurosci 2004;24:2708–2715.

20 Senin L, Al-Massadi O, Folgueira C, Castelao C, Pardo M, Barja-Fernandez S, Roca-Rivada A, Amil M, Crujeiras AB, Garcia-Caballero T, Gabellieri E, Leis R, Dieguez C, Pagotto U, Casanueva FF, Seoane LM: Gastric CB1 receptor modulates ghrelin production through the mTOR pathway to regulate food intake. PLoS One 2013;8:e80339.

21 Wullschleger S, Loewith R, Hall MN: TOR signaling in growth and metabolism. Cell 2006;124:471–484.

22 Khamzina L, Veilleux A, Bergeron S, Marette A: Increased activation of the mammalian target of rapamycin pathway in liver and skeletal muscle of obese rats: possible involvement in obesity-linked insulin resistance. Endocrinology 2005;146:1473–1481.

23 Xu G, Li Y, An W, Li S, Guan Y, Wang N, Tang C, Wang X, Zhu Y, Li X, Mulholland MW, Zhang W: Gastric mammalian target of rapamycin signaling regulates ghrelin production and food intake. Endocrinology 2009;150:3637–3644.

24 Li Z, Xu G, Li Y, Zhao J, Mulholland MW, Zhang W: mTOR-dependent modulation of gastric nesfatin-1/NUCB2. Cell Physiol Biochem 2012;29:493–500.

25 Gomez R, Navarro M, Ferrer B, Trigo JM, Bilbao A, Del Arco I, Cippitelli A, Nava F, Piomelli D, Rodriguez de Fonseca F: A peripheral mechanism for CB1 cannabinoid receptor-dependent modulation of feeding. J Neurosci 2002;22:9612–9617.

Felipe F. Casanueva, PhD
Laboratorio de Endocrinologia Molecular y Celular, Laboratorio 14
IDIS, CHUS/SERGAS, Travesia da Choupana s/n
ES–15706 Santiago de Compostela (Spain)
E-Mail felipe.casanueva@usc.es

Delhanty PJD, van der Lely AJ (eds): How Gut and Brain Control Metabolism.
Front Horm Res. Basel, Karger, 2014, vol 42, pp 93–106 (DOI: 10.1159/000358317)

Prader-Willi Syndrome as a Model of Human Hyperphagia

Maithe Tauber[a–c] · Gwenaelle Diene[a, b] · Emmanuelle Mimoun[a, b] ·
Sophie Çabal-Berthoumieu[a, b] · Carine Mantoulan[a, b] ·
Catherine Molinas[a–c] · F. Muscatelli[d] · Jean Pierre Salles[a–c]

[a]Centre de référence du syndrome de Prader-Willi, [b]Unité d'Endocrinologie, Hôpital des Enfants, CHU de
Toulouse, [c]Centre de Physiopathologie de Toulouse Purpan, INSERM UMR 1043/CNRS UMR 5282, Université
Paul Sabatier, Toulouse, and [d]Institut de Neurobiologie de la Méditerranée (INMED), INSERM U901, Parc
Scientifique de Luminy, Marseille, France

Abstract

Prader-Willi syndrome (PWS), first described in 1956, is considered as a paradigm of a neurodevelopmental disorder with severe and early obesity with hyperphagia and impaired satiety. The improved knowledge in the natural history and recent data on genetics offer new perspectives for understanding the metabolic and endocrine dysfunctions and possibly for treatment. Natural history of the disease has been described due to the early diagnosis performed in the first months of life and various nutritional phases have been described. In addition, there is clear evidence that the abnormal feeding behavior is included in the behavioral problems. Brain imaging studies have shown that some brain regions may be important in PWS. The role of SNORD116 gene cluster is detailed and its links with circadian rhythm and brain and hypothalamus development. Pathophysiology of the abnormal ghrelin levels and of OT dysfunction is documented. While no effect on appetite and weight regulation has been reported with ghrelin antagonists, OT has been shown to improve some of the behavioral problems in adults. We discuss our hypothesis of an abnormal ghrelin/OT/dopamine pathway which may explain the switch of nutritional phases and behavior. These new aspects offer an opportunity for therapeutic use and possible early intervention.

Prader-Willi syndrome (PWS) is a rare neurodevelopment genetic disorder arising from the lack of expression of paternally inherited imprinted genes on chromosome 15q11–q13. It is the first known example of a human disorder involving genomic imprinting. The phenotype, first described by Prader et al. [1] in 1956, includes neonatal hypotonia with suckling difficulties, facial dysmorphia with acromicria, early onset of morbid obesity with hyperphagia and impaired satiety, endocrine dysfunction including short stature, with growth hormone (GH) deficiency, hypogonadism and learning disabilities, behavioral problems with psychiatric phenotypes. This complex disease leads to severe consequences and difficult management issues for patients, families and carers [2]. The estimated birth incidence is at about 1 in 15–20,000, and the population prevalence at about 1 in 50,000. PWS is the more frequent cause of identified syndromic obesities. Other studies have highlighted the high rates and varied causes of morbidity and mortality throughout the natural history of the disease, mainly due to respiratory problems in infancy and obesity complications later on. Early diagnosis and an integrated multidisciplinary approach have completely changed the phenotype of children and also had a strong impact on the comorbidities seen in adults. Of note, hyperphagia was defined at the Hyperphagia Meeting organized by the PWS Association in Baton Rouge, La., USA in October 2012, and not only includes excess of eating but also a 'qualitative' abnormal eating behavior.

In this chapter, we enlighten the more recent and challenging data on hyperphagia in PWS opening new outcomes in understanding the pathophysiology and offering therapeutic perspectives.

An Improved Knowledge on Natural History of the Syndrome

PWS classically has two nutritional phases: Phase 1 ranges from birth to early infancy (6–9 months) when infants with PWS show severe hypotonia and a poor ability to suck, thus often requiring tube feeding. Failure to thrive refers to the lack of weight gain despite normal calorie intake. Phase 2 begins between 2 and 4 years with the onset of obesity and hyperphagia. Recent progress in early diagnosis has shed light on the natural history of this syndrome and has revealed more complex nutritional phases. Indeed, between 18 and 36 months of age, body weight and BMI increase excessively, in such a way that they cross one, two or even more weight percentiles without a significant increase in calorie intake or any change in eating behavior. Miller et al. [3] then delineated seven nutritional phases in PWS including the neonatal period. These phases are described in table 1.

In our opinion, it is as if PWS infants display anorexia and subsequently develop obesity with hyperphagia and impaired satiety. There is no data describing the underlying mechanisms for this switch from failure to thrive to excessive weight gain in PWS. An early postnatal critical period for implementing hypothalamic maturation has been described in rodents and has not been well documented in humans. The early postnatal implementation of the brain circuits involved in appetite regulation is not yet fully understood and appears to be very complex. PWS appears to be a unique model for decrypting this critical period.

Table 1. Clinical characteristics of the nutritional phases [from 5]

Phase 0	*Decreased fetal movements and lower birth weight* Full-term birth weight and BMI are about 15–20% less than the siblings Typically normal gestational age 85% have decreased fetal movements
Phase 1a	*Hypotonia with difficulty feeding (0–9 months)* Weak, uncoordinated suck. Usually cannot breastfeed Needs assistance with feeding either through feeding tubes (nasal/oral gastric tube, gastrostomy tube) or orally with special, widened nipples. Many would die without assisted feeding Oral feeds are very slow Severely decreased appetite. Shows little or no evidence of being hungry Does not cry for food or get excited at feeding time If feeding just occurred when baby 'acted hungry' then would have severe 'failure-to-thrive' Weak cry
Phase 1b	*No difficulty feeding and growing appropriately on growth curve (9–25 months)* No longer needs assisted feeding Growing steadily along growth curve with normal feeding Normal appetite
Phase 2a	*Weight increasing without an increase in appetite or excessive calories (2.1–4.5 years)* Infant starts crossing growth curve centile lines No increase in appetite Appetite appropriate for age Will become obese if given the recommended daily allowance (RDA) for calories or if eating a 'typical' toddler diet of 70% carbohydrates Typically needs to be restricted to 60–80% of RDA to prevent obesity
Phase 2b	*Weight increasing with an increase in appetite (4.5–8 years)* Increased interest in food. Frequently asking 'food-related' questions Preoccupied with food. Very concerned about the next meal/snack (e.g. 'Did you remember to pack my lunch?') Increased appetite Will eat more food than a typical child if allowed Will eat food within their line of sight if unattended Will become obese if allowed to eat what they want Can be fairly easily redirected about food Can feel full Will stop eating voluntarily
Phase 3	*Hyperphagic, rarely feels full (8 years' adulthood)* Constantly thinking about food While eating one meal they are already thinking about the next meal Will awaken from sleep early thinking about food Will continue eating if portion size is not limited Rarely (truly) feels full Will steal food or money to pay for food Can eat food from garbage and other unsavory/inedible sources (e.g. dog food, frozen food, crayons, etc.)

Table 1. Continued

Phase 3	Typically are not truthful about what they have eaten (i.e. amount and types of food)
	Will gain considerable amount of weight over a short period of time if not supervised
	Food typically needs to be locked up. Frequently the child will ask the parent to lock the food if the parent has forgotten
	Will break into neighbors' houses for food
	Temper tantrums and 'meltdowns' frequently related to food
	Needs to be placed on a diet that is approximately 50–70% of the RDA to maintain a healthy weight
Phase 4	Appetite is no longer insatiable (adulthood)
	Appetite may still be increased or may be normal or less than normal
	Previously in phase 3, but now a noticeable improvement in their appetite control
	Can feel full
	Appetite can fluctuate in this phase, but the key component is noticeable improvement in control of appetite compared to when they were younger
	Not as preoccupied with food
	Absence of major temper tantrums and 'meltdowns' related to food
	Onset in adulthood. Could be as early as 20s or as late as 40–50s
	Most adults have not gone into this phase and maybe some (most?) never will

A Precise Description of Eating Behavior

Individuals with PWS present a particular meal pattern with a slower initial eating rate but much longer meal duration (possibly to achieve satiation) and no decelerating eating curves. They also have an early return of hunger after the previous meal, with early meal initiation which defines an impaired satiety. The authors concluded that the eating behavior of patients with PWS might be due to decreased satiation and satiety rather than increased hunger.

Given free access to food, patients with PWS will consume approximately three times more than control subjects. The present authors examined food intake patterns in children with PWS and non-syndromic obesity by making standard chicken-salad sandwich quarters continuously available for 1 h. Moreover, this overeating occurs despite delayed gastric emptying, leading to extremely morbid obesity. Other authors elaborated a taste test with three types of foods (high carbohydrate, high protein and high fat) reduced to spread consistency. PWS subjects preferred high-carbohydrate foods over high-protein foods and high-protein foods over high-fat foods. Moreover, the preference for high-carbohydrate foods was significantly higher in PWS subjects than in obese controls. In addition, PWS patients are more likely than controls with and without mental retardation to eat non-food items (pica) and contaminated foods and to make inappropriate food combinations.

Overall, the drive for food remains a lifelong source of stress for individuals with PWS and their families. Complications of obesity remain the major cause of deaths in

Table 2. Eating behavior is part of general behavioral problems in PWS. Our hypothesis is that OT drives the behavior and sugar preference, and impaired satiation and satiety with prolonged duration of meal when ghrelin is possibly involved in obsession with food and food craving and storage

Behavioral problems	Eating behavior
Oxytocin – Emotional lability +++ – Deficit of understanding social codes – Lack of empathy and theory of mind – Anxiety, repetitions, stereotypies – Lack of trust in others – Temper tantrums	Ghrelin – Obsession with food, meal anticipation – Food craving and storaging Oxytocin – Food preference for sugar – Prolonged duration of meal – Deficit of satiation and satiety

adults with PWS in relation with cardiovascular or respiratory failures. These patients are also at risk of choking due to a swallowing defect combined with their abnormal voracity or gastric perforation after consuming high quantities of food, even in the absence of obesity.

Individuals with PWS display a permanent obsession with food and excessive food searching, food storage, foraging and hoarding. In our opinion, more than hunger, it is the obsession with food, particularly the timing of the meals and the hedonic part of food that are overexpressed. This behavior, mainly the drive for food, is much closer to the craving seen in patients with drug addiction. Of note, in our experience, individuals with PWS also have a propensity to excessively consume drugs like tobacco and to a lesser extent alcohol. They do not only display foraging and hoarding with food items but are prone to do so for many non-food items and may take things that belong to others without permission.

This specific eating behavior is a lifelong source of stress for individuals with PWS and their families and carers, and precludes their socialization. This eating behavior is in our opinion part of a general behavioral problem observed in these patients (table 2).

Behavioral and Psychiatric Problems

Patients with PWS present a greater overall behavioral disturbance than age-matched mentally-retarded patients, but score comparably to patients with psychiatric disorders. Indeed, they frequently display anxiety traits and an anxious mood comparable to those of patients presenting an anxiety disorder or schizophrenia. Skin-picking is linked with anxiety and is frequently observed in people with PWS with possible severe complications [2].

They also show pronounced emotional lability and a striking inability to control their emotions, which results in frequent temper outbursts. The anger often seems to be an expression of frustration and the feeling of not being understood, but it may also be due to an impaired capacity to understand the motivations of others in the social milieu, possibly indicating deficits in 'theory of mind' (the ability to attribute mental states to others) and empathy (the ability to infer emotional experiences). They also show poor social adjustment, with poor peer relationships, tendencies towards social withdrawal, and few attributions of feeling in social relationships compared with others with the same level of intellectual disabilities. They also display a lack of flexibility and difficulties in abstract understanding which worsen the social integration.

In our opinion, hyperphagia must be considered as part of this behavioral disturbance, which includes compulsive behaviors such as tantrums, skin-picking, hoarding, repetitions, stubbornness and concerns with exactness and sameness.

Brain Imaging Findings

Several morphological neuroimaging abnormalities have been described in PWS: ventriculomegaly, decreased volume of brain tissue in the parietal-occipital lobe, sylvian fissure polymicrogyria and incomplete insular closure, pituitary morphological abnormalities and smaller cerebellar volumes. Recent functional neuroimaging techniques, i.e. positron emission tomography and functional MRI (fMRI), in PWS have revealed abnormal brain activation patterns in corticolimbic structures such as the amygdala and the prefrontal, orbitofrontal (OFC) and insular cortex, in response to food stimuli after ingestion of oral glucose or a meal. These patterns suggest an abnormal reward and motivational responses to food that may underlie the hyperphagia in individuals with PWS.

In a published study using fMRIs, the authors showed that patients with PWS (8–38 years old) displayed a greater activation in the bilateral hypothalamus and right amygdala than controls for high-calorie foods. The OFC was more activated by high-calorie than low-calorie foods in the PWS subjects. The authors thus concluded to a hyperactivation of neural circuitry involving motivation, reward, taste and food-seeking behaviors (hypothalamus, amygdala, OFC).

The lack of satiety in patients with PWS has also been investigated using fMRI by examining the regions related to satiation (insula, ventromedial prefrontal cortex, and nucleus accumbens). The activation of these regions was delayed after a glucose oral load in PWS patients compared with obese and lean controls. Hyperphagia thus appears to be linked to at least two mechanisms, since patients with PWS (versus healthy weight controls) who were presented with visual food stimuli after eating a meal showed hyperfunction in limbic and paralimbic regions that drive eating behavior (e.g. the amygdala) and in regions that regulate food intake (e.g. the medial prefrontal cortex (mPFC)) [4]. Moreover, divergent neural mechanisms might be associated with behavioral phenotypes in genetic subtypes of PWS. In a study with a similar setting (e.g. fMRI pre-/post-meal with visual food stimuli), the same author compared 9 individuals with maternal uniparental disomy (UPD) and 9 matched individuals with type 2 deletion: the deletion subtype showed increased food motivation network activation both pre- and post-meal, especially in the mPFC, insula and amygdala. The mPFC is associated with integration of visceral and reward-based signaling. It is closely connected with the OFC, which is involved in stimulus reward evaluation and direct multisensory input. Thus, according to the authors, the hyperactivation of mPFC might be associated with greater preoccupation with food in PW. In contrast, the UPD group showed greater activation than the deletion subtype post-meal in the dorsolateral prefrontal cortex and parahippocampal gyrus: these are food-processing regions associated with higher cognition. The dorsolateral prefrontal cortex is involved in the integration of sensory and mnemonic information, reward signals and voluntary motor control and parahippocampal gyrus is associated with the recognition of spatial and social context. According to the authors, these patterns of activation match closely with behavioral evidence of decreased inhibition in the deletion subtype and greater restraint in the UPD group in situations involving food.

Interestingly, patients with UPD have a higher risk of presenting with affective psychosis; our personal experience suggests that the eating behavior profile differs according to whether or not psychotic traits are present [unpubl. data]. Moreover, the occurrence of such psychosis is often preceded by changes in eating patterns and can also induce them.

Although it has been clearly established that reward and motivation neural pathways and impaired satiation and satiety are involved in PWS hyperphagia, evidence has gradually emerged that the eating behavior of PWS patients arises from a complex mechanism combining insufficient neural development, hormonal dysfunctions and an overall behavioral disorder involving psychiatric manifestations of the syndrome.

Mechanisms Involved in Hyperphagia and Feeding Problems

Orexigenic and Anorexigenic Signals
Increased Ghrelin Levels
Over the past 10 years, the limited view of a few mainly hypothalamic centers involved in feeding behavior has gradually been modified by evidence of a much more complex distribution system that includes reward and prefrontal circuits. It is now acknowledged that cognitive (as decision-making circuits), hedonic and emotional neural processes play important roles in the regulation of food intake and energy expenditure and the resulting energy balance, and that hormones and neuropeptides modulate many of these processes.

Individuals with PWS, unlike those with other known causes of obesity, have high circulating levels of the orexigenic hormone ghrelin, which may explain obesity [5]. Most circulating ghrelin is released by the stomach into the general circulation and can cross the blood-brain barrier. In the CNS, ghrelin and its receptor GHSR1a are present in the four main hypothalamic nuclei involved in the regulation of food intake: the arcuate nucleus (ARC) and the dorsomedial, ventromedial and paraventricular (PVN) nuclei. Ghrelin receptors have also been identified in areas like the dorsovagal complex, which includes the nucleus tractus solitarius, area postrema and dorsal motor nucleus of the vagus. The vagal nerve obviously plays a crucial but not mandatory role in driving the central actions of ghrelin. Ghrelin stimulates NPY and AgRP release at the level of the ARC, thus demonstrating effects opposite to those of leptin by increasing appetite and decreasing energy expenditure. In addition, ghrelin activates dopamine neurons in the ventral tegmental area and increases dopamine turnover in the nucleus accumbens. These observations suggest that enhancement of reward processing in the mesolimbic dopamine system is an integrated part of endogenous ghrelin orexigenic action [6]. Moreover, ghrelin also interacts with lateral hypothalamic orexin neurons and magnocellular oxytocin neurons, which in turn modulate ghrelin action [7, 8]. More recent data suggest the role of ghrelin in meal anticipation as a factor of food-entrainable oscillator [9], with ghrelin bursts occurring after the peak of hunger and are related to habitual meal patterns and contents. Ghrelin has also been shown to be involved in food searching, food storage, foraging and hoarding in rodents, all of which are characteristic behaviors in PWS.

In addition, we demonstrated that ghrelin dysregulation in PWS occurs very early in life and precedes obesity, in line with the excessive weight gain with normal calorie intake shown in the first years of life [6]. Indeed, Steculorum and Bouret [10] in their recent review [10] enlighten the fact that the neonatal period is a critical period with an enhanced sensitivity to metabolic hormones such as leptin, ghrelin and insulin. These hormones appear to have a crucial role in the development of hypothalamus, axon growth and neuroplasticity during this period. This group had also shown that the blockade of ghrelin action early in life in neonate rats induces obesity, thereby demonstrating that ghrelin is an anorexigenic hormone at this age [unpubl. data]. Hyperghrelinemia may thus drive the decrease in appetite and the non-interest in food observed in infants with PWS during phase 1. In addition, these authors showed that induced hyperghrelinemia early in life predisposes to obesity later in life [unpubl. data].

Interestingly, various studies reported no benefit from acute [11] and chronic administration of a somatostatin analogue on weight or appetite in PWS despite the observed decrease in ghrelin levels. The lack of effect of decreased ghrelin levels obtained in patients with PWS (children and adults, not infants) by pharmacological agents may be due to the 'priming' effect of early elevated ghrelin levels, as described above. It may also be that the ratio unacylated/acylated ghrelin is important and there is no consistent data on the level of this ratio in PWS.

Nevertheless, hyperghrelinemia seems to play a role in PWS throughout life. Indeed a recent study by Kroemer et al. [12] showed using fMRI that ghrelin elevates the hedonic effects of food pictures regarding brain activation and subjective appetite ratings. Other studies have shown that elevated ghrelin levels are more consistent than plasma PYY and GLP-1 values in PWS individuals.

Tauber · Diene · Mimoun · Çabal-Berthoumieu · Mantoulan · Molinas · Muscatelli · Salles

Decreased Levels of Pancreatic Polypeptide

Levels of the anorexigenic gut hormone polypeptide pancreatic (PP) are reduced in PWS [13]. PP was discovered in 1975 and isolated from chicken pancreatic extracts. It is a 36-amino-acid peptide and a member of the PP-fold peptide family (also including NPY and PYY). The PP-fold family binds to receptors Y1–Y6, but PP binds with greatest affinity to the Y4 and Y5 receptors. It is produced in the endocrine type F cells, which are located in the peripheries of the pancreatic islets. PP cannot cross the blood-brain barrier and its central effects may thus be mediated in regions where the blood-brain barrier is incomplete such as the hypothalamus, AP and adjacent brainstem areas. In humans, intravenous infusion of PP reduced food intake by 21.8% at a free-choice buffet, but did not affect gastric emptying.

Basal PP levels are elevated in anorexia nervosa and in patients with advanced malignant disease. People with PWS had a blunted PP response to meals and short-term infusions of peripheral PP given to these subjects were shown to reduce subsequent food intake by 12%. The precise role of PP in appetite regulation is not yet elucidated. PP may be involved in the pathophysiology of obesity and dysregulation of body weight via effects on the parasympathetic nervous system which is also impaired in patients with PWS.

Interestingly, these two abnormal signals, one orexigenic (ghrelin) and the second involved in satiety control (PP), may explain the major feeding disturbances described in people with PWS. Part of their action requires an intact vagal nerve reflex and they both regulate gastric emptying. Both hormones are elevated in anorexia nervosa. A decreased parasympathetic tone has long been described in PWS together with a defect in gastric emptying and other gut dysfunctions possibly related to these hormone dysfunctions.

Decreased Oxytocin Neurons Number and Volume in the Hypothalamus

Quantitative neuroanatomical studies of postmortem human hypothalamic tissue from patients with PWS in The Netherlands Brain Bank were implemented and offer the opportunity to search for pathological abnormalities in orexigenic and anorexigenic peptides. A reduced oxytocin (OT) neuron number and volume in the hypothalamic PVN of adults with PWS in comparison with control were reported in 1994 [14]. Similarly, an alteration in the OT system was described in the Necdin knockout (KO) mouse model in 2000. Moreover, abnormalities in the maturation of OT neurons were also reported in 2010 in another PWS mouse model with the KO of the *Magel2* gene. Taken together, this information suggests that the abnormal OT neurons may be involved in the PWS phenotype.

OT is produced in two hypothalamic nuclei, the PVN and supraoptic nucleus, by magnocellular and parvocellular neurons. Besides its well-known peripheral effects on uterine contractions and milk secretion, OT is known as an anorexigenic hormone, the effects of which have been recently reported on the induction of satiety [15]. Very recently, we demonstrated in *Magel2* KO pups that a single OT injection before the first 5 h of life completely rescued 50% of the newborn mice from early death by the recovery of normal suckling [16]. Therefore, OT induces suckling in this period of life and decreases food intake thereafter. Furthermore, social interactions were significantly disturbed in adult *Magel2* KO mice and a single OT administration restored normal behavior within hours following injection [F. Muscatelli, unpubl. data]. Restricted production of mature OT was detected specifically in the hypothalamus of the mutant newborns, although the prohormone was normally produced [16].

Therefore, OT, like ghrelin, displays two opposite effects – inducing suckling in early life and controlling satiety in adulthood. Furthermore, OT neurons interact with ghrelin and dopaminergic circuits in particular but not only in the ventral tegmental area, with axon projections to the OFC cortex [17, 18]. Moreover, OT receptors are present in the serotoninergic neurons and may modulate their functions. Thus, the OT defect in PWS may explain the deficit in suckling postnatally and the impaired satiety later on. The exact mechanism is not well elucidated but it depends on neuronal plasticity and possibly involves early hyperghrelinemia.

In addition, OT was recently identified as a key neuropeptide in the social interactions of numerous species by enhancing peer recognition and bonding behavior. In humans, nasal OT administration improves emotion recognition and face processing in healthy and autistic individuals. We therefore hypothesized that the possible dysfunction in OT may also explain, at least in part, the poor social adjustment of patients with PWS and their inability to control emotions, which in turn might explain their unpredictable disruptive behaviors and frequent temper outbursts. In a double-blind, randomized, placebo-controlled study of 24 adult patients with PWS, we demonstrated that the group that received a single intranasal administration of 24 IU of OT displayed significantly increased trust in others and decreased sadness tendencies, with less disruptive behavior and a trend towards decreased food intake, than did patients who received placebo [19]. Complementary data from studies with repeated administrations of OT will start soon in our group.

Recent Genetic Data Support the Hypothesis of a Metabolic Disease Driven by an Abnormal Nycthemeral Pattern

The chromosomal region involved in PWS is very complex encompassing imprinted and non-imprinted genes. Figure 1 shows a schematic representation of the region. To date there is no animal model that completely reproduces the human PWS phenotype and particularly the nutritional phases which start with a deficit of suckling and failure to thrive and later on lead to early morbid obesity with hyperphagia and a deficit of satiation and satiety. The hypothetical minimal chromosomal deletion associated with PWS phenotype deduced from clinical cases with chromosomal translocations removes SNORD109A, the SNORD116 cluster (30 snoRNAs copies) and IPW, and is shown in figure 1 by the dotted frame. Increasing evidence from animal

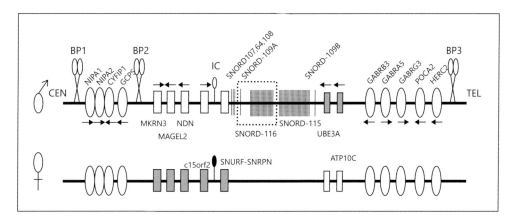

Fig. 1. The organization of the PWS locus on chromosome 15 is shown. Genes expressed from the paternal and maternal alleles are shown as white and grey squares, those expressed by both alleles are shown as ovals. snoRNA genes are shown as vertical bars, classical break points 1, 2 and 3 are indicated as BP1, 2 and 3. The imprinting center is shown as IC as an open circle when hypomethylated and black circle when hypermethylated. The critical minimum region for PWS is shown in the dotted frame [adapted from Tauber and Cavaillé, Obésité 2011;6:161–171].

and clinical data suggests that the loss of the paternally expressed snoRNA SNORD116 gene cluster plays a significant role in many of the features of the PWS phenotype [20–23]. Indeed, 3 human cases have been reported showing that the deletion of the SNORD116 gene cluster leads to PWS features including hyperphagia and obesity [21–23]. We presented an abstract at the endocrine meeting in 2013 with the preliminary report of a new case with the shortest microdeletion [unpubl. data] confirming the role of this critical minimal region in the PWS phenotype.

KO mice with deletion of only SNORD116 genes showed hyperphagia and decrease energy expenditure without the occurrence of obesity on regular and high-fat diets.

snoRNAs are a group of small RNAs ranging from 80 to 300 nucleotides in length that are located primarily in nucleoli and are required for the chemical modification and maturation of rRNAs. Animal studies have recently shown that the SNORD116 cluster is expressed in the hypothalamus [24]. In addition, it has been shown that the enhanced expression of SNORD116 in hypothalamic nuclei was observed at weaning and young adult stages, but was less obvious postnatally when expression was significantly more widespread, suggesting that the expression of the SNORD116 is regulated developmentally and may play a regulatory role on hypothalamic development and function.

The SNORD116 region encodes repeated C/D box snoRNAs (SNORD116) and a spliced long non-coding RNA (lncRNA) host gene (116HG) that is stably retained in the nucleus. While human and mouse genetics demonstrate the critical nature of the SNORD116 locus in PWS, the presence of multiple processed RNA products complicates a mechanistic understanding.

A very recent paper demonstrated that lncRNA 116HG regulates the transcription of genes important for regulation of diurnal transcription and metabolism and that loss of this lncRNA alters circadian energy homeostasis in SNORD116-deleted mice [25]. This lncRNA emerges in the brain in the first week of life as an RNA cloud in neuronal nuclei. Mice with *Snord116del* mice exhibited dysregulation of diurnally expressed *Mtor* and circadian genes *Clock*, *Cry1*, and *Per2*. The authors conclude that PWS is thus the first genetic disease due to the loss of a lncRNA. However, future studies will need to identify which of the RNAs generated from the *Snord116* locus are critically lost in PWS, and if loss of multiple RNAs underlies the complex phenotype of PWS.

Is PWS a Model of Hyperphagia?

It thus appears that most of the problem in PWS may be related to an impaired circadian pattern and particularly feeding behavior. Sleep problems in PWS patients, including shorter duration of nighttime sleep and excessive daytime sleepiness, should now be seen as a main feature consistent with a disruption in circadian metabolism, rather than a complication of obesity.

In humans, diurnal rhythms are not present at birth and become established further while the precise mechanisms and timing are not well understood. Indeed most hypothalamic and subsequently pituitary hormones show a circadian rhythm related or not with sleep pattern, i.e. GH, thyrotropin, prolactin, gonadotropins, corticotropin, all of them being impaired in PWS. Interestingly, an impaired metabolism with a higher body mass index and risk of obesity has been shown in night workers in humans together with a higher weight gain in mice fed during the day compared to those fed during the night with a comparable calorie intake. Alternatively, consumption of a high-calorie diet alters in turn the function of the mammalian circadian clock, thus leading to obesity and metabolic disorders and that timed restricted feeding provides a time cue and resets the circadian clock with better metabolic features and lower body weight gain. In addition, sleep deprivation induces a higher calorie intake with a preference for food with high energy content.

Interestingly, OT levels also display a circadian pattern which drives a circadian feeding behavior. Indeed changing the pattern of OT also results in changing the feeding pattern in rodents, while peripheral administration of OT rescues the abnormal feeding in rodents [26]. Conversely, the central administration of OT receptor antagonist within the PVN was shown to increase spontaneous food intake. From a neuroanatomical point of view, central OT appears to reduce food intake by acting mainly at the level of the NTS and adjacent dorsal motor nucleus of the vagus in the brainstem, through direct projections from parvocellular oxytocinergic neurons of the PVN.

Hypothesis

PWS is a genetic eating disorder linked to an abnormal circadian pattern and associated with behavioral problems. Our hypothesis is that there is an impaired oxytocin/ghrelin/dopamine pathway that explains at least partly the behavioral phenotype and the abnormal eating profile. We hypothesize that the early dysfunction in OT explains the suckling deficit at birth and early infancy while early excess of ghrelin may explain the decrease of motivation for food both hormones interacting with the reward dopaminergic pathways and neuroplasticity. Later in life the excess of ghrelin explains the permanent obsession with food and motivation for food, while the OT defect is involved in the lack of satiety and the deficit in understanding social codes. Overall the effects of these hormones on food intake are developmentally regulated with opposite effects in neonates and later in life. This integrated model thus drives what we may call 'the PWS nutritional phenotype' defined by the switch from an anorexic stage with a deficit in suckling and failure to thrive to excessive weight gain and severe obesity with hyperphagia, perspicaciously linked by Prader et al. [1] in 1956. Early neonatal diagnosis of this disease offers the possibility of implementing treatments within a reasonable window of opportunity, which may cure the primary defect and then perhaps part or the whole disease. We may also hypothesize that this approach may be suitable for babies with suckling difficulties of various origins and for other patients with eating disorders. We believe that our ongoing clinical trials will bring some important answers to these questions.

Disclosure Statement

M.T. received lecture fees from Pfizer and Novo Nordisk and is on the Ipsen Scientific and Advisory Board and received research funding from Pfizer, Ipsen and Sandoz. J.P.S. received lecture fees from Ipsen and is on the Novo Scientific Board and received research funding from Pfizer, Ipsen and Sandoz. The other authors have nothing to disclose.

References

1 Prader A, Labhart A, Willi H: Ein Syndrom von Adipositas, Kleinwuchs, Kryptorchidismus und Oligophrenie nach myotoniertigem Zustand im Neugeborenenalter. Schweiz Med Wochenschr 1956;6: 1260–1261.

2 Goldstone AP, Holland AJ, Hauffa BP, Hokken-Koelega AC, Tauber M: Speakers at the Second Expert Meeting of the Comprehensive Care of Patients with PWS: Recommendations for the diagnosis and management of Prader-Willi syndrome. J Clin Endocrinol Metab 2008;93:4183–4197.

3 Miller JL, Lynn CH, Driscoll DC, Goldstone AP, Gold JA, Kimonis V, Dykens E, Butler MG, Shuster JJ, Driscoll DJ: Nutritional phases in Prader-Willi syndrome. Am J Med Genet A 2011;155A:1040–1049.

4 Holsen LM, Zarcone JR, Brooks WM, Butler MG, Thompson TI, Ahluwalia JS, Nollen NL, Savage CR: Neural mechanisms underlying hyperphagia in Prader-Willi syndrome. Obesity (Silver Spring) 2006;14:1028–1037.

5   Feigerlova E, Diene G, Conte-Auriol F, Molinas C, Gennero I, Salles JP, Arnaud C, Tauber M: Hyperghrelinemia precedes obesity in Prader-Willi syndrome. J Clin Endocrinol Metab 2008;93:2800–2805.
6   Abizaid A: Ghrelin and dopamine: new insights on the peripheral regulation of appetite. J Neuroendocrinol 2009;21:787–793.
7   Olszewski PK, Bomberg EM, Martell A, Grace MK, Levine AS: Intraventricular ghrelin activates oxytocin neurons: implications in feeding behavior. Neuroreport 2007;18:499–503.
8   Coiro V, Saccani-Jotti G, Rubino P, Manfredi G, Vacca P, Volta E, Chiodera P: Oxytocin inhibits the stimulatory effect of ghrelin on circulating neuropeptide Y levels in humans. J Neural Transm 2008;115:1265–1267.
9   Carneiro BT, Araujo JF: The food-entrainable oscillator: a network of interconnected brain structures entrained by humoral signals? Chronobiol Int 2009;26:1273–1289.
10 Steculorum SM, Bouret SG: Developmental effects of ghrelin. Peptides 2011;32:2362–2366.
11 Tan TM, Vanderpump M, Khoo B, Patterson M, Ghatei MA, Goldstone AP: Somatostatin infusion lowers plasma ghrelin without reducing appetite in adults with Prader-Willi syndrome. J Clin Endocrinol Metab 2004;89:4162–4165.
12 Kroemer NB, Krebs L, Kobiella A, Grimm O, Pilhatsch M, Bidlingmaier M, Zimmermann US, Smolka MN: Fasting levels of ghrelin covary with the brain response to food pictures. Addict Biol 2013;18:855–862.
13 Berntson GG, Zipf WB, O'Dorisio TM, Hoffman JA, Chance RE: Pancreatic polypeptide infusions reduce food intake in Prader-Willi syndrome. Peptides 1993;14:497–503.
14 Swaab DF, Purba JS, Hofman MA: Alterations in the hypothalamic paraventricular nucleus and its oxytocin neurons (putative satiety cells) in Prader-Willi syndrome: a study of five cases. J Clin Endocrinol Metab 1995;80:573–579.
15 Olszewski PK, Klockars A, Schioth HB, Levine AS: Oxytocin as feeding inhibitor: maintaining homeostasis in consummatory behavior. Pharmacol Biochem Behav 2010;97:47–54.
16 Schaller F, Watrin F, Sturny R, Massacrier A, Szepetowski P, Muscatelli F: A single postnatal injection of oxytocin rescues the lethal feeding behaviour in mouse newborns deficient for the imprinted *Magel2* gene. Hum Mol Genet 2010;19:4895–4905.
17 Baskerville TA, Douglas AJ: Dopamine and oxytocin interactions underlying behaviors: potential contributions to behavioral disorders. CNS Neurosci Ther 2010;16:e92–e123.
18 Febo M: A bold view of the lactating brain: functional magnetic resonance imaging studies of suckling in awake dams. J Neuroendocrinol 2011;23:1009–1019.
19 Tauber M, Mantoulan C, Copet P, Jauregui J, Demeer G, Diene G, Roge B, Laurier V, Ehlinger V, Arnaud C, et al: Oxytocin may be useful to increase trust in others and decrease disruptive behaviours in patients with Prader-Willi syndrome: a randomised placebo-controlled trial in 24 patients. Orphanet J Rare Dis 2011;6:47.
20 Skryabin BV, Gubar LV, Seeger B, Pfeiffer J, Handel S, Robeck T, Karpova E, Rozhdestvensky TS, Brosius J: Deletion of the MBII-85 snoRNA gene cluster in mice results in postnatal growth retardation. PLoS Genet 2007;3:e235.
21 Duker AL, Ballif BC, Bawle EV, Person RE, Mahadevan S, Alliman S, Thompson R, Traylor R, Bejjani BA, Shaffer LG, et al: Paternally inherited microdeletion at 15q11.2 confirms a significant role for the SNORD116 C/D box snoRNA cluster in Prader-Willi syndrome. Eur J Hum Genet 2010;18:1196–1201.
22 Sahoo T, del Gaudio D, German JR, Shinawi M, Peters SU, Person RE, Garnica A, Cheung SW, Beaudet AL: Prader-Willi phenotype caused by paternal deficiency for the HBII-85 C/D box small nucleolar RNA cluster. Nat Genet 2008;40:719–721.
23 De Smith AJ, Purmann C, Walters RG, Ellis RJ, Holder SE, Van Haelst MM, Brady AF, Fairbrother UL, Dattani M, Keogh JM, et al: A deletion of the HBII-85 class of small nucleolar RNAs (snoRNAs) is associated with hyperphagia, obesity and hypogonadism. Hum Mol Genet 2009;18:3257–3265.
24 Zhang Q, Bouma GJ, McClellan K, Tobet S: Hypothalamic expression of snoRNA Snord116 is consistent with a link to the hyperphagia and obesity symptoms of Prader-Willi syndrome. Int J Dev Neurosci 2012;30:479–485.
25 Powell WT, Coulson RL, Crary FK, Wong SS, Ach RA, Tsang P, Alice Yamada N, Yasui DH, Lasalle JM: A Prader-Willi locus lncRNA cloud modulates diurnal genes and energy expenditure. Hum Mol Genet 2013;21:4318–4328.
26 Zhang G, Cai D: Circadian intervention of obesity development via resting-stage feeding manipulation or oxytocin treatment. Am J Physiol Endocrinol Metab 2011;301:E1004–E1012.

Maithe Tauber, MD
Unité d'Endocrinologie, Hôpital des Enfants, CHU de Toulouse
330, avenue de grande Bretagne, TSA 70034
FR–31059 Toulouse Cedex 9 (France)
E-Mail tauber.mt@chu-toulouse.fr

Delhanty PJD, van der Lely AJ (eds): How Gut and Brain Control Metabolism.
Front Horm Res. Basel, Karger, 2014, vol 42, pp 107–122 (DOI: 10.1159/000358320)

Interactions between the Gut, the Brain and Brown Adipose Tissue Function

Johanna C. van den Beukel · Aldo Grefhorst

Department of Internal Medicine, Erasmus MC, Rotterdam, The Netherlands

Abstract

Brown adipose tissue (BAT) has the unique ability to oxidize fatty acids to generate heat, a process termed thermogenesis. The mitochondrial uncoupling protein 1 is predominantly expressed in BAT and controls the thermogenetic properties of this tissue. Since activated BAT dissipates energy, it is considered beneficial in controlling metabolism, i.e. by combating obesity. Indeed, humans with a higher BMI have less active BAT. Many researchers attempt to uncover regulatory pathways in BAT activity in the pursuit for novel BAT modulators to control body weight. Endocrine factors such as thyroid hormone, sex steroid hormones and glucocorticoids can modulate BAT activity. Since the intestinal tract has emerged as an endocrine organ regulating energy balance and glucose homeostasis, this review will discuss how gut-derived hormones and other intestinal tract-related factors such as bile acids modulate BAT activity. Emphasis will be put on whether these hormones regulate BAT directly or via the central nervous system. In summary, it can be globally stated that anorexigenic gut hormones stimulate BAT while orexigenic gut hormones inhibit BAT activity. How these hormones modulate BAT and whether this is via a direct and/or central effect is largely unknown. Novel insights about gut-derived factors such as bile acids suggest that they also affect BAT activity. Altogether, effects of food intake per se on BAT activity are rather complex to interpret and depend on many (hormonal) factors.

Brown Adipose Tissue: Presence and Activity?

Mammals have two distinct types of adipose tissue. White adipose tissue (WAT) stores energy in the form of energy-dense triglycerides (TGs) and an excess intake of energy relative to energy dissipation will enhance TG storage in WAT and finally result in obesity. Brown adipose tissue (BAT), in contrast, dissipates energy since it has the unique ability to oxidize fatty acids released from TGs to generate heat, a process termed thermogenesis [1]. The mitochondrial uncoupling protein 1 (UCP1) is predominantly expressed in BAT and controls the thermogenetic properties of this tissue. When UCP1 is present and active in the mitochondrial membrane, it uncouples

ATP synthesis from oxidative phosphorylation in the mitochondria resulting in energy that is released as heat instead of being used for ATP synthesis. It has long been known that human babies and small animals have an active BAT depot, but it has only recently become clear that adult humans also harbor active BAT in the upper chest and neck regions, the activity of which can be enhanced by cold exposure [2, 3]. Human BAT is visualized by ^{18}F-deoxyglucose positron emission tomography scans since active BAT clears large amounts of glucose. The presence of UCP1 in these ^{18}F-deoxyglucose-positive areas revealed that humans indeed have active thermogenic adipose tissue.

Activation of BAT can attribute significantly to whole-body energy dissipation [4]. Laboratory animal models with genetically ablated BAT develop obesity [5], but also humans with a higher BMI have less active BAT [2, 3]. Activation of BAT is therefore considered an important modulator of weight and energy balance, and many researchers attempt to uncover regulatory pathways in BAT activity in the pursuit for novel BAT activators to combat obesity.

The most studied and presumably most important regulatory pathway activator of UCP1 and thereby BAT activity is the sympathetic innervation, i.e. effects of norepinephrine (NE) released by sympathetic nerves [1]. By binding to β-adrenergic receptors on the brown adipocyte, NE elevates intracellular cyclic AMP and hence TG lipolysis, fatty acid oxidation and enhanced UCP1 transcription and activity [1].

A number of recent studies have shown that endocrine factors found in the circulation can modulate and activate brown adipocytes [4]. Of these factors, thyroid hormone (3,3′,5-triiodothyronine (T$_3$)) has been the most studied, but also sex steroid hormones and glucocorticoids have been implicated in BAT activity regulation. Since the intestinal tract has emerged as an endocrine organ regulating energy balance and glucose homeostasis, this review will discuss how gut-derived hormones and other intestinal tract-related factors, such as bile acids, modulate BAT activity directly. In addition, since the gut hormones mediate their effects on satiety via the central nervous system (CNS) and BAT activity is predominantly regulated by the sympathetic nerves, the goal of this review is also to uncover whether the effects of the described gut hormones on the BAT are mediated via the CNS.

Gut Hormones in General: A Warning about Interpretation of Studies

Below we will describe many studies that address the role of gut hormones in BAT activity. Careful interpretation of the described results is needed because most studies draw straightforward conclusions without discussing possible confounders. Interplay between the different gut hormones can influence the effects found in vivo. For instance, infusion with glucagon-like peptide 1 (GLP-1) reduced, amongst others, plasma glucagon, gastric inhibitory polypeptide (GIP) and GLP-2 concentrations [6, 7]. In many studies, the effects of the intravenous, peripheral or central administration of a certain gut hormone on the other gut hormones is not investigated. Also, the combinatory effects of gut hormones on metabolism have hardly been studied, with the notable exception of the additional effects of the gut hormone amylin on the anti-obesity effects of the adipokine leptin in humans [8].

Although many gut hormones can regulate BAT activity via the CNS, the precise mechanisms by which the gut hormones mediate this effect in the brain are largely unknown. As recently discussed by López and Nogueiras [9], the role of the dorsomedial hypothalamic nucleus (DMH) in the regulation of BAT activity has been known for more than 30 years, but a start with uncovering the molecular mechanisms behind this activation has only very recently been made. A possible mechanism of action might be via neuropeptide Y (NPY) in the DMH which plays an inhibitory role on BAT activity [10]. Also the melanocortin (MC) system in the hypothalamic paraventricular nucleus (PVH) is presumably involved in regulation of BAT activity: injections with the MC receptor 3 and 4 agonist MTII into the PVH of hamsters increased the temperature in their intrascapular BAT [11]. Central effects of certain gut hormones might therefore be mediated via effects on NPY/MC activity, but other yet unknown factors can also be involved.

Cholecystokinin and Gastrin

Cholecystokinin (CCK) and gastrin were among the first gastrointestinal hormones to be discovered. Both are secreted by endocrine I cells of the duodenum and the jejunum upon a meal and suppress satiety. CCK and gastrin are encoded by two distinct genes and differ in length but share the 5-terminal amino acid sequence. The effects of both CCK and gastrin are mediated via the CCK1 and CCK2 receptor [12]. While CCK binds to both receptors with equal affinity, gastrin has a 1,000-fold higher affinity for the CCK2 receptor.

Studies with *Cck2r*-deficient mice might reveal the role of both CCK and gastrin on BAT activity, but these show conflicting results. Ten-week-old male *Cck2r*-deficient mice were not heavier than their male wild-type littermates, but female *Cck2r*-deficient mice of the same age were ~10% heavier than their sex- and age-matched wild-type littermates [13]. One-year-old *Cck2r*-deficient male mice are even ~40% heavier than their age-matched wild-type littermates [14]. These results might suggest that gastrin and CCK activate BAT activity. BAT depot weights do not support this since *Cck2r*-deficient mice of both sexes had smaller intrascapular BAT depots [13], which is suggestive of higher activity of the BAT depot. Another study showed no effect of absent CCK2 receptor on BAT activity since BAT deoxyglucose uptake was equal between 12-week-old *Cck2r*-deficient male mice and their sex- and age-matched wild-type littermates [14].

The Otsuka Long Evans Tokushima Fatty (OLETF) rats lack expression of functional CCK1 receptor and are therefore a perfect in vivo model to study the role of

CCK only on BAT activity. OLETF rats have a lower BAT mass at young age but a high BAT mass when they are ~4 months old [15]. In the BAT depot of adult OLETF rats, UCP1 mRNA expression is reduced [16], suggesting that CCK is needed to activate BAT. As with all satiety-regulating hormones, the effects on food intake might be a confounding factor. The OLETF rats are hyperphagic and therefore obese [15]. The effects of food intake per se on the BAT depot of OLETF rats was investigated by pair-feeding experiments: the OLETF rats were given the same amount of food as their lean wild-type littermates. Indeed, pair feeding of the OLETF rats resulted in BAT depots that had the same weight as control rats [17], suggesting that the reduced BAT activity in the OLETF rats is due to increased food intake per se. The effects in mice have been less well studied but it is evident that also the *Cck2r*-deficient mice eat more [14]. Thus, it is hard to extrapolate findings from experiments in these rats and mice to define the effects of CCK on the adipose tissue depots.

The most convincing studies that show an effect of CCK on BAT were performed by Yoshimatsu et al. [18] and show that the effects of CCK on the BAT depot are very likely due to the central effects of CCK. Yoshimatsu et al. investigated the central effects of CCK in rats on the firing of the sympathetic nerve in the region where it enters the BAT. The authors found that the localization of the central CCK application was of importance. Injection of CCK in the third ventricle, the ventromedial hypothalamic nucleus and the lateral hypothalamic area increased BAT sympathetic nerve activity while injections in the DMH, paraventricular nucleus and the preoptic area had no effect on BAT sympathetic activity. These experiments have not been performed for gastrin, but since gastrin preferentially binds to the CCK2 receptor and this subtype is found in the brain [19], it is very likely that gastrin will also induce sympathetic nerve firing into the BAT depot.

Altogether, we can conclude that CCK and gastrin very likely stimulate BAT via central mechanisms.

Glucagon

Already half a century ago it was shown that the pancreatic hormone glucagon activates BAT. Intravenously administrated glucagon enhanced oxygen consumption rates and elevated intrascapular BAT temperature [20]. The β-adrenergic antagonist propranolol did not block glucagon's effects on BAT in rabbits, making it plausible that glucagon activates BAT via mechanisms not involving a centrally regulated increase in sympathetic tone. In line with this is the fact that glucagon can activate BAT ex vivo: addition of glucagon to rat BAT slices dose-dependently induced oxygen consumption and fatty acid release [21]. These effects of glucagon on BAT ex vivo suggest that glucagon receptors are present on brown adipocytes, which was indeed found [22]. In line with the more potent actions of glucagon in WAT compared to BAT [21], Iwanij et al. [23] showed that glucagon receptor concentration in BAT is lower than in WAT.

van den Beukel · Grefhorst

The BAT-activating effects of glucagon raised the question whether glucagon might make it easier for animals to survive cold conditions. Indeed, when glucagon was given to cold-acclimated rats, BAT activity was potentiated [24]. In a more extreme condition, rats treated for 4 weeks with glucagon better withstood the extreme low temperature of –5°C [25]. It should however be noted that 3 of the 8 glucagon-treated rats but 6 out of the 8 control rats did not survive the –5°C. The same study showed that the long-term glucagon treatment led to induced BAT depot weights and enhanced the amount and size of mitochondria in this depot. Interestingly, exposure to –5°C itself also resulted in a ~6-fold rise in plasma glucagon concentrations. Even milder cold temperatures, e.g. 10°C, increased plasma glucagon concentrations in both rats and men [26]. It is very likely that the cold-induced elevation of plasma glucagon has functional effects on BAT since rats receiving a continuous glucagon infusion to reach levels comparable to what is seen upon cold exposure were able to induce BAT thermogenesis [27]. The rise in plasma glucagon might be the result of increased catecholamine concentrations upon cold exposure since NE injections increased glucagon concentrations in BAT and plasma in rats acclimatized to either warmth or cold [28].

An additional effect of cold is the modification of glucagon receptors in brown adipocytes although this might be an effect of stress because heat acclimation also changed glucagon receptors [29]. Stress in rats caused by either cold, warmth or immobilization all resulted in increased glucagon concentrations in plasma and BAT [30].

Most of these studies point out to a direct effect of glucagon on BAT activity but central effects of glucagon on BAT activity cannot be excluded and have also been proposed: injections of glucagon in the lateral hypothalamus resulted in an increased firing of sympathetic neurons into the intrascapular BAT [31]. Altogether, there is enough evidence to state that glucagon can activate the BAT depot, at least via a direct mechanism.

Glucagon-Like Peptide 1 and Oxyntomodulin

GLP-1 is secreted by intestinal L cells upon food intake and reduces blood glucose concentrations while stimulating pancreatic insulin secretion. GLP-1 mimetics are therefore used as antidiabetic drugs. It is known that GLP-1 receptors are present in the WAT depot [32]. Oxyntomodulin (OXM), a peptide hormone produced by the colonic oxyntic cells, is a ligand for both the glucagon receptor and the GLP-1 receptor and will also be discussed in this paragraph.

In the commonly used in vitro model of WAT, 3T3-L1 adipocytes, GLP-1 has multiple but conflicting effects. On the one hand, GLP-1 stimulates deoxyglucose uptake and potentiates insulin-mediated fatty acid incorporation in TGs [33]. In contrast, another study showed that GLP-1 enhances lipolysis in human adipocytes and 3T3-L1 cells [34].

Despite the effects of GLP-1 on WAT in vitro studies, the direct effects of GLP-1 on WAT are probably small compared to the central effects. A 2-day intracerebroventricular (ICV) GLP-1 infusion significantly reduced expression of genes encoding proteins involved in fatty acid and TG synthesis in WAT, while a 2-day peripheral GLP-1 infusion had only minor effects [35]. The latter study did not include analysis on the BAT depot, but Lockie et al. [36] showed that centrally administered GLP-1 almost completely abolished food intake but increased BAT activity in mice. The effects of GLP-1 on BAT were due to the increased firing of sympathetic nerves into the BAT depot. To test whether the GLP-1 receptor was involved, Lockie et al. [36] applied OXM ICV infusions to mice deficient for the GLP-1 receptor and found that OXM's thermogenic effects were absent in the GLP-1 receptor-deficient mice. Thus, the GLP-1 receptor has an important (central) role in stimulation of BAT activity by OXM (and GLP-1).

Apart from the above-described OXM ICV infusions [36], the effects of OXM on BAT have not been studied in detail. One study showed that ICV OXM led to lower body weight in rats and pair-feeding experiments showed that OXM's effect on body weight was not completely due to reduced food intake [37]. Thus, induction of BAT activity might have occurred in these rats, especially since the OXM infused rats had higher rectal temperature and reduced BAT and WAT mass.

Unfortunately, the above-mentioned studies by Lockie et al. [36] is one of just a few that report detailed information about the effects GLP-1 on BAT. Other similar mouse studies have been performed but did not investigate BAT in great detail. For instance, intraperitoneal injections with GLP-1 in obese mice resulted in reduced oxygen consumption, enhanced fatty acid utilization and enhanced BAT deoxyglucose uptake [38]. The GLP-1 receptor agonist Boc5 was given to mice fed a high-fat diet (HFD) and resulted in denser BAT independent of food intake [39].

Although it can be concluded from the above studies that central GLP-1 receptor agonism stimulates BAT activity, opposite effects are also reported. In lean and obese Zucker rats, central infusion of the GLP-1 mimetic exendin-4 reduced BAT temperature [40]. In humans, GLP-1 infusion reduces resting metabolic rate [6, 7], suggestive of reduced BAT activity. However, we have to be aware that GLP-1 infusion results in slower gastric emptying. The reduced resting metabolic rate might be due to slower uptake and thereby availability of substrates. Thus, despite the studies about the actions of GLP-1 in humans, we conclude that GLP-1 and OXM both increase BAT activity, mainly via central mechanisms.

Acylated and Des-Acyl Ghrelin

Ghrelin is predominantly produced by the stomach. To be able to bind to its receptor, growth hormone secretagogue receptor type 1a (GHSR1a), ghrelin has to be octanoylated by ghrelin O-acyltransferase at its third serine residue [41]. Thus, two subtypes of ghrelin can be distinguished: acylated ghrelin (AG) and des-acyl ghrelin (DAG). Different from the other gut hormones, AG induces satiety and stimulates food intake. The GHSR1a is ubiquitously expressed, but mainly in the hypothalamus where it induces release of growth hormone (GH) when activated by AG.

GHSR1a is only activated by AG and not by physiological concentrations of DAG [42]; the receptor for DAG is still unknown. Here we will discuss the effects of both AG and DAG on BAT activity. It is evident that administration of AG either centrally or in the periphery induces food intake and body weight [43]. The AG-mediated increase in the respiratory quotient (RQ) [43] is indicative for reduced fatty acid utilization and thus points towards reduced BAT activity. Indeed, intraperitoneal treatment with AG for 7 days decreased BAT *Ucp1* expression in mice [44] and ICV AG infusion resulted in decreased BAT sympathetic nerve activity and lower BAT temperatures [45]. These latter effects are not due to increased GH concentrations since ICV GH infusion did not decrease sympathetic nerve activity towards the adipose tissue depots. However, *Gshr1a*-deficient mice have denser BAT and higher BAT *Ucp1* mRNA and UCP1 protein content than their wild-type littermates, albeit only after 10 months of age [46]. In line with this are transgenic rats that express antisense GHSR mRNA under control of the tyrosine hydroxylase promoter that have reduced GHSR1a expression in the CNS and increased BAT NE content [47]. Another study showed that peripheral AG administration decreased the NE concentration in BAT that could be blocked by vagotomy [48], suggesting that peripheral administered AG exerts its effects on sympathetic nerve tone via the afferent vagal nerve. Altogether, peripheral and centrally administered AG inactivates BAT by diminishing the sympathetic tone towards BAT, by activating the central GHSR1a and by influencing the vagal afferent signalling.

AG is not stable in the circulation but can be converted in DAG. Since DAG is considered to be the inactive form of AG, it has not been studied in great detail. However, some studies suggest that DAG has an AG-opposing effect. Infusion of rodents with only DAG has shown beneficial effects on parameters associated with diabetes and obesity. For instance, infusion of mice with DAG for 4 weeks with mini-pumps partly prevented metabolic derangements due to HFD during the last 2 weeks of infusion. The DAG infusion stimulated expression of BAT *Ucp1* expression but also other mitochondrial markers in the BAT depot [49]. This beneficial effect of DAG might partially explain the increased BAT *Ucp1* mRNA and UCP1 protein content in *Ghsr1a* knockout animals.

BAT morphology and *Ucp1* expression do not differ between wild-type and *Ghrl*-deficient mice that lack both AG and DAG [46], underscoring the role of GHSR in BAT activity but complicating our understanding about the roles of AG and DAG in BAT activation. It could be that the deficiency of both AG and DAG results in normal BAT activity but that an excess of DAG, which is the case in *Ghsr* knockout animals, shifts the balance towards increased BAT activity.

In conclusion, AG inhibits BAT activity most likely via GHSR1a in the brain, while DAG activates BAT via a yet unknown mechanism.

Gastric Inhibitory Polypeptide

GIP is synthesized by K cells in the mucosa of the duodenum and the jejunum. The GIP receptor has been found in rat WAT [50] and all data considering WAT points towards lipogenic effects of this gut hormone in WAT. In rat WAT, GIP induces both fatty acid synthesis [51] and fatty acid incorporation in TGs [52]. Human studies confirmed the lipogenic properties of GIP in WAT. Infusion of healthy subjects with GIP increased their abdominal subcutaneous WAT blood flow, glucose uptake and fatty acid re-esterification under hyperinsulinemic conditions [53]. The lipogenic effects of GIP fits with the notion that obese type 2 diabetic patients [54] have increased plasma GIP concentrations. In addition, GIP inhibits glucagon and isoproterenol-induced lipolysis of WAT [55].

Mice deficient for the GIP receptor are protected against HFD-induced obesity and insulin resistance [56]. However, since GIP stimulates pancreatic insulin secretion upon absorption of nutrients [57], the lower insulin concentrations in the GIP receptor-deficient mice is also a crucial factor that regulates uptake of free fatty acids in adipose tissue and thereby adiposity.

Uptake of fatty acids from TGs from the circulation depends on the presence of lipoprotein lipase (LPL), a protein whose BAT gene expression is induced upon cold exposure [58]. Interestingly, GIP stimulates LPL activity in isolated white adipocytes [59] and potentiates insulin's effects on LPL activity [60]. The increased LPL activity is very likely of importance to warrant the availability of enough substrates in the white adipocytes and is thus in line with GIP-induced lipid synthesis in WAT.

We are unaware of studies addressing the effects of GIP on BAT. However, the whole profile of reduced lipolysis and enhanced lipogenic activity in WAT upon GIP make it very likely that GIP does not favor BAT activity. In line with this is the sole paper that describes a link between BAT and GIP. Treatment of HFD mice with Pro-3GIP, a GIP receptor antagonist, reduced the weight of the intrascapular BAT depot, suggesting increased BAT activity [61].

Pancreatic Polypeptide and Peptide YY

Pancreatic polypeptide (PP) and peptide YY (PYY) are both members of the PP-fold peptide family and will therefore be discussed together in this paragraph. PP is produced in the endocrine and exocrine pancreas, colon, and rectum. The entire but especially the distal part of the gastrointestinal tract can secrete PYY. PYY is present in two forms, the minor circulating form PYY(1–36) and the major circulating form PYY(3–36). PYY(1–36) and PYY(3–36) have opposite effects on food intake: PYY(1–36) is orexigenic whereas PYY(3–36) is anorexigenic [62]. This is very likely due to different affinities of the two forms for different receptors. While PYY(1–36) binds to all Y receptors, with a rank order of potency of Y2 > Y1 > Y5 >> Y4 > Y6, PYY(3–36) preferentially binds to Y2 receptors and to a lesser extent to Y5 receptors (reviewed by Blomqvist and Herzog [63]). According to a review of Lin et al. [64], the most important hypothalamic Y receptors are Y1, Y2 and Y5. Since BAT expresses Y5 but hardly any Y2 [65], the effects of PPY on BAT might be mediated by various hypothalamic Y receptors while in vitro effects are predominantly due to PYY's direct effects on Y5.

Since PYY is more capable of crossing the blood-brain barrier than PP [66], interpretation of both in vitro and in vivo data is of importance for PYY. *Pyy*-deficient mice are heavier at a younger age (14 weeks) but not when they are older (28 weeks) [67]. Compared to their wild-type littermates, *Pyy*-deficient mice ate less but had comparable locomotor activity. It is therefore tempting to speculate that deficiency of *Pyy* results in reduced BAT activity. Indeed, subcutaneous PYY(3–36) injections to mice immediately reduced food intake but also blunted the rise of RQ that occurs during feeding [68]. This is suggestive of enhanced fatty acid oxidation, an important process in BAT activation. In addition, a 1-week continuous subcutaneous PYY(3–36) infusion in diet-induced obese mice resulted in ~6% decline in body weight, an effect that could not be fully explained by the reduced food intake [69]. The total metabolic rate was not affected by PYY(3–36) infusion but it resulted in a declined RQ.

Not much evidence exists on the role of PP in adipocyte function. Pancreas-specific PP transgenic mice have higher circulating PP concentrations with a reduced body weight but this might be attributable to a reduced food intake and slower gastric emptying [70]. The effects of PP on BAT have been reported by Asakawa et al. [71] who found that peripheral PP administration to mice not only reduced food intake but also increased activity of sympathetic nerves innervating the BAT depot. When given a protein-rich meal, obese humans responded with severely blunted PP secretion [72]. Since PP increases BAT activity, the reduced PP secretion in obese subjects might have been attributed to their obese phenotype.

In conclusion, not much is known about the effects of PYY and PP on BAT. From the scarcely available data we can conclude that PYY likely activates BAT via a central mechanism since the preferred Y2 receptor is highly expressed in the brain but not in the BAT depot [65]. Also, PP likely increases BAT. Since PP cannot cross the blood-brain barrier, its effects on BAT are presumably direct.

Amylin

Amylin is co-secreted with insulin from the pancreatic β-cells in the ratio of approximately 100:1. In general, both systemic and brain-specific amylin treatment of laboratory animals results in a decline of body weight [73, 74] which can be attributed to the anorexogenic effects of amylin. However, Roth et al. [75] also showed that independent on effects on food intake, sustained subcutaneous infusion of amylin reduced the total body fat content of rats albeit that BAT *Ucp1* expression of the amylin-infused rats did not differ from that in control rats.

In contrast to the above study, chronic ICV infusion of amylin to rats reduced their RQ and increased their body temperature [76]. This CNS effect of amylin has recently gathered more attention since Fernandes-Santos et al. [77] showed that both intraperitoneal and ICV injected amylin increases the CNS activity that leads to increased BAT thermogenesis and weight loss. Thus, amylin acts via a central mechanism to acutely stimulate BAT.

In contrast to many of the other gut hormones, research has highlighted some of the key players in the modulation of amylin's effect on BAT via the CNS. Most of these studies have pointed towards an important role for an amylin receptor: receptor activity-modifying protein 1 (RAMP1). Mice with brain-specific overexpression of human RAMP1 have a higher energy expenditure, elevated body temperature and increased expression of *Ucp1* in BAT [78]. Of importance is the fact that the RAMP1 transgenic mice also had an increased sympathetic tone towards the BAT depot. Altogether, these data show that presumably via RAMP1, amylin activates BAT via the CNS.

Enterostatin

Enterostatin is a pancreatic gut hormone that reduces food intake and prevents body weight gain when fed a HFD [79]. Enterostatin has been thought to require the CCK1 receptor to regulate food intake [80].

Only one study has addressed the effect of enterostatin on BAT activity. Rippe et al. [81] investigated the effect of enterostatin on the BAT depot of mice on a HFD kept at different temperatures. They found that mice kept at 23 °C were protected against HFD-induced body weight concomitant with elevated BAT *Ucp1* mRNA concentrations. However, mice kept at a thermoneutral temperature of 29 °C became obese when fed the HFD and had a lack of BAT *Ucp1* mRNA induction with this diet. When enterostatin was added to the diet, BAT *Ucp1* expression was increased in HFD mice kept at 29 °C. This induction in BAT *Ucp1* expression is at least partly due to central effects since ICV injections of enterostatin in rats induced the sympathetic firing towards the BAT depot [82].

The direct effects of enterostatin on adipose tissue have, to our knowledge, not been investigated, but since CCK1 receptor is expressed in BAT, direct effects of enterostatin on BAT might not be ruled out. Altogether, only limited data are available on the effects of enterostatin on BAT, but it is clear that this gut hormone can induce BAT activity via a central effect.

Somatostatin

Somatostatin is predominantly secreted by the endocrine pancreas and can bind to five different subtypes of the somatostatin receptor (SSR). In 1988, Simón et al. [83] reported binding of somatostatin to rat adipocytes and later studies with primary human adipocytes showed that SSR1 and SSR2 are normally expressed in WAT while SSR3 and SSR4 are only detectable upon inflammation [84]. Such information is not available for brown adipocytes and thus the relative expression profiles of the SSRs in the BAT depot are not known.

Somatostatin has been linked to anti-obesity treatment since this hormone and its analogues octreotide and lanreotide bind to SSR5 on the β-cell membrane of the pancreas, thereby limiting insulin release and, consequently, decrease adipogenesis. Since somatostatin has equal affinity for SSR2 and SSR5, and octreotide and lanreotide bind preferentially to SSR2 [85], direct effects of these compounds on the WAT depot might also be expected. In humans, infusion of octreotide in the subcutaneous WAT depot resulted in a block of the actions of adrenaline, insulin and GH, and thus enhanced the exercise-induced lipid mobilization in this depot [86].

Somatostatin has been suggested to be a modulator of almost all gut hormones, thus it is unclear what the cumulative effect of all these modulations are on BAT activity. The sole study describing effects of somatostatin and/or the SSRs on BAT depots shows that *Ssr2*-deficient mice have smaller BAT depots despite similar food intake as their wild-type littermates [87]. Causes and consequences of the smaller BAT depot have however not been investigated. Thus, the effects of somatostatin on BAT are unknown.

Bile Acids

Bile acids are made from cholesterol by the liver in a process in which Cyp7a1 is the key enzyme. Upon digestion of food, bile acids are released in the bile to facilitate the uptake of fats from the intestinal tract. Recently, it has been shown that the bile acids also perform important signaling functions and might thus be considered gut hormones. For instance, bile acids activate the farnesoid X receptor (FXR) and inhibit their own synthesis in hepatocytes [88]. It has also recently been shown that bile acids induce BAT activity. Addition of the bile acid cholate to the HFD of mice resulted in more pronounced induction of *Ucp1* expression [89]. Cholate also induced expression of *Dio2* that encodes type 2 deiodinase that activates thyroxine to T_3, an endocrine factor that can activate brown adipocytes [4]. This suggests that bile acids stimulate the production of T_3 and thus activation of BAT. These direct actions of bile acids on BAT are not mediated by FXR, but by bile acid binding to the membrane receptor TGR5 [89]. Since TGR5 is ubiquitously expressed, other effects of the bile acids via TGR5 might also explain effects of increased bile acids in *Fxr*-deficient mice. Of interest here is that the TGR5 signaling pathway is critical in the regulation of intestinal GLP-1 secretion [90]. In addition, TGR5 is also expressed in the brain [91] and responds to the neurosteroid pregnanolone [92]. Thus, it is not unlikely that other TGR5 agonists might be pres-

Table 1. Effects of the gut hormones on BAT activity, being either via a direct mechanisms or via a central mechanism involving the CNS

Factor	Effect on BAT	Direct/central
CCK/gastrin	=/↑	Central?
Glucagon	↑	Direct (some central effects?)
GLP-1/OXM	↑	Central
AG	↓	Central
DAG	↑	Unknown
GIP	(↓/=)	(If any effect: presumably direct)
PP	↑?	Direct?
PYY	↑?	Central?
Amylin	↑	Central
Enterostatin	↑	Central
Somatostatin	?	?
Bile acids	↑	Direct

↑: Increasing BAT activity; ↓: decreasing BAT activity; =: no effect on BAT activity.

ent in the circulation and the CNS that activate BAT directly or via the CNS. This requires more research and dedicated studies.

In general, most data point towards an activating role of bile acids on BAT via a direct mechanism.

Conclusion

Different gut hormones have different effects on BAT activity. This is summarized in table 1. In general, however, anorexigenic gut hormones stimulate BAT and orexigenic gut hormones inhibit BAT activity. The mechanism via which the hormones modulate BAT is largely unknown and might be via a central mechanism, a direct mechanism or via both mechanisms. In addition, novel insights in gut-derived factors such as bile acids suggest that they might also affect BAT activity, making the interpretation of effects of food intake per se on BAT activity even more troublesome.

References

1 Cannon B, Nedergaard J: Brown adipose tissue: function and physiological significance. Physiol Rev 2004;84:277–359.
2 Van Marken Lichtenbelt WD, Vanhommerig JW, Smulders NM, Drossaerts JMAFL, Kemerink GJ, Bouvy ND, Schrauwen P, Teule GJJ: Cold-activated brown adipose tissue in healthy men. N Engl J Med 2009;360:1500–1508.
3 Cypess AM, Lehman S, Williams G, Tal I, Rodman D, Goldfine AB, Kuo FC, Palmer EL, Tseng Y-H, Doria A, Kolodny GM, Kahn CR: Identification and importance of brown adipose tissue in adult humans. N Engl J Med 2009;360:1509–1517.
4 Lee P, Swarbrick MM, Ho KKY: Brown adipose tissue in adult humans: a metabolic renaissance. Endocr Rev 2013;34:413–438.

5 Lowell BB, Susulic VS, Hamann A, Lawitts JA, Himms-Hagen J, Boyer BB, Kozak LP, Flier JS: Development of obesity in transgenic mice after genetic ablation of brown adipose tissue. Nature 1993;366: 740–742.

6 Flint A, Raben A, Rehfeld JF, Holst JJ, Astrup A: The effect of glucagon-like peptide-1 on energy expenditure and substrate metabolism in humans. Int J Obes Relat Metab Disord 2000;24:288–298.

7 Flint A, Raben A, Ersbøll AK, Holst JJ, Astrup A: The effect of physiological levels of glucagon-like peptide-1 on appetite, gastric emptying, energy and substrate metabolism in obesity. Int J Obes Relat Metab Disord 2001;25:781–792.

8 Moon H-S, Chamberland JP, Diakopoulos KN, Fiorenza CG, Ziemke F, Schneider B, Mantzoros CS: Leptin and amylin act in an additive manner to activate overlapping signaling pathways in peripheral tissues: in vitro and ex vivo studies in humans. Diabetes Care 2011;34:132–138.

9 López M, Nogueiras R: Firing up brown fat with brain amylin. Endocrinology 2013;154:2263–2265.

10 Chao P-T, Yang L, Aja S, Moran TH, Bi S: Knockdown of NPY expression in the dorsomedial hypothalamus promotes development of brown adipocytes and prevents diet-induced obesity. Cell Metab 2011;13:573–583.

11 Song CK, Vaughan CH, Keen-Rinehart E, Harris RBS, Richard D, Bartness TJ: Melanocortin-4 receptor mRNA expressed in sympathetic outflow neurons to brown adipose tissue: neuroanatomical and functional evidence. Am J Physiol Regul Integr Comp Physiol 2008;295:R417–R428.

12 Dufresne M, Seva C, Fourmy D: Cholecystokinin and gastrin receptors. Physiol Rev 2006;86:805–847.

13 Chen H, Kent S, Morris MJ: Is the CCK2 receptor essential for normal regulation of body weight and adiposity? Eur J Neurosci 2006;24:1427–1433.

14 Clerc P, Coll Constans MG, Lulka H, Broussaud S, Guigné C, Leung-Theung-Long S, Perrin C, Knauf C, Carpéné C, Pénicaud L, Seva C, Burcelin R, Valet P, Fourmy D, Dufresne M: Involvement of cholecystokinin 2 receptor in food intake regulation: hyperphagia and increased fat deposition in cholecystokinin 2 receptor-deficient mice. Endocrinology 2007; 148:1039–1049.

15 Schroeder M, Zagoory-Sharon O, Shbiro L, Marco A, Hyun J, Moran TH, Bi S, Weller A: Development of obesity in the Otsuka Long-Evans Tokushima Fatty rat. Am J Physiol Regul Integr Comp Physiol 2009; 297:R1749–R1760.

16 Rahman SM, Wang Y-M, Yotsumoto H, Cha J-Y, Han S-Y, Inoue S, Yanagita T: Effects of conjugated linoleic acid on serum leptin concentration, body-fat accumulation, and β-oxidation of fatty acid in OLETF rats. Nutrition 2001;17:385–390.

17 Schroeder M, Moran TH, Weller A: Attenuation of obesity by early-life food restriction in genetically hyperphagic male OLETF rats: peripheral mechanisms. Horm Behav 2010;57:455–462.

18 Yoshimatsu H, Egawa M, Bray GA: Effects of cholecystokinin on sympathetic activity to interscapular brown adipose tissue. Brain Res 1992;597:298–303.

19 Moran TH, Robinson PH, Goldrich MS, McHugh PR: Two brain cholecystokinin receptors: implications for behavioral actions. Brain Res 1986;362: 175–179.

20 Cockburn F, Hull D, Walton I: The effect of lipolytic hormones and theophylline on heat production in brown adipose tissue in vivo. Br J Pharmacol Chemother 1967;31:568–577.

21 Joel CD: Stimulation of metabolism of rat brown adipose tissue by addition of lipolytic hormones in vitro. J Biol Chem 1966;241:814–821.

22 Burcelin R, Li J, Charron MJ: Cloning and sequence analysis of the murine glucagon receptor-encoding gene. Gene 1995;164:305–310.

23 Iwanij V, Amos TM, Billington CJ: Identification and characterization of the glucagon receptor from adipose tissue. Mol Cell Endocrinol 1994;101:257–261.

24 Doi K, Kuroshima A: Modified metabolic responsiveness to glucagon in cold-acclimated and heat-acclimated rats. Life Sci 1982;30:785–791.

25 Yahata T, Ohno T, Kuroshima A: Improved cold tolerance in glucagon-treated rats. Life Sci 1981;28: 2603–2610.

26 Seitz HJ, Krone W, Wilke H, Tarnowski W: Rapid rise in plasma glucagon induced by acute cold exposure in man and rat. Pflugers Arch 1981;389:115–120.

27 Billington CJ, Briggs JE, Link JG, Levine AS: Glucagon in physiological concentrations stimulates brown fat thermogenesis in vivo. Am J Physiol Regul Integr Comp Physiol 1991;261:R501–R507.

28 Kuroshima A, Yahata T: Noradrenaline-induced changes in rat brown adipose tissue glucagon. Jpn J Physiol 1989;39:311–315.

29 Kuroshima A, Kurahashi M, Yahata T: Calorigenic effects of noradrenaline and glucagon on white adipocytes in cold- and heat-acclimated rats. Pflugers Arch 1979;381:113–117.

30 Yahata T, Kuroshima A: Cold-induced changes in glucagon of brown adipose tissue. Jpn J Physiol 1987; 37:773–782.

31 Shimizu H, Egawa M, Yoshimatsu H, Bray GA: Glucagon injected in the lateral hypothalamus stimulates sympathetic activity and suppresses monoamine metabolism. Brain Res 1993;630:95–100.

32 Mérida E, Delgado E, Molina LM, Villanueva-Peñacarrillo ML, Valverde I: Presence of glucagon and glucagon-like peptide-1(7–36) amide receptors in solubilized membranes of human adipose tissue. J Clin Endocrinol Metab 1993;77:1654–1657.

33 Egan JM, Montrose-Rafizadeh C, Wang Y, Bernier M, Roth J: Glucagon-like peptide-1(7–36) amide (GLP-1) enhances insulin-stimulated glucose metabolism in 3T3-L1 adipocytes: one of several potential extrapancreatic sites of GLP-1 action. Endocrinology 1994;135:2070–2075.

34 Vendrell J, El Bekay R, Peral B, García-Fuentes E, Megia A, Macias-Gonzalez M, Real JF, Jimenez-Gomez Y, Escoté X, Pachón G, Simó R, Selva DM, Malagón MM, Tinahones FJ: Study of the potential association of adipose tissue GLP-1 receptor with obesity and insulin resistance. Endocrinology 2011; 152:4072–4079.

35 Nogueiras R, Pérez-Tilve D, Veyrat-Durebex C, Morgan DA, Varela L, Haynes WG, Patterson JT, Disse E, Pfluger PT, López M, Woods SC, DiMarchi R, Diéguez C, Rahmouni K, Rohner-Jeanrenaud F, Tschöp MH: Direct control of peripheral lipid deposition by CNS GLP-1 receptor signaling is mediated by the sympathetic nervous system and blunted in diet-induced obesity. J Neurosci 2009;29:5916–5925.

36 Lockie SH, Heppner KM, Chaudhary N, Chabenne JR, Morgan DA, Veyrat-Durebex C, Ananthakrishnan G, Rohner-Jeanrenaud F, Drucker DJ, DiMarchi R, Rahmouni K, Oldfield BJ, Tschöp MH, Perez-Tilve D: Direct control of brown adipose tissue thermogenesis by central nervous system glucagon-like peptide-1 receptor signaling. Diabetes 2012;61: 2753–2762.

37 Dakin CL, Small CJ, Park AJ, Seth A, Ghatei MA, Bloom SR: Repeated ICV administration of oxyntomodulin causes a greater reduction in body weight gain than in pair-fed rats. Am J Physiol Endocrinol Metab 2002;283:E1173–E1177.

38 Gu W, Lloyd DJ, Chinookswong N, Komorowski R, Sivits G, Graham M, Winters KA, Yan H, Boros LG, Lindberg RA, Véniant MM: Pharmacological targeting of glucagon and glucagon-like peptide 1 receptors has different effects on energy state and glucose homeostasis in diet-induced obese mice. J Pharmacol Exp Ther 2011;338:70–81.

39 He M, Su H, Gao W, Johansson SM, Liu Q, Wu X, Liao J, Young AA, Bartfai T, Wang M-W: Reversal of obesity and insulin resistance by a non-peptidic glucagon-like peptide-1 receptor agonist in diet-induced obese mice. PLoS One 2010;5:e14205.

40 Al-Barazanji KA, Arch JR, Buckingham RE, Tadayyon M: Central exendin-4 infusion reduces body weight without altering plasma leptin in (fa/fa) Zucker rats. Obes Res 2000;8:317–323.

41 Yang J, Brown MS, Liang G, Grishin NV, Goldstein JL: Identification of the acyltransferase that octanoylates ghrelin, an appetite-stimulating peptide hormone. Cell 2008;132:387–396.

42 Gauna C, van de Zande B, van Kerkwijk A, Themmen APN, van der Lely AJ, Delhanty PJD: Unacylated ghrelin is not a functional antagonist but a full agonist of the type 1a growth hormone secretagogue receptor (GHS-R). Mol Cell Endocrinol 2007;274: 30–34.

43 Tschöp M, Smiley DL, Heiman ML: Ghrelin induces adiposity in rodents. Nature 2000;407:908–913.

44 Tsubone T, Masaki T, Katsuragi I, Tanaka K, Kakuma T, Yoshimatsu H: Ghrelin regulates adiposity in white adipose tissue and UCP1 mRNA expression in brown adipose tissue in mice. Regul Pept 2005;130: 97–103.

45 Yasuda T, Masaki T, Kakuma T, Yoshimatsu H: Centrally administered ghrelin suppresses sympathetic nerve activity in brown adipose tissue of rats. Neurosci Lett 2003;349:75–78.

46 Ma X, Lin L, Qin G, Lu X, Fiorotto M, Dixit VD, Sun Y: Ablations of ghrelin and ghrelin receptor exhibit differential metabolic phenotypes and thermogenic capacity during aging. PLoS One 2011;6:e16391.

47 Mano-Otagiri A, Iwasaki-Sekino A, Nemoto T, Ohata H, Shuto Y, Nakabayashi H, Sugihara H, Oikawa S, Shibasaki T: Genetic suppression of ghrelin receptors activates brown adipocyte function and decreases fat storage in rats. Regul Pept 2010;160:81–90.

48 Mano-Otagiri A, Ohata H, Iwasaki-Sekino A, Nemoto T, Shibasaki T: Ghrelin suppresses noradrenaline release in the brown adipose tissue of rats. J Endocrinol 2009;201:341–349.

49 Delhanty PJD, Huisman M, Baldeon-Rojas LY, van den Berge I, Grefhorst A, Abribat T, Leenen PJM, Themmen APN, van der Lely A-J: Des-acyl ghrelin analogs prevent high-fat-diet-induced dysregulation of glucose homeostasis. FASEB J 2013;27:1690–1700.

50 Usdin TB, Mezey E, Button DC, Brownstein MJ, Bonner TI: Gastric inhibitory polypeptide receptor, a member of the secretin-vasoactive intestinal peptide receptor family, is widely distributed in peripheral organs and the brain. Endocrinology 1993;133: 2861–2870.

51 Oben J, Morgan L, Fletcher J, Marks V: Effect of the enteropancreatic hormones, gastric inhibitory polypeptide and glucagon-like polypeptide-1(7–36) amide, on fatty acid synthesis in explants of rat adipose tissue. J Endocrinol 1991;130:267–272.

52 Beck B, Max JP: Gastric inhibitory polypeptide enhancement of the insulin effect on fatty acid incorporation into adipose tissue in the rat. Regul Pept 1983; 7:3–8.

53 Asmar M, Simonsen L, Madsbad S, Stallknecht B, Holst JJ, Bülow J: Glucose-Dependent insulinotropic polypeptide may enhance fatty acid re-esterification in subcutaneous abdominal adipose tissue in lean humans. Diabetes 2010;59:2160–2163.

54 Creutzfeldt W, Ebert R, Willms B, Frerichs H, Brown JC: Gastric inhibitory polypeptide and insulin in obesity: increased response to stimulation and defective feedback control of serum levels. Diabetologia 1978;14:15–24.

55 Getty-Kaushik L, Song DH, Boylan MO, Corkey BE, Wolfe MM: Glucose-dependent insulinotropic polypeptide modulates adipocyte lipolysis and re-esterification. Obes (Silver Spring) 2006;14:1124–1131.

56 Miyawaki K, Yamada Y, Ban N, Ihara Y, Tsukiyama K, Zhou H, Fujimoto S, Oku A, Tsuda K, Toyokuni S, Hiai H, Mizunoya W, Fushiki T, Holst JJ, Makino M, Tashita A, Kobara Y, Tsubamoto Y, Jinnouchi T, Jomori T, Seino Y: Inhibition of gastric inhibitory polypeptide signaling prevents obesity. Nat Med 2002;8:738–742.

57 Meier JJ, Nauck MA, Schmidt WE, Gallwitz B: Gastric inhibitory polypeptide: the neglected incretin revisited. Regul Pept 2002;107:1–13.

58 Bartelt A, Bruns OT, Reimer R, Hohenberg H, Ittrich H, Peldschus K, Kaul MG, Tromsdorf UI, Weller H, Waurisch C, Eychmüller A, Gordts PL, Rinninger F, Bruegelmann K, Freund B, Nielsen P, Merkel M, Heeren J: Brown adipose tissue activity controls triglyceride clearance. Nat Med 2011;17:200–205.

59 Eckel RH, Fujimoto WY, Brunzell JD: Gastric inhibitory polypeptide enhanced lipoprotein lipase activity in cultured preadipocytes. Diabetes 1979;28:1141–1142.

60 Knapper JME, Puddicombe SM, Morgan LM, Fletcher JM: Investigations into the actions of glucose-dependent insulinotropic polypeptide and glucagon-like peptide-1(7–36)amide on lipoprotein lipase activity in explants of rat adipose tissue. J Nutr 1995;125:183–188.

61 McClean PL, Irwin N, Cassidy RS, Holst JJ, Gault VA, Flatt PR: GIP receptor antagonism reverses obesity, insulin resistance, and associated metabolic disturbances induced in mice by prolonged consumption of high-fat diet. Am J Physiol Endocrinol Metab 2007;293:E1746–E1755.

62 Batterham RL, Cowley MA, Small CJ, Herzog H, Cohen MA, Dakin CL, Wren AM, Brynes AE, Low MJ, Ghatei MA, Cone RD, Bloom SR: Gut hormone PYY(3–36) physiologically inhibits food intake. Nature 2002;418:650–654.

63 Blomqvist AG, Herzog H: Y-receptor subtypes – how many more? Trends Neurosci 1997;20:294–298.

64 Lin S, Boey D, Herzog H: NPY and Y receptors: lessons from transgenic and knockout models. Neuropeptides 2004;38:189–200.

65 Shimada K, Ohno Y, Okamatsu-Ogura Y, Suzuki M, Kamikawa A, Terao A, Kimura K: Neuropeptide Y activates phosphorylation of ERK and STAT3 in stromal vascular cells from brown adipose tissue, but fails to affect thermogenic function of brown adipocytes. Peptides 2012;34:336–342.

66 Dumont Y, Moyse E, Fournier A, Quirion R: Distribution of peripherally injected peptide YY ([^{125}I] PYY(3–36)) and pancreatic polypeptide ([^{125}I] hPP) in the CNS: enrichment in the area postrema. J Mol Neurosci 2007;33:294–304.

67 Boey D, Lin S, Karl T, Baldock P, Lee N, Enriquez R, Couzens M, Slack K, Dallmann R, Sainsbury A, Herzog H: Peptide YY ablation in mice leads to the development of hyperinsulinaemia and obesity. Diabetologia 2006;49:1360–1370.

68 Van den Hoek AM, Heijboer AC, Voshol PJ, Havekes LM, Romijn JA, Corssmit EPM, Pijl H: Chronic PYY3–36 treatment promotes fat oxidation and ameliorates insulin resistance in C57BL6 mice. Am J Physiol Endocrinol Metab 2007;292:E238–E245.

69 Adams SH, Lei C, Jodka CM, Nikoulina SE, Hoyt JA, Gedulin B, Mack CM, Kendall ES: PYY(3–36) administration decreases the respiratory quotient and reduces adiposity in diet-induced obese mice. J Nutr 2006;136:195–201.

70 Ueno N, Inui A, Iwamoto M, Kaga T, Asakawa A, Okita M, Fujimiya M, Nakajima Y, Ohmoto Y, Ohnaka M, Nakaya Y, Miyazaki JI, Kasuga M: Decreased food intake and body weight in pancreatic polypeptide-overexpressing mice. Gastroenterology 1999;117:1427–1432.

71 Asakawa A, Inui A, Yuzuriha H, Ueno N, Katsuura G, Fujimiya M, Fujino MA, Niijima A, Meguid MM, Kasuga M: Characterization of the effects of pancreatic polypeptide in the regulation of energy balance. Gastroenterology 2003;124:1325–1336.

72 Lassmann V, Vague P, Vialettes B, Simon MC: Low plasma levels of pancreatic polypeptide in obesity. Diabetes 1980;29:428–430.

73 Chance WT, Balasubramaniam A, Stallion A, Fischer JE: Anorexia following the systemic injection of amylin. Brain Res 1993;607:185–188.

74 Chance WT, Balasubramaniam A, Zhang FS, Wimalawansa SJ, Fischer JE: Anorexia following the intrahypothalamic administration of amylin. Brain Res 1991;539:352–354.

75 Roth JD, Hughes H, Kendall E, Baron AD, Anderson CM: Antiobesity effects of the β-cell hormone amylin in diet-induced obese rats: effects on food intake, body weight, composition, energy expenditure, and gene expression. Endocrinology 2006;147:5855–5864.

76 Wielinga PY, Löwenstein C, Muff S, Munz M, Woods SC, Lutz TA: Central amylin acts as an adiposity signal to control body weight and energy expenditure. Physiol Behav 2010;101:45–52.

77 Fernandes-Santos C, Zhang Z, Morgan DA, Guo D-F, Russo AF, Rahmouni K: Amylin acts in the central nervous system to increase sympathetic nerve activity. Endocrinology 2013;154:2481–2488.

78 Zhang Z, Liu X, Morgan DA, Kuburas A, Thedens DR, Russo AF, Rahmouni K: Neuronal receptor activity-modifying protein 1 promotes energy expenditure in mice. Diabetes 2011;60:1063–1071.

79 Erlanson-Albertsson C, Yorkf D: Enterostatin-A peptide regulating fat intake. Obes Res 1997;5:360–372.

80 Lin L, Thomas SR, Kilroy G, Schwartz GJ, York DA: Enterostatin inhibition of dietary fat intake is dependent on CCK-A receptors. Am J Physiol Regul Integr Comp Physiol 2003;285:R321–R328.

81 Rippe C, Berger K, Böiers C, Ricquier D, Erlanson-Albertsson C: Effect of high-fat diet, surrounding temperature, and enterostatin on uncoupling protein gene expression. Am J Physiol Endocrinol Metab 2000;279:E293–E300.

82 Nagase H, Bray GA, York DA: Effect of galanin and enterostatin on sympathetic nerve activity to interscapular brown adipose tissue. Brain Res 1996;709: 44–50.

83 Simón MA, Romero B, Calle C: Characterization of somatostatin binding sites in isolated rat adipocytes. Regul Pept 1988;23:261–270.

84 Seboek D, Linscheid P, Zulewski H, Langer I, Christ-Crain M, Keller U, Müller B: Somatostatin is expressed and secreted by human adipose tissue upon infection and inflammation. J Clin Endocrinol Metab 2004;89:4833–4839.

85 Weckbecker G, Lewis I, Albert R, Schmid HA, Hoyer D, Bruns C: Opportunities in somatostatin research: biological, chemical and therapeutic aspects. Nat Rev Drug Discov 2003;2:999–1017.

86 De Glisezinski I, Larrouy D, Bajzova M, Koppo K, Polak J, Berlan M, Bulow J, Langin D, Marques MA, Crampes F, Lafontan M, Stich V: Adrenaline but not noradrenaline is a determinant of exercise-induced lipid mobilization in human subcutaneous adipose tissue. J Physiol 2009;587:3393–3404.

87 Singh V, Grötzinger C, Nowak KW, Zacharias S, Göncz E, Pless G, Sauer IM, Eichhorn I, Pfeiffer-Guglielmi B, Hamprecht B, Wiedenmann B, Plöckinger U, Strowski MZ: Somatostatin receptor subtype-2-deficient mice with diet-induced obesity have hyperglycemia, nonfasting hyperglucagonemia, and decreased hepatic glycogen deposition. Endocrinology 2007;148:3887–3899.

88 Kuipers F, Claudel T, Sturm E, Staels B: The farnesoid X receptor (FXR) as modulator of bile acid metabolism. Rev Endocr Metab Disord 2004;5:319–326.

89 Watanabe M, Houten SM, Mataki C, Christoffolete MA, Kim BW, Sato H, Messaddeq N, Harney JW, Ezaki O, Kodama T, Schoonjans K, Bianco AC, Auwerx J: Bile acids induce energy expenditure by promoting intracellular thyroid hormone activation. Nature 2006;439:484–489.

90 Thomas C, Gioiello A, Noriega L, Strehle A, Oury J, Rizzo G, Macchiarulo A, Yamamoto H, Mataki C, Pruzanski M, Pellicciari R, Auwerx J, Schoonjans K: TGR5-mediated bile acid sensing controls glucose homeostasis. Cell Metab 2009;10:167–177.

91 Vassileva G, Golovko A, Markowitz L, Abbondanzo SJ, Zeng M, Yang S, Hoos L, Tetzloff G, Levitan D, Murgolo NJ, Keane K, Davis HR, Hedrick J, Gustafson EL: Targeted deletion of Gpbar1 protects mice from cholesterol gallstone formation. Biochem J 2006;398:423–430.

92 Keitel V, Görg B, Bidmon HJ, Zemtsova I, Spomer L, Zilles K, Häussinger D: The bile acid receptor TGR5 (Gpbar-1) acts as a neurosteroid receptor in brain. Glia 2010;58:1794–1805.

Aldo Grefhorst, PhD
Department of Internal Medicine, Room Ee532
Erasmus MC, PO Box 2040
NL–3000 CA Rotterdam (The Netherlands)
E-Mail a.grefhorst@erasmusmc.nl

Delhanty PJD, van der Lely AJ (eds): How Gut and Brain Control Metabolism.
Front Horm Res. Basel, Karger, 2014, vol 42, pp 123–133 (DOI: 10.1159/000358321)

Gut Sweet Taste Receptors and Their Role in Metabolism

A.C. Meyer-Gerspach · B. Wölnerhanssen · C. Beglinger

Department of Biomedicine and Division of Gastroenterology and Hepatology, University Hospital Basel, Basel, Switzerland

Abstract

Obesity is caused by an imbalance between food intake and energy expenditure. In recent decades the gastrointestinal tract has received growing attention as a control parameter for the regulation of appetite and food intake, however regulatory circuits and their interactions are complex. The basic understanding on the role of the gut starts with the notion 'we are what we eat'. Food enters the gastrointestinal tract, which then triggers specific mechanisms or a sensing machinery that respond to specific components of food. Enteroendocrine cells in the small intestine are the anatomical basis for the sensing machinery, which act as neural triggers or as intestinal satiation peptide-secreting cells. These cells express chemosensory receptors that respond to luminal stimuli. The understanding of each gastrointestinal mechanism that might be involved in the process of eating provides a basis for the assessment of the potential of the gastrointestinal tract in the fight against obesity. This review discusses the function of the gut sweet taste receptor T1R2/T1R3 in sensing sweet compounds, as well as its role in gastrointestinal peptide secretion and glucose metabolism.

© 2014 S. Karger AG, Basel

In recent decades knowledge of the gustatory system has greatly improved. Especially the understanding of the mechanisms by which the gut senses luminal nutrients and induces gastrointestinal (GI) peptide secretion has witnessed remarkable advances. Specific receptor and transporter systems, which are located in the membrane of specialized epithelial cells such as enteroendocrine cells (EECs), are able to sense ingested food in the gut lumen. The GI gustatory system consists of a neural-epithelial machinery linking the sensory epithelial cells of the gut to the first gustatory relay center in the brain. The gut epithelial machinery includes neuroactive peptides like glucagon-like peptide-1 (GLP-1), peptide tyrosine-tyrosine (PYY) and cholecystokinin (CCK), which are secreted upon specific nutrient stimulation. G protein-coupled receptors (GPCRs) and solute transporters expressed on the apical end of taste receptor cells function as the receptors for luminal nutrients and induce specific secretion of signaling molecules such as GLP-1 and PYY. The main ligands for these receptor and transporter systems in the gut are the three macronutrients (proteins, fats and carbohydrates) as well as their breakdown products, including amino acids and proteolytic products, fatty acids and glucose.

Enteroendorine Cells

EECs are dispersed among mucosal cells of the GI tract and although they represent less than 1% of the gut epithelial population they constitute the largest endocrine organ of the human body. They produce and secrete more than 20 different peptides or signaling molecules. The secretion products are located in secretory granules and after stimulation they are secreted by exocytosis at the basolateral membrane into the lamina propria where they either act locally on vagal afferents (paracrine manner) or enter directly into the bloodstream (endocrine manner). The stimulation of exocytosis is mediated through activation of GPCRs (located at the apical membrane of EECs) by ingested foods. There are at least 10 discrete cell types that make up the enteroendocrine family – each classically described by a distinct localization along the gut and a different hormonal profile. Many EECs include microvilli extending to the lumen, leading to their description as 'open cells', which enable direct sensing of luminal factors (nutrients). In contrast, 'closed cells' do not reach the lumen and are believed to respond to luminal content indirectly through mechanical stimuli and neuronal or humoral factors. Together, EECs can be regarded as primary chemoreceptors, capable of responding to luminal contents by releasing secretory molecules, which act locally, centrally and in the periphery [1, 2].

G Protein-Coupled Receptors

In recent years, GPCRs have been identified as obvious nutrient sensors in the intestine. GPCRs, also known as seven-transmembrane receptors, are subdivided into six families based on sequence homology and functional similarity: family A (rhodopsin-like receptors), family B (secretin receptors), family C (metabotropic glutamate receptors), family D (fungal mating pheromone receptors), family E (cyclic AMP receptors) and family F (frizzled/smoothed receptors) [3]. A role in nutrient sensing was shown for family A and C receptors. Family A receptors include the GPR93 (responsive to protein degradation products) and the free fatty acid receptors (FFAR1–3). Family C receptors are characterized by a large extracellular Venus flytrap ligand-binding domain and include metabotropic glutamate (mGlut) receptors, calcium-sensing receptors (CaR), family 1 taste receptors (T1Rs) and GPCR family C, group 6, subtype A (GPRC6A) [2].

Meyer-Gerspach · Wölnerhanssen · Beglinger

Extracellular binding of nutrients or their breakdown products to GPCRs induces conformational changes of the receptor that results in a separation of the membrane-bound heterotrimeric guanine nucleotide-binding G-protein subunits (α, β and γ). Subsequently, these subunits stimulate their respective effector pathways: (i) stimulation of phospholipase C (PLC), leading to the generation of inositol triphosphate (IP_3) and diacylglycerol (DAG), which activate protein kinase (PK) C; (ii) stimulation of adenylate cylase (AC), which results in an elevation of cyclic adenosine monophosphate (cAMP) concentrations; (iii) stimulation of phospholipase C $\beta2$ (PLC $\beta2$). Each pathway results in an increase of cytoplasmic Ca^{2+} that activates transient receptor potential channel type 5 (TRPM-5) and with this the entry of cations. The resulting depolarization triggers the generation of action potentials and in turn the release of gut peptides [2, 4].

T1R2/T1R3 – The Sweet Taste Receptor

Recent findings document that populations of intestinal cells can 'taste' sugars or sweet compounds by sensory pathways similar to those described in lingual taste cells. In the gustatory buds of the tongue, the sensation of sweet taste is mediated by the GPCR heterodimer T1R2/T1R3 (sweet taste receptor). Glucose and artificial sweeteners bind to T1R2/T1R3 that is coupled to the heterotrimeric G-protein (α-gustducin, G$\beta3$ and G$\gamma13$) [1]. Through activation, the G-protein subunits separate to α-gustducin and $\beta\gamma$-unit (G$\beta3$-G$\gamma13$); the latter activates PLC $\beta2$ to generate IP_3 and DAG. IP_3 activates type III IP_3 receptors, which results in the release of Ca^{2+} from internal stores and in turn activate TRPM-5. The influx of cations induces taste cell depolarization and subsequent signaling to other taste cells and gustatory afferent nerves [1] (fig. 1).

Sweet Taste Receptor Expression in the Gut
The expression of signaling components of the sweet taste receptor in extragustatory regions was first described by Höfer et al. [5]. They found that α-gustducin is expressed in the stomach, duodenum and pancreatic duct of rats. In mice it was shown that the α-gustducin-containing cells are scattered throughout the epithelium of the gut and show structural features similar to the cells of the tongue [6]. In 2005, the expressions of T1R2, T1R3 and α-gustducin in mouse duodenum and small intestine at mRNA and protein levels were noted [7]. In humans, Rozengurt et al. [8] showed that α-gustducin is localized in enteroendocrine L-cells in the colonic mucosa; they also found expression of T1R3 and α-gustducin in the human colon. Furthermore, most α-gustducin-positive cells contained chromogranin A, a marker of EECs, which indicates that α-gustducin is expressed in EECs; the observed co-localization of α-gustducin with PYY and GLP-1 in human colonic cells confirms these findings [8]. In human duodenal biopsy sections, α-gustducin expression was shown by indirect immunofluorescence in GLP-1-expressing L-cells, GIP-expressing K-cells and GIP and GLP-1 co-expressing K/L-cells [9]. Confirmation of the expression of α-gustducin in human

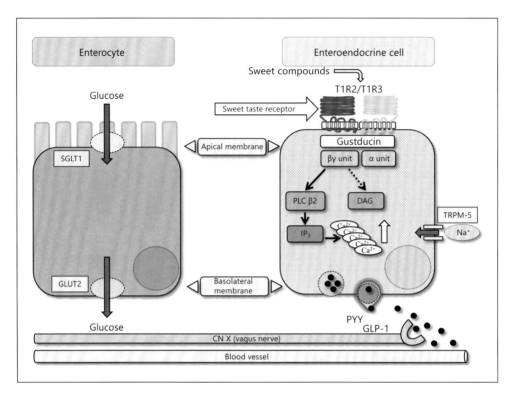

Fig. 1. Simplified model of the pathways involved in the sensing of sweet compounds in the GI tract. Glucose and other sweet compounds are sensed by the sweet taste receptor (T1R2/T1R3). T1R2/T1R3 induces, via gustducin, the release of second messengers that lead to the release of GI peptides which can communicate directly (via the bloodstream) or indirectly (via the vagus nerve) with the brain to control food intake. SGLT1 = Sodium-dependent glucose co-transporter; GLUT2 = glucose transporter 2; PLC β2 = phospholipase C β2; DAG = diacylglycerol; IP$_3$ = inositol triphosphate; TRPM-5 = transient receptor potential channel type 5; PYY = peptide tyrosine-tyrosine; GLP-1 = glucagon-like peptide-1.

enteroendocrine K- and L-cells came from laser capture followed by reverse transcriptase-polymerase chain reaction [9]. In addition, T1R2, T1R3, Gβ3, Gγ13, PLC β2 and TRPM-5 were found to be co-expressed with α-gustducin and GLP-1 in human duodenal L-cells [9]. The expression pattern of the taste-signaling elements in the human gut was shown by several groups: whereas the expression of T1R3 is nearly equally distributed throughout the gut, α-gustducin predominantly exists in the proximal part of the GI tract and expression for T1R2 is only low; no sex-specific differences were found [10].

In addition, it seems that glucose availability regulates the expression and/or membrane localization of sweet taste receptors: intrajejunal glucose infusion decreased the expression of T1R2 and T1R3 at the apical membrane in rats [11]; in mice, intrajejunal glucose infusion decreased T1R2 expression [12]. Together these findings support a feedback mechanism for the receptor expression, at least in animals.

Meyer-Gerspach · Wölnerhanssen · Beglinger

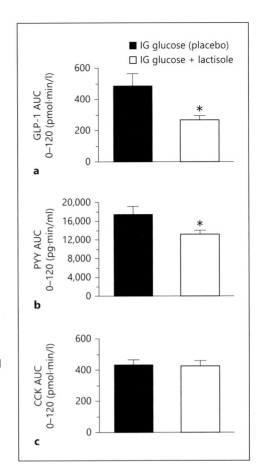

Fig. 2. Area under the concentration time curve (AUC) of (**a**) glucagon-like peptide-1 (GLP-1), (**b**) peptide tyrosine-tyrosine (PYY), and (**c**) cholecystokinin (CCK) after an intragastric load of 75 g glucose with or without 450 ppm lactisole. Data are expressed as means ± SE. * p < 0.05, statistically significant difference vs. placebo (IG glucose). Reported data are from 26 healthy subjects (13 males and 13 females).

Role of Sweet Taste Receptors in Glucose Sensing

To date a number of findings indicate that sweet taste receptors may underlie glucose sensing in gut EECs, particularly those releasing GLP-1 and PYY. Activation of cell lines (GLUTag and NCI-H716) with glucose, sucrose or the artificial sweetener sucralose resulted in the secretion of GLP-1; this release was blocked by the sweet taste receptor antagonists gurmarin and lactisole [9, 13]. In vivo, Jang et al. [9] showed that plasma GLP-1 levels following glucose gavage were reduced in α-gustducin (α-gust$^{-/-}$) or T1R3 ($T1R3^{-/-}$) *knockout* mice compared to wild-type mice. In addition, an impaired insulin release and elevated blood glucose levels were found – results that were recently confirmed by Geraedts et al. [14]. We performed experiments to determine the functional importance of sweet taste receptors in glucose-stimulated secretions of GLP-1, PYY and CCK in humans [15]. We used lactisole (competitive inhibitor of the sweet taste receptor subunit T1R3) to block the sweet taste receptors in the gut. In parallel to the in vitro data of Jang et al. [9], we could demonstrate that lactisole attenuated the glucose-stimulated secretion of GLP-1 and PYY (fig. 2). In contrast, CCK secretion was unaffected by lactisole,

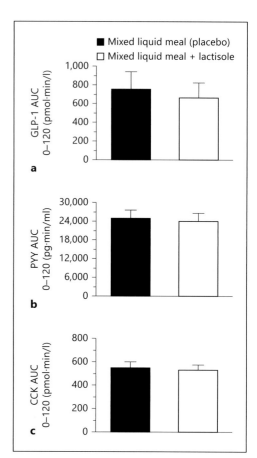

Fig. 3. Area under the concentration time curve (AUC) of (**a**) glucagon-like peptide-1 (GLP-1), (**b**) peptide tyrosine-tyrosine (PYY), and (**c**) cholecystokinin (CCK) after an intragastric infusion of a mixed liquid meal (500 ml Ensure Plus®; 17% protein, 29% fat and 54% carbohydrate; 1.5 kcal/ml) with or without 450 ppm lactisole. Data are expressed as means ± SE. Reported data are from 16 healthy subjects (8 males and 8 females).

indicating that glucose-induced CCK secretion is not mediated by the sweet taste receptor and that other glucose-sensing receptors must be involved. Furthermore, lactisole had no effect on mixed liquid meal-stimulated GI peptide secretion (fig. 3) [15]. Besides glucose, the liquid meal also consists of proteins, fats, and other complex carbohydrates. The lack of effect of lactisole suggests that these nutrients induce the release of satiation peptides via other mechanisms; more importantly, these mechanisms seem to outweigh the effect of sweet receptor blockade. This raises the question of the physiological importance of the sweet taste receptor system in regulating GLP-1 release and associated functions. Long-chain fatty acids, apart from glucose, are also potent luminal secretagogues for GLP-1 release [16]. Thus, the fast response to glucose is based on tasting and activation of the sweet receptor system, whereas the effects of a mixed meal are also mediated by lipids and perhaps proteins. A number of receptors were identified that possibly act as free fatty acid or amino acid sensors; the multiplicity of different receptors suggests that the sweet taste receptor T1R2/T1R3 alone is not responsible for the regulation of GLP-1 release and associated functions.

Meyer-Gerspach · Wölnerhanssen · Beglinger

Role of Sweet Taste Receptors in Glucose Absorption

Dietary glucose is absorbed across the enterocytes of the intestinal wall via the sodium-dependent glucose co-transporter (SGLT1) on the apical membrane and the glucose transporter 2 (GLUT2) on the basolateral membrane of the enterocyte (fig. 1). It seems that glucose sensing via the sweet taste receptor in the GI tract regulates the transport of dietary glucose via these transporters [7, 13]. The hypothesis is that luminal glucose activates the sweet taste receptors on intestinal EECs, which results in the secretion of GLP-1 and GIP, and in turn these peptides may act as neural or paracrine signals to enterocytes, causing upregulation of SGLT1 [17]. In addition, Kellett et al. [18] have proposed that glucose absorption can be further increased at high glucose concentrations (>30 mM) by insertion of GLUT2 at the apical membrane of the enterocyte. Indeed, SGLT1 [13] and GLUT2 [19] transcript and protein are rapidly upregulated in response to luminal glucose which resulted in an increase in SGLT1- as well as GLUT2-mediated glucose transport in mice and rats. The upregulation of SGLT1 and GLUT2 was not observed in $T1R3^{-/-}$ and $\alpha\text{-}gust^{-/-}$ rodents, implying a strong correlation between taste receptor activation and the modulation of glucose transporter expression [13, 19]. At the current time, the observed relationships between sweet taste receptors and SGLT1/GLUT2 expression in rodents are not apparent in humans.

Role of Sweet Taste Receptors in Artificial Sweetener Sensing

As it is well established that both non-nutritive (artificial) and caloric sweeteners bind to the oral sweet taste receptors resulting in the conscious sensation of sweetness, it is logical to hypothesize that artificial sweeteners could bind to the sweet taste receptors located on EECs and cause signal transduction and downstream actions such as GI peptide secretion. This possibility has been explored in multiple models with inconsistent results.

Studies with the human L-cell line, NCI-H716, as well as with the mouse GLUTag cell line showed that the secretion of GLP-1 was induced by sucralose (artificial sweetener) and was blocked by the sweet taste receptor antagonist lactisole or by siRNA targeting α-gustducin [9, 13]. However, these results were not confirmed in two other studies (reviewed by Brown and Rother [20]): sucralose as well as acesulfame-K (another artificial sweetener) failed to increase GLP-1 and GIP secretion in isolated mouse EECs. In addition, studies in rodents failed to find an artificial sweetener-induced release of incretins in vivo. Negative results were also reported in healthy humans: there was no effect of oral sucralose or intragastric sucralose, aspartame, or acesulfame-K on GLP-1, PYY, ghrelin, or GIP secretion [20, 21]. Taken together, these data support the notion that artificial sweeteners in isolation are not a sufficient stimulus for sweet taste receptors to induce GI peptide secretion in vivo.

Nevertheless, de Ruyter et al. [22] found that masked replacement of sugar-containing beverages with non-nutritive beverages reduced weight gain and fat accumulation in normal-weight children. In a study by Brown et al. [23] it was shown that artificial sweeteners in a commercially available diet soda can change the secretion of GLP-1 in combination with caloric sugars (oral glucose load): consumption of that diet soda enhanced (presumably via the artificial sweeteners) glucose-stimulated GLP-1 secretion in healthy adolescents and young adults; it is not clear from the experiment whether this effect was mediated via sweet taste receptors on EECs, lingual sweet taste receptors, or another mechanism. Furthermore, the clinical significance of these findings is not clear as insulin levels were not statistically different and other GLP-1 effects, such as appetite perceptions or gastric emptying were not measured. In addition, these findings were not confirmed by another study, which examined the effects of sucralose before a solid meal (powdered potatoes with 20 g glucose and egg yolk) and reported no effect on GIP or GLP-1 secretion [24].

Together, although most in vitro data support the idea that artificial sweeteners can increase GI peptide secretion by EECs, the available in vivo data have generally not supported this.

Other Gut Sweet Sensory Systems

The T1R2/T1R3 sweet taste receptor is most likely not the only sweet sensory system. The closure of K_{ATP} channels in the cell membrane could be another possible mechanism by which glucose is sensed in EECs. Metabolic regulation of K_{ATP} channel activity has been described in glucose-sensitive tissues, such as pancreatic β-cells and the brain. In pancreatic β-cells metabolism of glucose generates ATP which results in the closure of K_{ATP} channels. The reduction in K^+ triggers membrane depolarization, action potential generation, voltage-gated Ca^{2+} entry and subsequently the release of insulin [25]. This pathway was also described in GLUTag and NCI-H716 cells, both of which secrete GLP-1 [26]. Studies with native EECs isolated from mouse intestine confirmed a role for K_{ATP} channels in the release of GLP-1 and GIP [27]. Moreover, the expression of the K_{ATP} channel subunit Kir6.2 was detected by immunostaining in L- and K-cells of the human intestine [28, 29]. However, despite the clear presence of K_{ATP} channels in human K- and L-cells, there is little evidence that K_{ATP} channel closure causes the secretion of GLP-1 and GIP: sulfonylureas, which stimulate insulin release through closing of K_{ATP} channels in type 2 diabetes patients failed to trigger the release of GLP-1 or GIP [1].

Furthermore, a number of monosaccharide transporters, both sodium-coupled (such as SGLT1, SGLT3) and facilitative (such as GLUT2) mechanisms were suggested as glucose sensors. The role of SGLT1 in glucose sensing by EECs was demonstrated in GLP-1-secreting GLUTag cells: Gribble et al. [30] showed that these cells expressed mRNA for SGLT1 and that glucose triggered the secretion of GLP-1; the release of GLP-1 was blocked by phloridzin, the specific antagonist of SGLT1. The same was shown in vivo in mice, co-administration of phloridzin with glucose in the upper intestine blocked glucose absorption and glucose-induced secretion of GLP-1 and GIP [31]. In addition, mice deficient in SGLT1 exhibit a loss of incretin responsiveness to glucose both in vitro and in vivo [32]. Together these findings provide evidence for a role of SGLT1 in glucose sensing and subsequent GI peptide secretion. The role of SGLT3 in intestinal glucose sensing is less clear. Its expression has been shown in GLUTag cells and in the intestinal epithelium of rodents [30, 33]. Diez-Sampedro et al. [34] reported that human SGLT3 lacks glucose transport capacity and rather acts as glucose sensor. In fact, when human SGLT3 was transfected into oocytes, glucose was not transported but depolarized the membrane – this depolarization was blocked by phloridzin. GLUT2 also plays an important role in glucose-induced secretion of GI peptides by affecting membrane depolarization through closure of K_{ATP} channels [35]. In addition, an involvement of GLUT2 in glucose-induced secretion of GI peptides was described by Cani et al. [36] – *GLUT2$^{-/-}$ knockout* mice showed impaired GLP-1 secretion in response to oral glucose. Furthermore, glucose-stimulated release of GLP-1 and PYY in the small intestine of rats was reduced with inhibitors of GLUT2 [35].

Summary and Conclusion

The expression of the sweet taste receptor as well as its downstream signaling components in EECs of the GI tract is well established. The sweet taste receptor system is involved in glucose-stimulated secretion of GI peptides such as GLP-1 and PYY; the release of both peptides was significantly reduced in healthy subjects by using the specific sweet taste receptor antagonist lactisole. Furthermore, in vitro cell models as well as in vivo animal studies suggested that glucose sensing via the sweet taste receptor in the GI tract regulate the transport of dietary glucose via SGLT1 on the apical membrane and GLUT2 on the basolateral membrane of the enterocytes. However, these observed relationships between sweet taste receptors and SGLT1/GLUT2 expression in animals need further investigation in humans.

Most in vitro data support the idea that artificial sweeteners can bind to the sweet taste receptors located on EECs and cause signal transduction and downstream actions such as GI peptide secretion, however the available in vivo human data have generally not supported that artificial sweeteners in isolation are a sufficient stimulus to activate sweet taste receptors in the gut to induce peptide secretion.

Blocking the sweet taste receptor by lactisole had no inhibitory effect on mixed liquid meal-stimulated GI peptide secretion in healthy humans. These findings indicate that proteins, fats, and other complex carbohydrates in the mixed liquid meal induce the release of GI peptides via other gut receptor mechanisms.

The physiological conclusions of these findings seem to indicate that the sweet taste receptor in the gut is not alone responsible for peptide release, rather it is a complex interaction between different receptor mechanisms, including free fatty acid, amino acid or even other glucose sensory systems.

Acknowledgments

This research is supported by a grant of the Swiss National Science Foundation (Grant No. 320030-132960/1) and the affiliated Marie Heim-Vögtlin Foundation (Grant No. NMS1793).

References

1 Tolhurst G, Reimann F, Gribble FM: Intestinal sensing of nutrients. Handb Exp Pharmacol 2012;209: 309–335.

2 Reimann F, Tolhurst G, Gribble FM: G-protein-coupled receptors in intestinal chemosensation. Cell Metab 2012;15:421–431.

3 Tuteja N: Signaling through G protein-coupled receptors. Plant Signal Behav 2009;4:942–947.

4 Prezeau L, Rives ML, Comps-Agrar L, Maurel D, Kniazeff J, Pin JP: Functional crosstalk between GPCRs: with or without oligomerization. Curr Opin Pharmacol 2010;10:6–13.

5 Höfer D, Puschel B, Drenckhahn D: Taste receptor-like cells in the rat gut identified by expression of α-gustducin. Proc Natl Acad Sci USA 1996;93:6631–6634.

6 Wu SV, Rozengurt N, Yang M, Young SH, Sinnett-Smith J, Rozengurt E: Expression of bitter taste receptors of the T2R family in the gastrointestinal tract and enteroendocrine STC-1 cells. Proc Natl Acad Sci USA 2002;99:2392–2397.

7 Dyer J, Salmon KS, Zibrik L, Shirazi-Beechey SP: Expression of sweet taste receptors of the T1R family in the intestinal tract and enteroendocrine cells. Biochem Soc Trans 2005;33:302–305.

8 Rozengurt N, Wu SV, Chen MC, Huang C, Sternini C, Rozengurt E: Colocalization of the α-subunit of gustducin with PYY and GLP-1 in L-cells of human colon. Am J Physiol Gastrointest Liver Physiol 2006; 291:G792–G802.

9 Jang HJ, Kokrashvili Z, Theodorakis MJ, Carlson OD, Kim BJ, Zhou J, Kim HH, Xu X, Chan SL, Juhaszova M, et al: Gut-expressed gustducin and taste receptors regulate secretion of glucagon-like peptide-1. Proc Natl Acad Sci USA 2007;104:15069–15074.

10 Steinert RE, Gerspach AC, Gutmann H, Asarian L, Drewe J, Beglinger C: The functional involvement of gut-expressed sweet taste receptors in glucose-stimulated secretion of glucagon-like peptide-1 (GLP-1) and peptide YY (PYY). Clin Nutr 2011;30:524–532.

11 Mace OJ, Lister N, Morgan E, Shepherd E, Affleck J, Helliwell P, Bronk JR, Kellett GL, Meredith D, Boyd R, et al: An energy supply network of nutrient absorption coordinated by calcium and T1R taste receptors in rat small intestine. J Physiol 2009;587: 195–210.

12 Young RL, Sutherland K, Pezos N, Brierley SM, Horowitz M, Rayner CK, Blackshaw LA: Expression of taste molecules in the upper gastrointestinal tract in humans with and without type 2 diabetes. Gut 2009;58:337–346.

13 Margolskee RF, Dyer J, Kokrashvili Z, Salmon KS, Ilegems E, Daly K, Maillet EL, Ninomiya Y, Mosinger B, Shirazi-Beechey SP: T1R3 and gustducin in gut sense sugars to regulate expression of Na⁺-glucose cotransporter 1. Proc Natl Acad Sci USA 2007;104: 15075–15080.

14 Geraedts MC, Takahashi T, Vigues S, Markwardt ML, Nkobena A, Cockerham RE, Hajnal A, Dotson CD, Rizzo MA, Munger SD: Transformation of postingestive glucose responses after deletion of sweet taste receptor subunits or gastric bypass surgery. Am J Physiol Endocrinol Metab 2012;303:E464–E474.

15 Gerspach AC, Steinert RE, Schonenberger L, Graber-Maier A, Beglinger C: The role of the gut sweet taste receptor in regulating GLP-1, PYY, and CCK release in humans. Am J Physiol Endocrinol Metab 2011;301:E317–E325.

16 Beglinger S, Drewe J, Schirra J, Goke B, D'Amato M, Beglinger C: Role of fat hydrolysis in regulating glucagon-like peptide-1 secretion. J Clin Endocrinol Metab 2010;95:879–886.

17 Shirazi-Beechey SP, Moran AW, Batchelor DJ, Daly K, Al-Rammahi M: Glucose sensing and signalling; regulation of intestinal glucose transport. Proc Nutr Soc 2011;70:185–193.

18 Kellett GL, Brot-Laroche E, Mace OJ, Leturque A: Sugar absorption in the intestine: the role of GLUT2. Annu Rev Nutr 2008;28:35–54.

19 Mace OJ, Affleck J, Patel N, Kellett GL: Sweet taste receptors in rat small intestine stimulate glucose absorption through apical GLUT2. J Physiol 2007; 582:379–392.

20 Brown RJ, Rother KI: Non-nutritive sweeteners and their role in the gastrointestinal tract. J Clin Endocrinol Metab 2012;97:2597–2605.

21 Steinert RE, Frey F, Topfer A, Drewe J, Beglinger C: Effects of carbohydrate sugars and artificial sweeteners on appetite and the secretion of gastrointestinal satiety peptides. Br J Nutr 2011;105:1320–1328.

22 De Ruyter JC, Olthof MR, Seidell JC, Katan MB: A trial of sugar-free or sugar-sweetened beverages and body weight in children. N Engl J Med 2012;367: 1397–1406.

23 Brown RJ, Walter M, Rother KI: Ingestion of diet soda before a glucose load augments glucagon-like peptide-1 secretion. Diabetes Care 2009;32:2184–2186.

24 Wu T, Zhao BR, Bound MJ, Checklin HL, Bellon M, Little TJ, Young RL, Jones KL, Horowitz M, Rayner CK: Effects of different sweet preloads on incretin hormone secretion, gastric emptying, and postprandial glycemia in healthy humans. Am J Clin Nutr 2012;95:78–83.

25 Rorsman P: The pancreatic β-cell as a fuel sensor: an electrophysiologist's viewpoint. Diabetologia 1997; 40:487–495.

26 Tolhurst G, Reimann F, Gribble FM: Nutritional regulation of glucagon-like peptide-1 secretion. J Physiol 2009;587:27–32.

27 Parker HE, Habib AM, Rogers GJ, Gribble FM, Reimann F: Nutrient-dependent secretion of glucose-dependent insulinotropic polypeptide from primary murine K cells. Diabetologia 2009;52:289–298.

28 Theodorakis MJ, Carlson O, Michopoulos S, Doyle ME, Juhaszova M, Petraki K, Egan JM: Human duodenal enteroendocrine cells: source of both incretin peptides, GLP-1 and GIP. Am J Physiol Endocrinol Metab 2006;290:E550–E559.

29 Nielsen LB, Ploug KB, Swift P, Orskov C, Jansen-Olesen I, Chiarelli F, Holst JJ, Hougaard P, Porksen S, Holl R, et al: Co-localisation of the Kir6.2/SUR1 channel complex with glucagon-like peptide-1 and glucose-dependent insulinotrophic polypeptide expression in human ileal cells and implications for glycaemic control in new onset type 1 diabetes. Eur J Endocrinol 2007;156:663–671.

30 Gribble FM, Williams L, Simpson AK, Reimann F: A novel glucose-sensing mechanism contributing to glucagon-like peptide-1 secretion from the GLUTag cell line. Diabetes 2003;52:1147–1154.

31 Moriya R, Shirakura T, Ito J, Mashiko S, Seo T: Activation of sodium-glucose cotransporter 1 ameliorates hyperglycemia by mediating incretin secretion in mice. Am J Physiol Endocrinol Metab 2009;297: E1358–E1365.

32 Gorboulev V, Schurmann A, Vallon V, Kipp H, Jaschke A, Klessen D, Friedrich A, Scherneck S, Rieg T, Cunard R, et al: Na⁺-D-glucose cotransporter SGLT1 is pivotal for intestinal glucose absorption and glucose-dependent incretin secretion. Diabetes 2012;61:187–196.

33 Freeman SL, Bohan D, Darcel N, Raybould HE: Luminal glucose sensing in the rat intestine has characteristics of a sodium-glucose cotransporter. Am J Physiol Gastrointest Liver Physiol 2006;291:G439–G445.

34 Diez-Sampedro A, Hirayama BA, Osswald C, Gorboulev V, Baumgarten K, Volk C, Wright EM, Koepsell H: A glucose sensor hiding in a family of transporters. Proc Natl Acad Sci USA 2003;100: 11753–11758.

35 Mace OJ, Schindler M, Patel S: The regulation of K- and L-cell activity by GLUT2 and CasR in rat small intestine. J Physiol 2012;590:2917–2936.

36 Cani PD, Holst JJ, Drucker DJ, Delzenne NM, Thorens B, Burcelin R, Knauf C: GLUT2 and the incretin receptors are involved in glucose-induced incretin secretion. Mol Cell Endocrinol 2007;276:18–23.

Christoph Beglinger, MD
Division of Gastroenterology and Hepatology
University Hospital Basel, Petersgraben 4
CH–4031 Basel (Switzerland)
E-Mail beglinger@tmr.ch

Delhanty PJD, van der Lely AJ (eds): How Gut and Brain Control Metabolism.
Front Horm Res. Basel, Karger, 2014, vol 42, pp 134–146 (DOI: 10.1159/000358322)

What Is the Role of Metabolic Hormones in Taste Buds of the Tongue

Huan Cai · Stuart Maudsley · Bronwen Martin

Metabolism Unit, Laboratory of Clinical Investigation, National Institute on Aging, National Institutes of Health, Baltimore, Md., USA

Abstract

Gustation is one of the important chemical senses that guides the organism to identify nutrition while avoiding toxic chemicals. An increasing number of metabolic hormones and/or hormone receptors have been identified in the taste buds of the tongue and are involved in modulating taste perception. The gustatory system constitutes an additional endocrine regulatory locus that affects food intake, and in turn whole-body energy homeostasis. Here we provide an overview of the main metabolic hormones known to be present in the taste buds of the tongue; discuss their potential functional roles in taste perception and energy homeostasis and how their functional integrity is altered in the metabolic imbalance status (obesity and diabetes) and aging process. Better understanding of the functional roles of metabolic hormones in flavor perception as well as the link between taste perception and peripheral metabolism may be vital for developing strategies to promote healthier eating and prevent obesity or lifestyle-related disorders. © 2014 S. Karger AG, Basel

Taste is one of the sensory modalities that guides the organism to detect and consume nutrients while avoiding toxic substances. The basic taste modalities are essential for the survival and evolution of organisms, for example sweet taste signals the presence of carbohydrates, umami taste can detect protein content in food, salty taste governs intake of Na^+ and other salts, sour taste reflects dietary acids, and bitter taste warns organisms of toxic chemicals. In addition, fat taste is considered as the sixth taste quality that senses the lipid components in food [1]. Taste perception begins with chemical activation of oral taste cells by tastant molecules. Upon reception of tastants, transmitters are released by taste cells to activate associated gustatory nerve fibers. Taste cells are organized into onion-shaped structures known as taste buds, within three types of papillae in the tongue, i.e. the circumvallate, foliate and fungiform papillae (fig. 1). According to the distinct functions, different differentiation stages, taste cells can be classified into four types. Type I cells, the most abundant cells present in taste buds, are recognized as glial-like cells that maintain taste bud structure and terminate synaptic transmission. Type II cells, also known as receptor cells, express many taste-related G protein-coupled receptors (GPCRs) which are responsible for sweet, bitter and umami taste detection. Type III cells, considered presynaptic cells, express synaptic proteins and can generate depolarization-dependent Ca^{2+} transients. Type IV cells are non-polarized, undifferentiated basal cells. Taste bud cells have an average lifespan of approximately 10 days and are constantly generated from these basal cells [1].

Gustatory Regulation by Metabolic Hormones

The gustatory system is the first biochemical gateway that identifies and controls food intake and thereby helps maintain somatic energy homeostasis. There is increasing evidence that demonstrates the presence of several metabolic hormones and their cognate receptors in subsets of taste cells and that these receptor/ligand systems are involved in modulating taste responsiveness. These findings therefore suggest a strong link between taste perception and somatic metabolic control. Here we provide an overview of the main metabolic hormones and receptor systems present within the gustatory system and summarize their potential functions in regulating taste modalities (fig. 1, 2).

Glucagon-Like Peptide 1/Glucagon
Stimulated by nutrient ingestion, glucagon-like peptide 1 (GLP-1) is mainly secreted by enteroendocrine L cells located in the distal ileum and colon. Besides its main function of regulating blood glucose by amplifying postprandial insulin synthesis and secretion, GLP-1 exerts multiple effects throughout the body including regulation of pancreatic β-cell survival and function, regulation of food intake and satiety, promotion of neuronal cell survival, regulation of gastric emptying and bowel motility as well as cardioprotection [2]. It is reported that in enteroendocrine L cells of the gut, α-gustducin and the sweet taste receptor subunit T1R3 mediate the glucose-dependent secretion of GLP-1 [3]. Similarly, functional GLP-1 is also expressed in two distinct subsets of taste cells: a subset of type II cells that co-express T1R3 and a subset of type III cells. The cognate GLP-1 receptor is expressed on adjacent intragemmal afferent nerve fibers [4, 5]. GLP-1 receptor knockout mice demonstrate dramatically reduced taste responses to both nutritive (sucrose) and non-nutritive (sucralose) sweeteners, indicating that GLP-1 signaling acts to maintain or enhance sweet taste sensitivity [4]. In addition, GLP-1 receptor null mice also exhibit enhanced sensitivity to umami-tasting stimuli [6]. Taste stimuli also elicit unique patterns of neuropeptide secretion from taste buds that are correlated with those perceptive qualities. Sweet and umami stimuli were reported recently to elicit GLP-1 secretion from

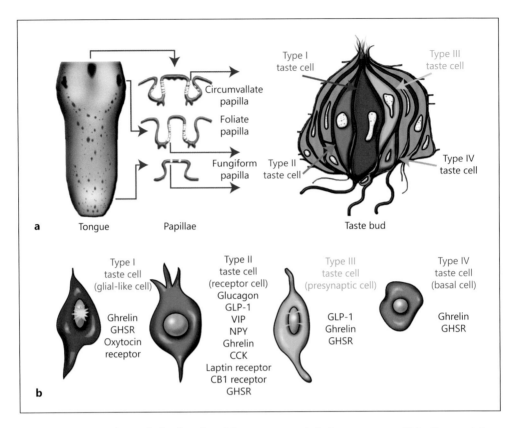

Fig. 1. Location of metabolically-related hormones and their receptors within the gustatory system. **a** Various papillae on the tongue and different types of taste cells within taste buds. **b** Distribution of metabolic hormones and hormone receptors in type I, II, III and IV taste cells. CB1 receptor = Cannabinoid receptor type 1; CCK = cholecystokinin; GHSR = growth hormone secretagogue receptor; GLP-1 = glucagon-like peptide 1; NPY = neuropeptide Y; VIP = vasoactive intestinal peptide.

circumvallate papillae [7]. However this effect is abolished in T1R3$^{-/-}$ mice, indicating an obligatory role for the T1R3 subunit common to the sweet and umami taste receptors. The presence, as well as secretion, of GLP-1 from taste cells highlights an interesting parallel between gustatory and intestinal epithelia. GLP-1 is produced from proglucagon though enzymatic cleavage by prohormone convertase (PC)1/3, while glucagon is derived from proglucagon via the alternate processing enzyme PC2 [8]. Similar to GLP-1 expression, glucagon and PC2 are also found in mouse taste cells [4]. Further work has confirmed that glucagon and its receptor are co-expressed in a subset of mouse taste receptor cells which also express the T1R3 [9]. Both genetic and pharmacological disruption of glucagon signaling in mice resulted in reduced sweet taste responsiveness without affecting salty, sour or bitter taste responsiveness, indicating a role also for local glucagon signaling in the peripheral modulation of sweet taste responsiveness [9].

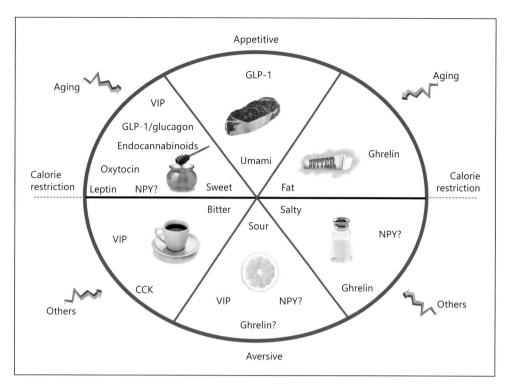

Fig. 2. Overview of the modulation of different taste modalities by metabolically-related hormones. Six taste modalities are shown: umami, sweet, bitter, sour, salty, and fat. Aging, diet and other factors may affect taste perception and metabolic hormones in taste cells. CCK = Cholecystokinin; GLP-1 = glucagon-like peptide 1; NPY = neuropeptide Y; VIP = vasoactive intestinal peptide.

Vasoactive Intestinal Peptide

Vasoactive intestinal peptide (VIP), the 28-amino-acid peptide first isolated from pig small intestine, has a diverse range of effects including increasing vasodilatation, reducing arterial blood pressure, smoothing muscle relaxation and stimulating electrolyte secretion in the gut [10]. Due to the sequence similarity with peptides such as secretin and glucagon, VIP and pituitary adenylate cyclase-activating polypeptide (PACAP) have been classified as members of the 'secretin family' of peptides. VIP/PACAP preferentially stimulates adenylate cyclase in recipient cells and increases intracellular cAMP through three common GPCRs (VPAC1, VPAC2 and PAC1R) [11]. VIP demonstrates a widespread cellular distribution and has also been identified in taste cells in rat, hamster, carp and human tongue [12]. Shen et al. [13] delineated the location and potential functional role of VIP in taste buds by demonstrating the co-expression of VIP with α-gustducin (which is involved in bitter and sweet transduction cascades) and T1R2 (sweet taste receptor subunit). Our recent study also deepens the understanding of the VIP's role in taste perception and regulation of energy homeostasis. VIP receptors (VPAC1/2) were found primarily expressed in phospholipase C-β_2-positive cells (type II taste cells), and VIP knockout mice showed altered taste perception of sweet, bitter and sour stimuli. Interestingly, we also found reduced leptin receptor and increased GLP-1 expression in VIP knockout mice taste cells, indicating the potential functional interactions between VIP, GLP-1 and the leptin receptor [14].

Cholecystokinin

Cholecystokinin (CCK) is a gastrointestinal peptide secreted by endocrine cells in the proximal portion of the small intestine upon ingestion of a meal. CCK is expressed in endocrine cells of the duodenum as well as in peripheral and central neurons. CCK can exert many actions such as slowing gastric emptying and motility, and stimulating pancreatic and gallbladder secretions [15]. CCK mediates these actions through the stimulation of its cognate GPCRs, the CCK-A and the CCK-B receptors. The CCK-A receptor is primarily distributed in gastrointestinal tract while the CCK-B receptor is mainly located in the central nervous system [16]. Herness et al. [17] first observed CCK (both mRNA and protein) expression in a subset of taste receptor cells. These cells were able to respond, via CCK-A receptor activation, to the exogenous application of CCK with altered cellular potassium currents or elevated intracellular calcium levels [17]. CCK-responsive cells were also demonstrated to be sensitive to either bitter stimuli or to cholinergic stimulation [18]. Subsequent research has demonstrated that more than half (56%) of the CCK-expressing taste receptor cells coexpressed α-gustducin whereas far fewer (15%) co-expressed T1R2 mRNA, suggesting that CCK may be involved in bitter taste-signaling transduction [13]. It is thought that CCK operates in an autocrine manner in the taste buds since CCK and CCK receptors are mostly expressed in the same subsets of taste cells [19].

Ghrelin

The gastrointestinal peptide hormone ghrelin was discovered in 1999 as the endogenous ligand for the growth hormone secretagogue receptor (GHSR) [20]. Ghrelin is considered a key pleiotropic hormone regulating systemic energy metabolism via its ability to stimulate food intake, decrease energy expenditure and fat utilization, stimulate gut motility and gastric acid secretion as well as regulate glucose metabolism and modulate taste sensation [21]. Interestingly, prepro-ghrelin, PC1/3, ghrelin, its cognate receptor (GHSR), and ghrelin-O-acyltransferase (GOAT, the enzyme that activates ghrelin) are expressed in type I, II, III and IV taste cells of mouse taste buds. The co-localization of ghrelin and GHSR in the same taste cells suggests that ghrelin may work in a strong autocrine manner. In addition, GHSR null mice exhibit significantly reduced taste responsivity to sour (citric acid) and salty (sodium chloride) tastants [22]. However, there is compelling evidence showing that there are likely other ghrelin subtype receptor(s) apart from GHSR and other as-yet-unidentified GHSR ligand(s) besides ghrelin [23]. Although O-*n*-octanoylation by GOAT at serine 3 is important for acyl ghrelin binding to its receptor, the GHSR1a, mouse lines with genetic deletion of ghrelin and GOAT exhibited differential phenotypes [24]. Thus the examination and comparison of different genetic modification animal models will help better explain the precise mechanisms of ghrelin ligand-mediated gustation. We also recently found that both ghrelin and GOAT null mice possessed reduced lipid taste responsivity. However, salty taste responsivity was attenuated in ghrelin$^{-/-}$ mice, yet potentiated in GOAT$^{-/-}$ mice compared to wild-type mice indicating that acyl ghrelin and des-acyl ghrelin may exert distinct functions in taste sensation [25].

Neuropeptide Y

Neuropeptide Y (NPY) is a 36-amino-acid neuropeptide possessing structural similarities to peptide YY and pancreatic polypeptide. NPY is widely distributed throughout the central and peripheral nervous systems. Five NPY receptor subtypes (Y1, Y2, Y4, Y5 and Y6) mediate NPY's actions upon food intake, blood pressure, circadian rhythms, stress, hormone secretion and reproduction [26]. In addition to CCK and VIP, NPY is another neuropeptide selectively expressed in a subset of taste cells. NPY expression overlaps nearly 100% with CCK- or VIP-positive taste cells, although the number of NPY-positive cells is less than those for CCK or VIP [27]. NPY specifically enhances an inwardly rectifying potassium current via NPY-Y1 receptors which is antagonistic to the actions of CCK, suggesting that NPY may play a complimentary role to that of CCK in taste buds [19]. Pharmacological evidence strongly suggests that the modulatory effect of NPY upon gustation is mediated by activation of the NPY-1 receptor (NPY-1R) subtype. NPY-1R-immunopositive cells were observed in the taste buds and lingual epithelium. However, NPY-immunopositive cells and NPY-1R-immunopositive cells are non-overlapping in the taste bud, suggesting NPY plays a paracrine signaling role [19]. Appetitive (sweet and umami) stimuli were recently demonstrated to elicit GLP-1 and NPY secretion from taste cells and both sour (citric acid) and salty (NaCl) increased NPY secretion as well [7]. However, the exact functional role of NPY in gustation has yet to be determined.

Oxytocin

Oxytocin, a neuropeptide hormone best known for its role in lactation and parturition, is primarily synthesized in magnocellular neurons of the paraventricular and supraoptic nuclei of the hypothalamus. The oxytocin receptor belongs to the rhodopsin-type (class I) GPCR superfamily and is coupled to phospholipase C through G$_{\alpha q11}$ [28]. Oxytocin is involved in the regulation of a wide variety of social (social memory and attachment, sexual and maternal behavior, aggression, bonding and trust, autism) and non-social (learning, anxiety, feeding, pain perception) behaviors [29]. With respect to feeding behavior, oxytocin regulates the intake of food and other nutrients, such as NaCl and sucrose [30]. Oxytocin knockout mice overconsume solutions of saccharin and carbohydrates including sucrose, but have a normal appetite for palatable, energy-rich lipid emulsions [31]. Interestingly, a recent study demonstrated that the oxytocin receptor, but not the oxytocin peptide, was expressed in a subset of glial-like taste cells and also in cells on the periphery of taste buds [32]. Oxytocin was found to evoke Ca^{2+} mobilization in a subset of taste cells and this response was readily inhibited by the addition of an oxytocin receptor antagonist [32]. These findings therefore suggest that peripheral taste organs may be an important locus for the oxytocin-mediated regulation of food ingestion.

Leptin
Leptin, one of the most important adipose-derived hormones, plays a key role in regulating energy intake and expenditure. Leptin has been shown to control appetite, food intake, energy metabolism, body weight, and behavior. The leptin or obesity (Ob) receptor is a member of class I cytokine receptor family, and the full-length isoform (Ob-Rb) which is a single-transmembrane-domain receptor, is able to fully transduce activation signal [33]. The functional leptin receptor (Ob-Rb) is abundantly expressed in several hypothalamic nuclei as well as peripheral organs such as the lymph nodes, liver, pancreas, adipose tissue, lung, uterus, and kidney [33]. The *db/db* mouse, in much the leptin receptor is rendered ineffective by mutation, is a model of obesity, diabetes and dyslipidemia [34]. Enhanced gustatory neural responses and lower thresholds for sugars were reported in diabetic *db/db* mice as early as 7 days of age, suggesting that these characteristics may be genetically induced by the action of the *db* locus [35]. In addition, *db/db* mice also showed enhanced responses of the chorda tympani nerve to non-sugar sweeteners [36]. Similar to its action on pancreatic β-cells and hypothalamic neurons, leptin was also demonstrated to activate outward K^+ currents of taste receptor cells, which resulted in hyperpolarization of taste cells; in addition the leptin receptor was also found expressed in these taste cells [37]. These observations suggest that taste cells are peripheral sites of leptin action and that leptin may be a sweet-sensing suppressor that may take part in the regulation of food intake. Furthermore, the presence of the leptin receptor (Ob-Rb) and STAT3 (signal transducers and activators of transcription-3), which is considered to be involved in the leptin signaling via Ob-Rb, in the mouse taste bud cells confirms the involvement of leptin in the control of sweet taste sensitivity [38].

Endocannabinoids
Endocannabinoids are endogenous lipid-signaling mediators capable of binding to and functionally activating the endocannabinoid GPCR system. N-arachidonoylethanolamine (anandamide) and 2-arachidonoylglycerol (2-AG) are two well-established endocannabinoids identified in animal tissues [39]. The cannabinoid CB1 receptors are abundantly distributed in the central nervous system and are responsible for the central actions of natural cannabinoid (Δ^9-tetrahydrocannabinol) found in marijuana, while the cannabinoid CB2 receptors are largely restricted to immune and hematopoietic cells mediating some of the immunomodulatory actions of Δ^9-tetrahydrocannabinol. The endocannabinoid system can potentially regulate energy metabolism and energy homeostasis at both central and peripheral sites. The

endocannabinoid system plays a dual role in the regulation of food intake by hedonic and homeostatic energy regulation in the central nervous system. With the widespread expression of the CB1 receptor in pancreas, adipose tissue, skeletal muscle and liver, the endocannabinoid system can reduce energy expenditure and can direct energy balance towards energy storage into fat at the peripheral level [40]. Endocannabinoids are known as orexigenic mediators stimulating food intake thus opposing plasma leptin, the anorexigenic mediator that reduces food intake [41]. Endocannabinoids can increase gustatory nerve responses to sweeteners (which oppose the actions of leptin) without affecting responses to salty, sour, bitter and umami compounds. Furthermore, the effects of endocannabinoids on sweet taste responses are abolished in mice genetically lacking the CB1 receptor and are diminished by the administration of CB1 receptor antagonists. In addition, CB1 receptors are found in type II taste cells that also express the T1R3 sweet taste receptor component [42]. It is therefore likely that endocannabinoids and leptin can reciprocally regulate peripheral sweet taste perception via activation of their cognate receptors in the tongue and in turn help orchestrate energy homeostasis.

Factors That Affect Taste Perception and Metabolic Hormones in Taste Cells

It is becoming clear from recent studies that taste functional integrity is altered in several physiological and pathological states. Aging and obesity are two relatively well-studied factors that affect taste perception. In the following section we will provide an overview of how taste functional integrity and metabolic hormones in taste cells are changed in the aging process and obese/calorie-restricted states. These findings may help generate a better understanding of the effects of metabolic context on taste perception as well as suggest potential strategies for the pharmacological manipulation of aging and obesity associated disorders.

Aging
The aging process is a dynamic and highly integrative process characterized by accumulating multiple changes over time including reduced chemical sense of smell and taste. There are a large number of studies that have demonstrated that taste sensitivity decreases with aging and that the elderly require the presence of more molecules or ions to detect and recognize a specific tastant [43]. This age-related reduction in the sense of taste and smell may, in part, contribute to the prevalence of loss of appetite, anorexia and weight loss in the elderly population [44]. Therefore the study of age-related changes in taste perception is important to help improve the consumption of nutrients or ameliorate the lifestyle-related metabolic disorders in older adults. Compelling evidence of human studies found that the detection thresholds of salt, sour, bitter, umami and sweet are increased in older adults, suggesting the taste perception declines with age. However, the effect of age on taste perception is complex,

and the extent and significance of this decline varies between taste modalities, tastants and research studies [45]. The decreasing sensitivity to taste with age may be due to certain degenerative anatomical changes in the tongue such as reductions in numbers of papillae and taste buds during aging [46]. In addition, fungiform papillae and blood vessel density is decreased in older men and women than younger individuals [47]. Besides the large body of human studies, investigations of animal models have also demonstrated that taste sensitivities decline with aging, which is accompanied by a delayed cell renewal and highly vacuolated cytoplasm in taste buds [48]. Furthermore, our recent study demonstrated a significant reduction in taste bud size and number of taste cells per bud accompanied with altered sweet taste responsivity in older mice compared with younger counterparts [49]. Since several hormones play important roles in modulating taste responsiveness via autocrine, paracrine or endocrine mechanisms, these hormones may change in accordance with taste alterations. We have previously shown that the metabolic hormones GLP-1, ghrelin as well as the sweet taste receptor subunit T1R3, protein gene product 9.5 and sonic hedgehog are significantly decreased in taste buds of the older rodents, and that all of these factors combined are likely to be involved in altered taste perception during advanced aging [49].

Obesity and Diet

A number of observations in humans and rodents revealed that obesity is associated with alterations in taste responsiveness and food reward functions [50]. For example, obese and non-obese children and adolescents differ in their taste perception, in which obese subjects could identify taste qualities less precisely than children and adolescents of a normal weight [50]. In addition, specific populations of African-Americans that are prone to obesity have been shown to have an elevated desire for sweet diets [51]. Not only sweet taste perception, but also monosodium glutamate, bitter, sour and salty taste perceptions were also reported to be altered in obese adults [51]. Besides the five basic taste modalities, i.e. sweet, sour, bitter, salty and umami, compelling evidence from rodent and human studies has suggested that lipid perception is an additional sixth taste modality, and that fat taste is tightly linked to lipid consumption and in turn can affect body adiposity [52]. It has been reported that high-fat diet-induced obese rats shift sucrose and corn oil preference towards higher concentrations compared to lean control rats [53]. Furthermore, obesity alters oral perception of dietary lipids in the mouse via a CD36-mediated mechanism [54]. Decreased expression of CD36 in circumvallate taste buds of high-fat diet-induced obese rats may be associated with diminished fatty taste sensitivity [55]. The evidence that the levels of metabolic hormones such as ghrelin, leptin, GLP-1, CCK, and PYY are also changed in obese subjects, suggests that these metabolic hormones may also be involved in altered gustatory perception in obesity [56]. It has recently been demonstrated that high-fat diet-induced obese rats exhibit reduced sweet taste receptor T1R3, increased GLP-1 and decreased leptin receptor in taste buds, which may be involved in inducing the greater preference for sweet taste in high-fat diet-induced obese rats [57]. Furthermore, CCK type A receptor-deficient Otsuka Long-Evans Tokushima Fatty (OLETF) rats display an increased preference for sucrose compared with lean control rats, and this effect was partially influenced by the orosensory-stimulating effect of sucrose [51]. In contrast, calorie restriction-induced or bariatric surgery-induced weight loss was found to have effects on taste responsiveness in human and animal studies [51]. For example, dieters rated 20 and 40% sucrose solutions less pleasant than non-dieters both before and after an oral glucose load [58]. Calorie restriction of the high-fat diet-induced obese rats was found to change the performance of brief-access licking responses to sucrose and corn oil [53]. Our recent study found that 30-month-old calorie-restricted rats showed reduced taste cell T1R3, α-gustducin and GLP-1 levels, and increased taste cell leptin receptor expression compared with age-matched ad libitum rats. The coordinated alterations of sweet taste receptor (T1R3), taste-signaling transducer (α-gustducin), GLP-1 and leptin receptor in taste cells of calorie-restricted rats may therefore shed some light on the mechanism of taste perception alteration in calorie-restricted subjects [59].

Concluding Remarks

The gustatory system plays important roles in identifying and governing food intake, which in turn affects whole-body physiological function and energy homeostasis, and this functional integrity is attenuated in the status of accumulating deterioration (aging) and energy imbalance (obesity/metabolic syndrome). The increasing number of metabolic hormones identified in the taste buds suggests that the tongue is likely another important peripheral organ, in addition to stomach, intestine, pancreas, and adipose tissue, that is vitally involved in orchestrating metabolic homeostasis. It seems multiple layers of physiological systems utilize conserved regulatory mechanisms to attain whole-body physiological integrity and the gustatory system may be the first biochemical gateway in this process. However, we are still in the beginning of uncovering the exact functional roles of these hormones in taste modulation. It is clear that a better grasp of the functional mechanisms in taste modulation will pave the way for an enhanced understanding and pharmacological manipulation of metabolic disorders associated with obesity, diabetes and aging.

Acknowledgements

The authors are supported by the Intramural Research Program of the National Institute on Aging, NIH. We thank Jimmy Burrill for his expert assistance with the artwork for the figures.

References

1 Chaudhari N, Roper SD: The cell biology of taste. J Cell Biol 2010;190:285–296.

2 Janssen P, Rotondo A, Mule F, Tack J: Review article: a comparison of glucagon-like peptides 1 and 2. Aliment Pharmacol Ther 2013;37:18–36.

3 Jang HJ, Kokrashvili Z, Theodorakis MJ, Carlson OD, Kim BJ, Zhou J, Kim HH, Xu X, Chan SL, Juhaszova M, Bernier M, Mosinger B, Margolskee RF, Egan JM: Gut-expressed gustducin and taste receptors regulate secretion of glucagon-like peptide-1. Proc Natl Acad Sci USA 2007;104:15069–15074.

4 Shin YK, Martin B, Golden E, Dotson CD, Maudsley S, Kim W, Jang HJ, Mattson MP, Drucker DJ, Egan JM, Munger SD: Modulation of taste sensitivity by GLP-1 signaling. J Neurochem 2008;106:455–463.

5 Feng XH, Liu XM, Zhou LH, Wang J, Liu GD: Expression of glucagon-like peptide-1 in the taste buds of rat circumvallate papillae. Acta Histochem 2008;110:151–154.

6 Martin B, Dotson CD, Shin YK, Ji S, Drucker DJ, Maudsley S, Munger SD: Modulation of taste sensitivity by GLP-1 signaling in taste buds. Ann NY Acad Sci 2009;1170:98–101.

7 Geraedts MC, Munger SD: Gustatory stimuli representing different perceptual qualities elicit distinct patterns of neuropeptide secretion from taste buds. J Neurosci 2013;33:7559–7564.

8 Rouille Y, Kantengwa S, Irminger JC, Halban PA: Role of the prohormone convertase PC3 in the processing of proglucagon to glucagon-like peptide 1. J Biol Chem 1997;272:32810–32816.

9 Elson AE, Dotson CD, Egan JM, Munger SD: Glucagon signaling modulates sweet taste responsiveness. FASEB J 2010;24:3960–3969.

10 Said SI, Mutt V: Polypeptide with broad biological activity: isolation from small intestine. Science 1970;169:1217–1218.

11 Dickson L, Finlayson K: VPAC and PAC receptors: from ligands to function. Pharmacol Ther 2009;121:294–316.

12 Martin B, Maudsley S, White CM, Egan JM: Hormones in the naso-oropharynx: endocrine modulation of taste and smell. Trends Endocrinol Metab 2009;20:163–170.

13 Shen T, Kaya N, Zhao FL, Lu SG, Cao Y, Herness S: Co-expression patterns of the neuropeptides vasoactive intestinal peptide and cholecystokinin with the transduction molecules α-gustducin and T1R2 in rat taste receptor cells. Neuroscience 2005;130:229–238.

14 Martin B, Shin YK, White CM, Ji S, Kim W, Carlson OD, Napora JK, Chadwick W, Chapter M, Waschek JA, Mattson MP, Maudsley S, Egan JM: Vasoactive intestinal peptide-null mice demonstrate enhanced sweet taste preference, dysglycemia, and reduced taste bud leptin receptor expression. Diabetes 2010;59:1143–1152.

15 Dockray GJ: Cholecystokinin. Curr Opin Endocrinol Diabetes Obes 2012;19:8–12.

16 Dufresne M, Seva C, Fourmy D: Cholecystokinin and gastrin receptors. Physiol Rev 2006;86:805–847.

17 Herness S, Zhao FL, Lu SG, Kaya N, Shen T: Expression and physiological actions of cholecystokinin in rat taste receptor cells. J Neurosci 2002;22:10018–10029.

18 Lu SG, Zhao FL, Herness S: Physiological phenotyping of cholecystokinin-responsive rat taste receptor cells. Neurosci Lett 2003;351:157–160.

19 Herness S, Zhao FL: The neuropeptides CCK and NPY and the changing view of cell-to-cell communication in the taste bud. Physiol Behav 2009;97:581–591.

20 Kojima M, Hosoda H, Date Y, Nakazato M, Matsuo H, Kangawa K: Ghrelin is a growth-hormone-releasing acylated peptide from stomach. Nature 1999;402:656–660.

21 Muller TD, Tschöp MH: Ghrelin – a key pleiotropic hormone-regulating systemic energy metabolism. Endocr Dev 2013;25:91–100.

22 Shin YK, Martin B, Kim W, White CM, Ji S, Sun Y, Smith RG, Sevigny J, Tschöp MH, Maudsley S, Egan JM: Ghrelin is produced in taste cells and ghrelin receptor null mice show reduced taste responsivity to salty (NaCl) and sour (citric acid) tastants. PLoS One 2010;5:e12729.

23 Ma X, Lin Y, Lin L, Qin G, Pereira FA, Haymond MW, Butte NF, Sun Y: Ablation of ghrelin receptor in leptin-deficient ob/ob mice has paradoxical effects on glucose homeostasis when compared with ablation of ghrelin in ob/ob mice. Am J Physiol Endocrinol Metab 2011;303:E422–E431.

24 Kang K, Zmuda E, Sleeman MW: Physiological role of ghrelin as revealed by the ghrelin and GOAT knockout mice. Peptides 2011;32:2236–2241.

25 Cai H, Cong WN, Daimon CM, Wang R, Tschöp MH, Sevigny J, Martin B, Maudsley S: Altered lipid and salt taste responsivity in ghrelin and GOAT null mice. PLoS One 2013;8:e76553.

26 Gehlert DR: Introduction to the reviews on neuropeptide Y. Neuropeptides 2004;38:135–140.

27 Zhao FL, Shen T, Kaya N, Lu SG, Cao Y, Herness S: Expression, physiological action, and coexpression patterns of neuropeptide Y in rat taste-bud cells. Proc Natl Acad Sci USA 2005;102:11100–11105.

28 Young WS 3rd, Gainer H: Transgenesis and the study of expression, cellular targeting and function of oxytocin, vasopressin and their receptors. Neuroendocrinology 2003;78:185–203.

29 Lee HJ, Macbeth AH, Pagani JH, Young WS 3rd: Oxytocin: the great facilitator of life. Prog Neurobiol 2009;88:127–151.

30 Leng G, Onaka T, Caquineau C, Sabatier N, Tobin VA, Takayanagi Y: Oxytocin and appetite. Prog Brain Res 2008;170:137–151.

31 Miedlar JA, Rinaman L, Vollmer RR, Amico JA: Oxytocin gene deletion mice overconsume palatable sucrose solution but not palatable lipid emulsions. Am J Physiol Regul Integr Comp Physiol 2007;293: R1063–R1068.

32 Sinclair MS, Perea-Martinez I, Dvoryanchikov G, Yoshida M, Nishimori K, Roper SD, Chaudhari N: Oxytocin signaling in mouse taste buds. PLoS One 2010;5:e11980.

33 Gorska E, Popko K, Stelmaszczyk-Emmel A, Ciepiela O, Kucharska A, Wasik M: Leptin receptors. Eur J Med Res 2010;15(suppl 2):50–54.

34 Hummel KP, Dickie MM, Coleman DL: Diabetes, a new mutation in the mouse. Science 1966;153:1127–1128.

35 Ninomiya Y, Sako N, Imai Y: Enhanced gustatory neural responses to sugars in the diabetic *db/db* mouse. Am J Physiol 1995;269:R930–R937.

36 Ninomiya Y, Imoto T, Yatabe A, Kawamura S, Nakashima K, Katsukawa H: Enhanced responses of the chorda tympani nerve to non-sugar sweeteners in the diabetic *db/db* mouse. Am J Physiol 1998;274: R1324–R1330.

37 Kawai K, Sugimoto K, Nakashima K, Miura H, Ninomiya Y: Leptin as a modulator of sweet taste sensitivities in mice. Proc Natl Acad Sci USA 2000; 97:11044–11049.

38 Shigemura N, Miura H, Kusakabe Y, Hino A, Ninomiya Y: Expression of leptin receptor (Ob-R) isoforms and signal transducers and activators of transcription (STATs) mRNAs in the mouse taste buds. Arch Histol Cytol 2003;66:253–260.

39 Sugiura T, Waku K: Cannabinoid receptors and their endogenous ligands. J Biochem 2002;132:7–12.

40 Matias I, Cristino L, Di Marzo V: Endocannabinoids: some like it fat (and sweet too). J Neuroendocrinol 2008;20(suppl 1):100–109.

41 Cota D, Marsicano G, Tschöp M, Grübler Y, Flachskamm C, Schubert M, Auer D, Yassouridis A, Thöne-Reineke C, Ortmann S, Tomassoni F, Cervino C, Nisoli E, Linthorst AC, Pasquali R, Lutz B, Stalla GK, Pagotto U: The endogenous cannabinoid system affects energy balance via central orexigenic drive and peripheral lipogenesis. J Clin Invest 2003; 112:423–431.

42 Yoshida R, Ohkuri T, Jyotaki M, Yasuo T, Horio N, Yasumatsu K, Sanematsu K, Shigemura N, Yamamoto T, Margolskee RF, Ninomiya Y: Endocannabinoids selectively enhance sweet taste. Proc Natl Acad Sci USA 2010;107:935–939.

43 Schiffman SS: Taste and smell losses in normal aging and disease. JAMA 1997;278:1357–1362.

44 Kmieć Z, Pétervári E, Balaskó M, Székely M: Anorexia of aging. Vitam Horm 2013;92:319–355.

45 Methven L, Allen VJ, Withers CA, Gosney MA: Ageing and taste. Proc Nutr Soc 2012;71:556–565.

46 Arey LB, Tremaine MJ, Monzingo FL: The numerical and topographical relations of taste buds to human circumvallate papillae throughout the life span. Anat Rec 1935;64:9–25.

47 Pavlidis P, Gouveris H, Anogeianaki A, Koutsonikolas D, Anogianakis G, Kekes G: Age-related changes in electrogustometry thresholds, tongue tip vascularization, density, and form of the fungiform papillae in humans. Chem Senses 2013;38: 35–43.

48 Fukunaga A: Age-related changes in renewal of taste bud cells and expression of taste cell-specific proteins in mice (in Japanese). Kokubo Gakkai Zasshi 2005;72:84–89.

49 Shin YK, Cong WN, Cai H, Kim W, Maudsley S, Egan JM, Martin B: Age-related changes in mouse taste bud morphology, hormone expression, and taste responsivity. J Gerontol A Biol Sci Med Sci 2011;67:336–344.

50 Overberg J, Hummel T, Krude H, Wiegand S: Differences in taste sensitivity between obese and nonobese children and adolescents. Arch Dis Child 2012; 97:1048–1052.

51 Donaldson LF, Bennett L, Baic S, Melichar JK: Taste and weight: is there a link? Am J Clin Nutr 2009;90: 800S–803S.

52 Newman L, Haryono R, Keast R: Functionality of fatty acid chemoreception: a potential factor in the development of obesity? Nutrients 2013;5:1287–1300.

53 Shin AC, Townsend RL, Patterson LM, Berthoud HR: 'Liking' and 'wanting' of sweet and oily food stimuli as affected by high-fat diet-induced obesity, weight loss, leptin, and genetic predisposition. Am J Physiol Regul Integr Comp Physiol 2011;301:R1267–R1280.

54 Chevrot M, Bernard A, Ancel D, Buttet M, Martin C, Abdoul-Azize S, Merlin JF, Poirier H, Niot I, Khan NA, Passilly-Degrace P, Besnard P: Obesity alters the gustatory perception of lipids in the mouse: plausible involvement of the lingual CD36. J Lipid Res 2013.

55 Zhang XJ, Zhou LH, Ban X, Liu DX, Jiang W, Liu XM: Decreased expression of CD36 in circumvallate taste buds of high-fat diet-induced obese rats. Acta Histochem 2011;113:663–667.

56 Huda MS, Wilding JP, Pinkney JH: Gut peptides and the regulation of appetite. Obes Rev 2006;7:163–182.

57 Zhang XJ, Wang YQ, Long Y, Wang L, Li Y, Gao FB, Tian HM: Alteration of sweet taste in high-fat diet-induced obese rats after 4 weeks treatment with exenatide. Peptides 2013;47:115–123.

58 Esses VM, Herman CP: Palatability of sucrose before and after glucose ingestion in dieters and non-dieters. Physiol Behav 1984;32:711–715.

59 Cai H, Daimon CM, Cong WN, Wang R, Chirdon P, de Cabo R, Sevigny J, Maudsley S, Martin B: Longitudinal analysis of calorie restriction on rat taste bud morphology and expression of sweet taste modulators. J Gerontol A Biol Sci Med Sci 2013, Epub ahead of print.

Bronwen Martin, PhD
Metabolism Unit, Laboratory of Clinical Investigation
National Institute on Aging, National Institutes of Health
251 Bayview Blvd, Suite 100, Baltimore, MD 21224 (USA)
E-Mail martinbro@mail.nih.gov

Delhanty PJD, van der Lely AJ (eds): How Gut and Brain Control Metabolism.
Front Horm Res. Basel, Karger, 2014, vol 42, pp 147–154 (DOI: 10.1159/000358343)

Protein PYY and Its Role in Metabolism

Samantha L. Price · Stephen R. Bloom

Division of Diabetes, Endocrinology and Metabolism, Department of Medicine, Imperial College London,
London, UK

Abstract

The hormone PYY is released from the distal gut in response to nutrient ingestion. Numerous studies have shown that PYY3–36, the most abundant circulating isoform of PYY, reduces food intake when given to obese rodents and humans. Its infusion to mimic postprandial levels in fasting subjects inhibits appetite, suggesting a physiological role in postprandial satiety. However, the mechanisms underlying this effect remain unclear. Neuronal activity within several brain areas appears to be modified following peripheral administration of PYY3–36 and a direct effect on the central nervous system is possible. Several studies suggest that PYY3–36 levels are reduced in obesity and are elevated following gastric bypass surgery, possibly contributing to the increased feelings of satiety following this procedure. Whether PYY has a role in the regulation of energy expenditure is currently unclear. However, due to the clear appetite-inhibitory effect of PYY, this hormone continues to be investigated as a potential therapeutic agent in the treatment of obesity.

© 2014 S. Karger AG, Basel

Protein tyrosine-tyrosine (PYY) is a 36-amino-acid peptide released from L-cells in the distal gut in response to nutrient ingestion. PYY is part of a larger family of proteins which also includes neuropeptide Y (NPY) and pancreatic polypeptide (PP). All three peptides contain a hairpin turn within the amino acid backbone and hence are known as PP-fold proteins. PYY circulates in two biologically active forms: PYY1–36, which is secreted by the L-cells, and the truncated PYY3–36 which is the predominant circulating form produced by dipeptidyl-peptidase IV (DPP-IV) cleavage of PYY1–36 [1]. This removal of the N-terminal tyrosine-proline residues alters the receptor specificity and hence the biological actions of PYY3–36.

The biological effects of the PP-fold proteins are mediated via five G-protein-coupled 'Y receptors' (Y1, Y2, Y4, Y5 and Y6) which are classified according to their differing affinities for NPY, PP and PYY. PYY1–36 binds with differing affinity to all five receptors whereas PYY3–36 selectively binds to Y2 receptors (Y2r) and with lower affinity to Y5 receptors (Y5r) [2]. Although PYY is a gut hormone it crosses the blood-brain barrier and acts as a neuropeptide via central Y receptors which are widely expressed within the brain.

Plasma PYY levels increase postprandially and remain elevated for several hours. Release occurs within 15 min of meal onset which is before nutrients reach the PYY-secreting L-cells in the distal gastrointestinal tract, suggesting the involvement of other hormonal or neural signals in triggering PYY release. Adrian et al. [3] found that PYY levels peak at around 1–2 h after meal onset and the temporal response and peak levels are proportional to caloric content, macronutrient composition and consistency of the food consumed. Additionally, PYY levels remain elevated for several hours after meal termination, suggesting PYY could play a role in nutrient metabolism and satiety. It was initially thought that the major function of PYY was as a mediator of the 'ileal brake', a feedback mechanism triggered by the presence of nutrients in the small intestine. The 'ileal brake' increases stomach to caecum transit time by reducing gastric motility in the small intestine, delaying gastric emptying and reducing gastric and pancreatic secretions, all of which increase and prolong feelings of satiety. However, subsequent investigations suggest PYY may play a more direct role in the regulation of appetite and energy metabolism. Indeed, its use as a potential treatment for obesity has been explored.

PYY and Food Intake

Batterham et al. [4] first demonstrated that PYY3–36 dose dependently reduced food intake in rats. A number of groups initially claimed that they could not replicate these results. However the anorectic effects of PYY3–36 are now widely accepted and several different groups have since replicated the findings. The inconsistency is attributed to poor stress acclimatization as stress inhibits food intake, probably by inhibiting the action of NPY in the hypothalamic appetite circuits, and may thus mask the inhibitory effects of PYY3–36 [5]. Transgenic PYY knockout mice are hyperphagic and do not respond to the satiating effects of dietary protein; they also develop obesity and demonstrate an increase in both subcutaneous and visceral fat. However, this phenotype is reversed by the administration of exogenous PYY3–36. Food intake is inhibited to a greater extent in PYY-deficient animals compared to controls, suggesting they are actually hypersensitive to the anorectic effects of PYY3–36 [1]. Boey et al. [6] demonstrated that overexpression of PYY prevented diet-induced obesity in their transgenic mouse model, as well as protecting against obesity when these animals were crossed onto a genetically obese leptin-deficient ob/ob background. Le Roux et al. [7] observed that PYY levels in both the fasted and fed state were reduced in diet-induced obese mice fed a high-fat diet when compared to normal weight mice fed regular chow. Their findings suggested this was due to a reduction in the release of PYY and that this might be a contributory factor in the development of obesity.

In humans, PYY3–36 infusion in normal-weight subjects reduces appetite and food intake over 24 h [4]. Unlike with leptin, where obesity produces resistance, the anorectic effect of peripheral PYY3–36 is retained in obese subjects [8], although they have reduced basal circulating levels of endogenous PYY and a blunted postprandial rise. It has been suggested that a reduction in PYY-induced satiety could possibly contribute to the maintenance of obesity [7]. This is supported by several studies which have demonstrated a temporal association between circulating postprandial PYY levels and satiety scores [5]. Both basal and nutrient stimulated plasma PYY levels are increased after gastric bypass surgery and this is thought to contribute to the increased feelings of satiety experienced after this procedure. Interestingly, fasting levels of circulating PYY are significantly elevated in Anorexia Nervosa and could act to further inhibit appetite [5]. In both obese and normal weight humans a diet high in protein is reported to be more satiating than a high-fat or high-carbohydrate diet. A high-protein meal elicits the greatest increase in postprandial PYY. Mice fed high-protein diets gain less weight and have reduced adiposity as well as increased plasma PYY levels and the finding that this is abrogated in PYY knockout mice [1] indicates a critical role for PYY in protein metabolism.

Several studies have demonstrated the importance of the Y2r in mediating the anorectic effects of both endogenous and exogenous PYY3–36. Transgenic Y2r knockout mice are hyperphagic with increased body weight and fat deposition and they do not demonstrate a reduction in feeding after peripheral PYY3–36 administration [4]. The administration of the Y2-specific antagonist BIIE0246 blocks the anorectic effects of exogenous PYY3–36 [9]. Although PYY3–36 is often referred to as being 'Y2-selective' it also possesses moderate affinity for the Y5r but binds less well to the Y1 receptor (Y1r) [2]. The effects of exogenous PYY1–36 on appetite and energy metabolism have been largely ignored due to its high affinity for Y1r and Y5r, activation of the latter being claimed to induce hyperphagia and weight gain. Additionally, PYY3–36 is the most abundant isoform present in the circulation in both the fed and fasted state [1, 7]. Although administration of PYY1–36 in rodents was shown to inhibit feeding, albeit less potently than PYY3–36, this effect was reportedly abolished in DPP-IV-deficient animals suggesting that the conversion of PYY1–36 to PYY3–36 was responsible for the anorectic effects. Sloth et al. [10] found no effect of PYY1–36 on energy metabolism in either obese or lean human subjects.

Current evidence from both human and rodent studies strongly indicates that PYY3–36 plays an essential role in the regulation of energy homeostasis.

Central Mechanisms of Action

The Hypothalamus
The hypothalamus is one of the main brain areas involved in regulating feeding behaviour and there is evidence that PYY3–36 exerts its anorectic effects by acting

directly upon hypothalamic neurons. Administering PYY3–36 directly into the arcuate nucleus (ARC) of the hypothalamus reduces food intake [4] and peripheral administration of an anorectic dose of PYY3–36 increases the expression of c-Fos, a marker of neuronal activation, in the ARC [4, 11]. Injecting the Y2r antagonist BIIE0246 into the ARC prevents the anorectic effects of peripheral PYY3–36 [9]. PYY3–36 is able to cross the blood-brain barrier via a non-saturable mechanism and the ARC is located in close proximity to the median eminence, which is a circumventricular organ and hence has a partial blood-brain barrier. It is therefore possible that peripheral PYY3–36 could directly access the ARC. Within the ARC, Y2r mRNA is expressed in more than 80% of orexigenic NPY neurons [12]. It has been postulated that PYY3–36 inhibits food intake by acting via presynaptic Y2r to directly inhibit NPY neurons which reduces the tonic inhibition of adjacent anorectic proopiomelanocortin (POMC) neurons by NPY. This subsequently stimulates feeding due to increased α-MSH signalling via MC4 receptors [4, 13]. Indeed, administration of Y2r-selective agonists reduces NPY release from hypothalamic explants [4], whereas the Y2r antagonist BIIE0246 increases NPY release [14]. Several groups have shown that peripheral administration of PYY3–36 induces c-Fos expression in 20% of POMC neurons [4] or neurons expressing α-MSH, the signalling product of POMC [13]. However, other groups have found that PYY3–36 inhibits both NPY and POMC ARC neurons [15] and moreover that the anorectic response to PYY3–36 is maintained in POMC-null mice [16] suggesting that melanocortin signalling is not necessary for the anorectic effects of PYY3–36. Therefore, either the anorectic actions of PYY3–36 are mainly due to the reduction in NPY neuron activity, or PYY3–36 may reduce the overall input of ARC signalling to feeding behaviour. Alternatively, the majority of POMC neurons also co-express the neuropeptide cocaine- and amphetamine-regulated transcript (CART) and central administration of CART suppresses feeding independently of melanocortin signalling. PYY3–36 administration could therefore increase the release of CART which could enhance the anorectic effects of NPY neuron inhibition although this has not currently been investigated [13].

The Vagus and Brainstem

The anorectic effects of peripheral PYY3–36 also require intact vagal afferent signalling from the gut to the brainstem. The dorsal vagal complex within the brainstem is the termination site of afferent vagal nerve fibres and comprises the area postrema (AP), the dorsal motor nucleus of the vagus and the nucleus tractus solitarius (NTS). Vagal information is relayed to the hypothalamus via the brainstem, particularly via projections from the NTS. In rats, vagotomy or transectioning of the brainstem-hypothalamic pathway abolishes the reduction in food intake observed after peripheral PYY3–36 administration and prevents the associated increase in ARC c-Fos expression [13, 17]. Y2r mRNA is also expressed in the nodose ganglion and peripheral vagal afferent terminals and administration of peripheral PYY3–36 increases vagal afferent firing [13], as well as increasing the expression of c-Fos in the NTS and AP [18].

However, in mice neither vagotomy [18] nor degeneration of the nodose ganglion and vagus nerve [9] prevented the anorectic effects of peripheral PYY3–36. Food intake reduction was prolonged in mice subjected to subdiaphragmatic vagotomy suggesting that vagal signalling modulates the duration of the anorectic actions of PYY3–36 [18].

As a circumventricular organ the AP has an incomplete blood-brain barrier. It is located in close proximity to the 4th ventricle and densely expresses the Y2r; therefore, peripheral PYY3–36 could also act directly on neurons in the AP. However, Cox and Randich [19] found that AP ablation actually enhances the reduction in food intake caused by peripheral PYY3–36, suggesting that the direct actions of PYY3–36 in the AP may oppose the anorectic actions in the hypothalamus, possibly via Y5r activity. There are currently no studies examining the effects of PYY3–36 administration directly into the brainstem or the 4th ventricle. However, administration of PYY3–36 into the lateral ventricles has been shown to increase food intake and this effect is diminished in Y5 knockout mice and surprisingly, also in Y1 knockout mice [2]. Therefore it is possible that the actions of PYY3–36 within the brain could be both anorectic and orexigenic and the effects are dependent upon which receptor type is available in different brain areas.

Halatchev and Cone [18] found that peripheral PYY3–36 administration caused conditioned taste aversion in mice. They suggested that PYY3–36 activated a specific subset of neurons in the NTS that were previously shown to be associated with the response to aversive stimuli such as lithium chloride (LiCl). Although another group did not replicate these findings [9], it is possible that part of the anorectic effect of PYY3–36 may be due to an aversive response. Indeed, human studies have reported that high PYY3–36 levels are associated with nausea and vomiting, although this does not correlate with an effect on food intake [10].

Recently, several groups have demonstrated that PYY-expressing neurons are solely located within the gigantocellular reticular nucleus (Gi) of the rostral medulla [20, 21]. These neurons project abundantly to the dorsal vagal complex, with the highest density seen in the NTS. Thus some of the Yr activity in the brainstem that has been attributed to the effects of peripheral PYY may actually be mediated by central PYY. In the periphery, PYY3–36 is the predominant isoform in both the fed and fasted state, however Gelegen et al. [21] found that in the brainstem PYY1–36 is the predominant form in the fed state. Conversion of PYY1–36 to PYY3–36 increases in the fasted state until levels of both isoforms are similar, although overall PYY mRNA levels are reduced. This seems counterintuitive if the actions of PYY3–36 within the brainstem are anorectic, however it is possible that it is the ratio of PYY1–36 to PYY3–36 activity which is important in brainstem-mediated regulation of food intake. Interestingly, Parkinson et al. [22] found that although peripheral administration of PYY3–36 was associated with an acute anorectic response, it was also associated with a later orexigenic response. This was independent of any previous reduction in food intake and was also observed with a PYY3–36 analogue, though not with other anorectic gut peptides or LiCl. The study only measured PYY3–36 levels, which were decreased prior to the period of orexigenic activity; therefore it is unclear whether there was also a concomitant increase in PYY1–36 levels which may have contributed to the increased food intake along with the increase in ghrelin levels shown.

Gi expression of PYY has been seen in river lamprey, primates and rodents, suggesting conservation throughout evolution and implying a functional importance of this central PYY system. Neuronal outputs from the Gi and caudal brainstem have been implicated in the motor and visceral aspects of feeding, including chewing, licking and swallowing and also control of gastric motility and pancreatic function [20, 21]. A possible mechanism behind the 'ileal brake' could be vagal activation of these areas by peripheral PYY.

Other Brain Areas

The hypothalamus and brainstem are the main brain areas involved in the regulation of energy homeostasis. However, due to the relative abundance of calorie-rich foods in the Western world, non-homeostatic factors like emotion and reward have become more salient when deciding upon the nutrient composition and volume of food intake. Current evidence from a limited number of studies suggests that PYY3–36 also modulates neuronal activity in higher cortical and corticolimbic areas, particularly the obitofrontal cortex which is the main brain area involved in reward, emotion and decision-making [23, 24]. Batterham et al. [23] found that when PYY3–36 levels are high, for example in the postprandial state, changes in obitofrontal cortex activity predicts subsequent food intake, whereas in the fasted state hypothalamic activity is a better predictor of feeding behaviour. They postulated that the presence of a postprandial satiety factor like PYY3–36 switches the regulation of food intake from homeostatic-hypothalamic control to hedonic-corticolimbic control.

Thus, current evidence indicates that PYY plays a major role in energy metabolism via the modulation of food intake and that this occurs via actions in the central nervous system. The mechanisms underlying the effects of PYY on food intake remain to be clarified. Further investigation is necessary to determine the role of central PYY and also whether the actions of the two PYY isoforms, PYY1–36 and PYY3–36, are consistent across different brain areas.

Energy Expenditure

Several studies have suggested an association between PYY and energy expenditure and substrate partitioning. Transgenic mice that overexpress PYY have an increased core body temperature which could be indicative of an increase in thermogenesis [6]. Similarly in humans, postprandially increased PYY levels are associated with the thermic effect of food [25]. Sloth et al. [10] showed that peripheral infusion of PYY3–36 in humans was associated with an increase in energy expenditure, and Doucet et al. [25] found that postprandial PYY levels were also associated with energy expenditure.

The PYY-immunoreactive fibres in the Gi are closely associated with MCH- and orex-in-expressing neurons, both of which are involved in regulation of sympathetic and parasympathetic outflow from the brainstem, including projections to brown adipose tissue, activation of which has been linked to thermogenesis in both rodents and humans. MCH and orexin neuronal projections from the Gi have also been postulated to be involved in the regulation of cardiovascular and respiratory function [20, 21] which supports the finding that infusion of PYY3–36 in humans was associated with an increase in heart rate [10]. Additionally, both human and animal studies have found that levels of PYY3–36 are associated with respiratory quotient values and indicate an alteration in substrate partitioning in favour of fat oxidation [10, 26]. Initial studies suggest that PYY3–36 regulates energy homeostasis by increasing energy expenditure as well as reducing food intake. However, further investigation is necessary to elucidate the mechanism underlying these energy expenditure effects.

Conclusions

PYY3–36 is released into the circulation from endocrine cells in the distal gut in response to nutrients and plays a physiological role in inhibiting appetite. The exact mechanism underlying this action is unclear but a direct central nervous system effect seems possible. PYY3–36 levels are elevated after the gastric bypass procedure for obesity, and are also raised in a number of conditions associated with appetite reduction. It is not currently clear if PYY has some role in regulating energy expenditure. However, due to the clear inhibition of appetite, PYY is being explored as a possible therapeutic agent for the treatment of obesity.

References

1 Batterham RL, Heffron H, Kapoor S, Chivers JE, Chandarana K, Herzog H, Le Roux CW, Thomas EL, Bell JD, Withers DJ: Critical role for peptide YY in protein-mediated satiation and body-weight regulation. Cell Metab 2006;4:223–233.

2 Kanatani A, Mashiko S, Murai N, Sugimoto N, Ito J, Fukuroda T, Fukami T, Morin N, MacNeil DJ, Van der Ploeg LH, Saga Y, Nishimura S, Ihara M: Role of the Y1 receptor in the regulation of neuropeptide Y-mediated feeding: comparison of wild-type, Y1 receptor-deficient, and Y5 receptor-deficient mice. Endocrinology 2000;141:1011–1016.

3 Adrian TE, Ferri GL, Bacarese-Hamilton AJ, Fuessl HS, Polak JM, Bloom SR: Human distribution and release of a putative new gut hormone, peptide YY. Gastroenterology 1985;89:1070–1077.

4 Batterham RL, Cowley MA, Small CJ, Herzog H, Cohen MA, Dakin CL, Wren AM, Brynes AE, Low MJ, Ghatei MA, Cone RD, Bloom SR: Gut hormone PYY(3–36) physiologically inhibits food intake. Nature 2002;418:650–654.

5 Ashby D, Bloom SR: Recent progress in PYY research – an update report for 8th NPY meeting. Peptides 2007;28:198–202.

6 Boey D, Lin S, Enriquez RF, Lee NJ, Slack K, Couzens M, Baldock PA, Herzog H, Sainsbury A: PYY transgenic mice are protected against diet-induced and genetic obesity. Neuropeptides. 2008;42:19–30.

7 Le Roux CW, Batterham RL, Aylwin SJ, Patterson M, Borg CM, Wynne KJ, Kent A, Vincent RP, Gardiner J, Ghatei MA, Bloom SR: Attenuated peptide YY release in obese subjects is associated with reduced satiety. Endocrinology 2006;147:3–8.

8 Batterham RL, Cohen MA, Ellis SM, Le Roux CW, Withers DJ, Frost GS, Ghatei MA, Bloom SR: Inhibition of food intake in obese subjects by peptide YY3–36. N Engl J Med 2003;349:941–948.

9 Talsania T, Anini Y, Siu S, Drucker DJ, Brubaker PL: Peripheral exendin-4 and peptide YY(3–36) synergistically reduce food intake through different mechanisms in mice. Endocrinology 2005;146:3748–3756.

10 Sloth B, Holst JJ, Flint A, Gregersen NT, Astrup A: Effects of PYY1–36 and PYY3–36 on appetite, energy intake, energy expenditure, glucose and fat metabolism in obese and lean subjects. Am J Physiol Endocrinol Metab 2007;292:E1062–E1068.

11 Abbott CR, Monteiro M, Small CJ, Sajedi A, Smith KL, Parkinson JR, Ghatei MA, Bloom SR: The inhibitory effects of peripheral administration of peptide YY(3–36) and glucagon-like peptide-1 on food intake are attenuated by ablation of the vagal-brainstem-hypothalamic pathway. Brain Res 2005;1044: 127–131.

12 Broberger C, Landry M, Wong H, Walsh JN, Hokfelt T: Subtypes Y1 and Y2 of the neuropeptide Y receptor are respectively expressed in proopiomelanocortin- and neuropeptide-Y-containing neurons of the rat hypothalamic arcuate nucleus. Neuroendocrinology 1997;66:393–408.

13 Koda S, Date Y, Murakami N, Shimbara T, Hanada T, Toshinai K, Niijima A, Furuya M, Inomata N, Osuye K, Nakazato M: The role of the vagal nerve in peripheral PYY3–36-induced feeding reduction in rats. Endocrinology 2005;146:2369–2375.

14 King PJ, Williams G, Doods H, Widdowson PS: Effect of a selective neuropeptide Y Y(2) receptor antagonist, BIIE0246 on neuropeptide Y release. Eur J Pharmacol 2000;396:R1–R3.

15 Acuna-Goycolea C, van den Pol AN: Peptide YY(3–36) inhibits both anorexigenic proopiomelanocortin and orexigenic neuropeptide Y neurons: implications for hypothalamic regulation of energy homeostasis. J Neurosci 2005;25:10510–10519.

16 Challis BG, Coll AP, Yeo GS, Pinnock SB, Dickson SL, Thresher RR, Dixon J, Zahn D, Rochford JJ, White A, Oliver RL, Millington G, Aparicio SA, Colledge WH, Russ AP, Carlton MB, O'Rahilly S: Mice lacking pro-opiomelanocortin are sensitive to high-fat feeding but respond normally to the acute anorectic effects of peptide-YY(3–36). Proc Natl Acad Sci USA 2004;101:4695–4700.

17 Abbott CR, Monteiro M, Small CJ, Sajedi A, Smith KL, Parkinson JR, Ghatei MA, Bloom SR: The inhibitory effects of peripheral administration of peptide YY(3–36) and glucagon-like peptide-1 on food intake are attenuated by ablation of the vagal-brainstem-hypothalamic pathway. Brain Res 2005;1044:127–131.

18 Halatchev IG, Cone RD: Peripheral administration of PYY(3–36) produces conditioned taste aversion in mice. Cell Metab 2005;1:159–168.

19 Cox JE, Randich A: Enhancement of feeding suppression by PYY(3–36) in rats with area postrema ablations. Peptides 2004;25:985–989.

20 Glavas MM, Grayson BE, Allen SE, Copp DR, Smith MS, Cowley MA, Grove KL: Characterization of brainstem peptide YY (PYY) neurons. J Comp Neurol 2008;506:194–210.

21 Gelegen C, Chandarana K, Choudhury AI, Al-Qassab H, Evans IM, Irvine EE, Hyde CB, Claret M, Andreelli F, Sloan SE, Leiter AB, Withers DJ, Batterham RL: Regulation of hindbrain PYY expression by acute food deprivation, prolonged caloric restriction, and weight loss surgery in mice. Am J Physiol Endocrinol Metab 2012;303:E659–E668.

22 Parkinson JR, Dhillo WS, Small CJ, Chaudhri OB, Bewick GA, Pritchard I, Moore S, Ghatei MA, Bloom SR: PYY3–36 injection in mice produces an acute anorexigenic effect followed by a delayed orexigenic effect not observed with other anorexigenic gut hormones. Am J Physiol Endocrinol Metab 2008;294: E698–E708.

23 Batterham RL, Ffytche DH, Rosenthal JM, Zelaya FO, Barker GJ, Withers DJ, Williams SC: PYY modulation of cortical and hypothalamic brain areas predicts feeding behaviour in humans. Nature 2007;450: 106–109.

24 De Silva A, Salem V, Long CJ, Makwana A, Newbould RD, Rabiner EA, Ghatei MA, Bloom SR, Matthews PM, Beaver JD, Dhillo WS: The gut hormones PYY 3–36 and GLP-1 7–36 amide reduce food intake and modulate brain activity in appetite centers in humans. Cell Metab 2011;14:700–706.

25 Doucet E, Laviolette M, Imbeault P, Strychar I, Rabasa-Lhoret R, Prud'homme D: Total peptide YY is a correlate of postprandial energy expenditure but not of appetite or energy intake in healthy women. Metabolism 2008;57:1458–1464.

26 Adams SH, Lei C, Jodka CM, Nikoulina SE, Hoyt JA, Gedulin B, Mack CM, Kendall ES: PYY3–36 administration decreases the respiratory quotient and reduces adiposity in diet-induced obese mice. J Nutr 2006;136:195–201.

Prof. Stephen R. Bloom
Division of Diabetes, Endocrinology and Metabolism, Department of Medicine
6th Floor Commonwealth Building, Hammersmith Hospital, Imperial College London
Du Cane Road, London W12 0NN (UK)
E-Mail s.bloom@imperial.ac.uk

Delhanty PJD, van der Lely AJ (eds): How Gut and Brain Control Metabolism.
Front Horm Res. Basel, Karger, 2014, vol 42, pp 155–162 (DOI: 10.1159/000358344)

Nutropioids Regulate Gut-Brain Circuitry Controlling Food Intake

Gilles Mithieux

National Institute of Health and Medical Research, U855, and University of Lyon, Lyon, and University Lyon 1, Villeurbanne, France

Abstract

The modulation of hunger sensations by the μ-opioid receptor (MOR) present in the brain is an established fact. That MORs expressed in the periphery could have a similar role was outstanding. Using portal infusions of agonists and/or antagonists of MOR in conscious rodents, we have shown that MORs present in the walls of the portal vein nervous system control a gut-brain circuit of induction of intestinal gluconeogenesis (IGN), a function controlling hunger sensations. Then, we have shown that peptides and proteins promote a MOR-dependent induction of IGN. Peptides have no effect in mice knockout for MOR. MOR-KO mice are also insensitive to satiety induced by protein-enriched diets. In addition, portal infusions of MOR modulators have no effect on food intake in mice deficient for IGN. Thus, the regulation by portal MORs and peptides of a gut-brain neural circuit of induction of IGN is a causal link in the phenomenon of satiety induced by dietary protein.

As part of the worldwide efforts for a better understanding of the mechanisms of energy homeostasis, an increasingly important area relates to the search for hormonal and metabolic signals produced by the intestine in response to nutrient uptake and which modulate hunger. This concerns in particular the gastrointestinal hormones such as cholecystokinin, glucagon-like peptide 1 or peptide YY. It is interesting to note that the enteric nervous system plays an important role in the detection and transmission of hormonal signals to the brain [1–3].

In this context, intestinal gluconeogenesis (IGN) is a newly described function [4–8] that interferes with the control of energy homeostasis in the postabsorptive state [for a review, see 9]. An induced IGN results in a release of glucose into the portal vein, which collects blood from the whole intestine. Its detection by a portal glucose sensor, recently identified as the glucose receptor SGLT3 [10] and the transmission of this signal to the brain via the peripheral nervous system induces a decrease in hunger and an increased sensitivity to insulin of hepatic glucose production. This pathway is of particular importance in two special nutritional situations, protein-enriched diets (PED) [11–13], and obesity surgery of the type gastric bypass [14].

A long known property of proteins is that a number of them, particularly of interest in human nutrition as milk caseins, encompass oligopeptides having a μ-opioid activity in vitro after partial proteolytic digestion [15]. In addition, extensive literature on the subject mentions the μ-opioid activity of numerous oligopeptides [16]. It is also recognized that modulation of μ-opioid receptor (MOR) in the central nervous system may interfere with the control of food intake. Agonists increase food intake, while antagonists inhibit it [17]. Interestingly, MORs are expressed in the small intestine neural system, where they control intestinal motility [18, 19]. Food proteins are absorbed from the intestinal lumen after incomplete proteolysis and thus may play a role in systemic signaling via the peptidic residues they release [15]. However, that they can reach the brain after oral ingestion is precluded by the proteolytic activity of the liver [20]. This led us to test the hypothesis of a role of intestinal MOR in the satiety effect of dietary protein via the induction of IGN.

Periportal MOR Regulates IGN via a Gut-Brain Circuitry

To test the role of the gastrointestinal and/or periportal nervous system in the induction of IGN gene expression by dietary protein, we first investigated the effect of a PED in rats after periportal treatment by capsaicin, a substance that inactivates afferent nerves. No induction of the activity of glucose-6-phosphatase (G6Pase) or the phosphoenolpyruvate carboxykinase-cytosolic form (PEPCK-C), two key regulatory enzymes of IGN, was observed in capsaicin-treated rats, in contrast to control animals where IGN enzymes were markedly induced. To test the putative role of MOR in this induction, we infused MOR regulators in the portal vein of conscious rats. Two agonists, β_{1-7} casomorphin (derived from β-casein) and DAMGO reduced the intestinal G6Pase activity (fig. 1a). Instead, two MOR antagonists (casoxin C, from κ-casein, and naloxone (Nalox)) increased G6Pase activity (fig. 1a). Similar results were obtained for the expression of PEPCK-C protein. Intestinal glucose production, quantified at the end of the Nalox infusion using a glucose metabolic tracer (tritiated on carbon 3), represented 25–30% of the total endogenous glucose production. Instead, no appearance of glucose was observed in rats infused with DAMGO. Consistent with what might be expected from the effect of MOR effectors on IGN, rats infused with a MOR antagonist (Caso-C) in the portal vein decreased their food intake, whereas those infused with a MOR agonist (β_{1-7}) increased their food ingestion [16].

We used three methods to document the role played by the portal MORs. Firstly, immunohistochemical studies combining the detection of MOR and of the neuronal marker PGP9.5 revealed the presence of MOR in the neuronal fibers of the walls of the rat portal vein (fig. 1b). We observed a comparable co-localization of MOR and

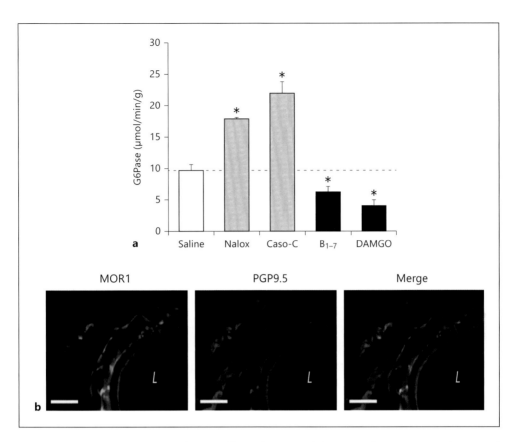

Fig. 1. Portal MORs and control of IGN. **a** Effect of MOR modulators on the expression of intestinal G6Pase: MOR modulators were infused for 8 h in the portal vein of conscious rats. The G6Pase activity is measured in a sample of middle jejunum at the end of the infusion (mean ± SEM, n = 6). * p < 0.05 (Tukey's post hoc test). **b** Expression of MOR in the neural periportal system: MORs are visualized by a specific antibody (green fluorescence), the neuronal marker PGP9.5 is displayed in red fluorescence. The merging of the two signals reveals in yellow-orange the presence of both markers in some neuronal structures in the portal vein of rats.

PGP9.5 in the portal branches irrigating the portal spaces of the human liver. We then studied the effect of β_{1-7} or Caso-C on gene expression of IGN in rats treated with capsaicin. There was no effect on the enzymes of gluconeogenesis, strongly suggesting that the periportal neural system is crucial for MOR signal transmission. Finally, we evaluated the effect of β_{1-7} and Nalox on the brain regions involved in the reception of gastroenteric signals: the dorsal vagal complex, which connects the vagus nerve, and the parabrachial nucleus, which connects afferents from the spinal cord [1]. By immunohistochemistry, we studied the expression of the protein c-Fos, a well-known marker of neuronal activation. The infusion of the antagonist Nalox induced the expression of c-Fos in both the dorsal vagal complex and the parabrachial nucleus, strongly suggesting that both the vagal and spinal pathways were involved in the signal transmission to the brain. A comparable c-Fos activation took place in the main hypothalamic regions, which control food intake (e.g. the arcuate and paraventricular nuclei). Confirming the role of peripheral nerves in the signal transmission, no activation occurred in rats with portal vein treated with capsaicin at the time of surgery for the implantation of the catheter [16].

Protein Digests and Oligopeptides Act as MOR Antagonists

To document the hypothesis that dietary protein could induce IGN via a MOR-dependent process, we combined several approaches.

First, we infused a proteolytic digest (peptone) or selected oligopeptides (di- or tri-peptides) in the portal mesenteric vein of rats. In all cases, a marked induction of G6Pase was observed in both the jejunum and ileum. In addition, glucose tracer dilution revealed that intestinal glucose production took place after the portal infusion of Tyr-Ala or peptones. Finally, as previously observed for MOR antagonists, no induction of intestinal G6Pase by oligopeptides occurred in rats with the periportal area denervated by capsaicin. Second, in rats infused with the dipeptide Tyr-Ala, there was a threefold increase in the expression of c-Fos in the dorsal vagal complex and in all the brain regions previously studied, as in rats infused with Nalox (see above). Moreover, no increase in c-Fos took place after the inactivation of portal afferent nerves. Third, we tested whether the oligopeptides may behave as MOR antagonists in cultured neuroblastoma cells constitutively expressing MOR [21, 22]. Notably, we studied the effect of oligopeptides on MOR coupling to adenylate cyclase. Because MORs are coupled to adenylate cyclase via inhibitory G-protein, DAMGO (a MOR agonist) significantly decreased the intracellular cAMP content. In contrast, Caso-C and Nalox (MOR antagonists) significantly increased the intracellular cAMP content. It was noteworthy that all oligopeptides increased the cAMP content and prevented the DAMGO-induced decrease in cAMP in co-incubation experiments [16]. This strongly suggests that oligopeptides may behave as MOR antagonists both in vivo and in vitro.

MOR-Dependent Induction of IGN Is a Causal Link in the Satiety Effect of Dietary Proteins

To demonstrate the causal role of MOR in the induction of IGN by protein during their assimilation and its role in the associated satiety, we performed experiments of portal perfusion in MOR-knockout mice (MOR-KO) and in mice with deletion of the G6Pase catalytic subunit (G6PC) specifically in the intestine (I-G6PC-KO). When infused in wild-type mice (WT), the di-and tri-peptides and peptones induced G6Pase activity in the gut. In contrast, DAMGO suppressed the G6Pase activity and this was

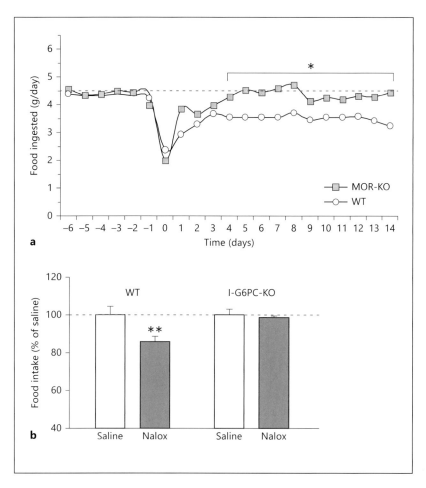

Fig. 2. Control of food intake in the absence of MOR or of IGN. **a** Effect of PED in WT and MOR-KO mice: food intake was measured before and after passage (day 0) from a conventional high-carbohydrate diet to a PED. Mean ± SEM, n = 8 mice per group. * $p < 0.05$ (Student's t test for unpaired values). **b** Effect of portal Nalox infusion on food intake in WT and I-G6PC-KO mice: the mice were infused into the portal vein for 24 h alternately with saline or Nalox and their food intake quantified. Mean ± SEM of 6 mice in each condition. ** $p < 0.01$ vs. saline (Student's t test for paired values).

reversed by peptones in co-infusion experiments. It should be noted that none of these effectors induced any effect on IGN in MOR-KO mice [16]. In addition, we studied the food intake of MOR-KO mice and WT mice after switching from the standard diet rich in starch (SED) to PED. Food intake per day for the two groups did not differ with the SED. After a transient decrease, a classic response to changes in the type of food in rodents, food intake was reduced by approximately 20% in WT mice fed the PED. Instead, KO mice resumed their previous food intake (fig. 2a). This was associated with a lack of modulation of intestinal G6Pase in MOR-KO mice, differing significantly from the induction observed in WT mice [16]. Lastly, we studied food ingestion in WT mice and I-G6PC-KO mice perfused with a MOR antagonist in the portal vein. There was a 15% decrease in food intake in WT mice infused with Nalox (fig. 2b), i.e. mice exhibiting increased IGN (see above). In contrast, no effect was observed during the infusion of Nalox in I-G6PC-KO mice, i.e. in the absence of IGN (fig. 2b). Comparable results were obtained when Tyr-Ala was infused instead of Nalox. These data strongly suggest that the modulation of IGN by the portal MOR and the effect of portal MOR on hunger are closely related phenomena, and that they could account for the satiety effect of dietary protein.

Final Remarks

It is worth noting that to demonstrate that MOR associated with portal neuronal fibers control a gut-brain neural circuitry of induction of IGN, we combined infusions of MOR effectors in the portal vein in conscious rats and effects of denervation of the walls of the portal vein. This method of infusion was preferred to infusions into the intestinal lumen. Indeed, the production and flow of native peptide metabolites from the intestinal lumen is difficult to control due to its high content of various proteases. Diverging from the actual in vivo context, the nervous system immediately surrounding the intestinal mucosa (the so-called intrinsic gastrointestinal system or enteric neural system) is shunted during mesenteric-portal infusions. Therefore, even if the detection of metabolites in the neural system of the portal vein (belonging to the so-called extrinsic gastrointestinal nervous system) were involved in the experimental conditions studied by Duraffourd et al. [16], it cannot be excluded that a MOR-dependent pathway could also occur upstream (i.e. in the enteric neural system [18, 23]) outside this experimental context.

It is established that proteins are incompletely digested within the gut lumen and that they release peptidic fragments composed mainly of di- or tri-peptides [24]. These oligopeptides are then transported through the enterocytes via a specific carrier (PEPT1) to the luminal membrane [25, 26]. A fraction of these undergo further proteolysis to amino acids to supply intestinal metabolism, which is known to be very intense. It is less known that another fraction is released into the portal blood, with amino acids, via a presently unknown mechanism [27]. A number of proteins release peptides with μ-opioid activity. Often, this relates to an agonist activity, as for β-casomorphin (see above). However, the assumption that any type of food protein can induce IGN via a MOR-dependent pathway implies that protein digests from all backgrounds should globally exert a MOR antagonist activity. This inference is strongly supported by the observation that all peptides studied by Duraffourd et al. [16], either alone or in mixture (peptones), behave as MOR antagonists both in vivo to induce NGI and in vitro in experiments of coupling to adenylate cyclase.

An interesting question relates to the complexity of the sequence of events that allows food proteins to exert their final effect on satiety. Indeed, intestinal factors released by the intestine in response to meals are supposed to modulate food intake by directly binding to their receptors in the hypothalamus. In the case of dietary protein, a series of events initiate first the IGN gene expression program via a reflex arc within the brain. This is progressive and takes place during the postprandial period. After that the glucose released can initiate its central action via the mechanisms deriving from portal glucose sensing [10, 11]. Since this is a process based on the induction of genes, it can therefore continue after the assimilation of food. This is consistent with the fact that PED are well known to reduce hunger following the complete digestion of a previous meal, which is the definition of the phenomenon called 'satiety' [28, 29].

In conclusion, MOR expressed in the mesenteric-portal area control a gut-brain neural circuit regulating IGN, which controls food intake [11, 13, 14]. So far, the regulatory role of MOR in the control of food intake was documented in the central nervous system. Moreover, food proteins initiate their satiety effects through the μ-opioid antagonist activity of the peptidic residues of proteolytic digestion by acting on this previously unsuspected gut-brain neural circuitry. Remarkably, several MOR antagonists administered orally reduced hunger in humans [17]. In addition, the satiety effect of dietary protein concerns rodents and humans as well [11, 28, 29]. Therefore, the new knowledge summarized here could pave the way for future approaches of treatment and/or prevention of metabolic diseases.

Acknowledgement

The author thanks the team members who have been involved in the acquisition of these results.

Disclosure Statement

The author has no conflicts of interest to disclose.

References

1 Berthoud HR: Anatomy and function of sensory hepatic nerves. Anat Rec A Discov Mol Cell Evol Biol 2004;280:827–835.

2 Moran TH: Cholecystokinin and satiety: current perspectives. Nutrition 2000;16:858–865.

3 Vahl TP, Tauchi M, Durler TS, Elfers EE, Fernandes TM, Bitner RD, Ellis KS, Woods SC, Seeley RJ, Herman JP, D'Alessio DA: Glucagon-like peptide-1 (GLP-1) expressed receptors on nerve terminals in the portal vein mediate the effects of endogenous GLP-1 on glucose tolerance in rats. Endocrinology 2007;148:4965–4973.

4 Croset M, Rajas F, Zitoun C, Hurot JM, Montano S, Mithieux G: Rat small intestine is an insulin-sensitive gluconeogenic organ. Diabetes 2001;50:740–746.

5 Mithieux G, Rajas F, Gautier-Stein A: A novel role for glucose-6-phosphatase in the small intestine in the control of glucose homeostasis. J Biol Chem 2004;279:44231–44234.

6 Mithieux G, Bady I, Gautier A, Croset M, Rajas F, Zitoun C: Induction of control genes in intestinal gluconeogenesis is sequential falling on fasting and maximal in diabetes. Am J Physiol Endocrinol Metab 2004;286:E370–E375.

7 Rajas F, Croset M, Zitoun C, Montano S, Mithieux G: Induction of PEPCK gene expression in insulinopenia in rat small intestine. Diabetes 2000;49:1165–1168.

8 Rajas F, Bruni N, Montano S, Zitoun C, Mithieux G: The glucose-6-phosphatase gene is expressed in human and rat small intestine: regulation of speech in fasted and diabetic rats. Gastroenterology 1999;117:132–139.

9 Mithieux G, Magnan C: Intestinal gluconeogenesis: a new player in the control of food intake. Cah Nutr Diet 2006;41:211–215.

10 Delaere F, Duchampt A, Mounien L, Seyer P, Duraffourd C, Zitoun C, Thorens B, Mithieux G: The role of sodium-coupled glucose co-transporter-3 in the satiety effect of portal glucose sensing. Mol Metab 2012;2:47–53.

11 Mithieux G, Misery P, Magnan C, Pillot B, Gautier-Stein A, Bernard C, Rajas F, Zitoun C: Portal sensing of intestinal gluconeogenesis is a mechanistic link in the diminution of food intake induced by diet protein. Cell Metab 2005;2:321–329.

12 Pillot B, Soty M, Gautier-Stein A, Zitoun C, Mithieux G: Protein feeding promotes redistribution of endogenous glucose output to the kidney and potentiates its suppression by insulin. Endocrinology 2009;150:616–624.

13 Penhoat A, Mutel E, Amigo-Correig M, Pillot B, Stefanutti A, Rajas F, Mithieux G: Protein-induced satiety is abolished in the lack of intestinal gluconeogenesis. Physiol Behav 2011;105:89–93.

14 Troy S, Soty M, Ribeiro L, Laval L, Migrenne S, Fioramonti X, Pillot B, Fauveau V, Aubert R, Viollet B, Foretz M, Leclerc J, Duchampt A, Zitoun C, Thorens B, Magnan C, Mithieux G, Andreelli F: Intestinal gluconeogenesis is a key factor for early metabolic changes after gastric bypass but not after gastric lap-band in mice. Cell Metab 2008;8:201–211.

15 Zioudrou C, Streaty RA, Klee WA: Opioid peptides derived from food proteins. The exorphins. J Biol Chem 1979;254:2446–2449.

16 Duraffourd C, De Vadder F, Goncalves D, Delaere F, Penhoat A, Brusset B, Rajas F, Chassard D, Duchampt A, Stefanutti A, Gautier-Stein A, Mithieux G: Mu-opioid receptors and dietary protein stimulate a gut-brain neural circuitry limiting food intake. Cell 2012;150:377–388.

17 Yeomans MR, Gray RW: Opioid peptides and the control of human ingestive behavior. Biobehav Rev Neurosci 2002;26:713–728.

18 Hedner T, Cassuto J: Opioids and opioid receptors in peripheral tissues. Scand J Gastroenterol 1987;130(suppl):27–46.

19 Sternini C, Patierno S, Selmer IS, Kirchgessner A: The opioid system in the gastrointestinal tract. Neurogastroenterol Motil 2004;16:3–16.

20 Kreil G, Umbach M, Brantl V, Teschemacher H: Studies on the enzymatic degradation of β-casomorphins. Life Sci 1983;33(suppl 1):137–140.

21 Lorentz M, Hedlund B, Arhem P: Morphine Activates cloned calcium channels in mouse neuroblastoma cell lines. Brain Res 1988;445:157–159.

22 Yang JC, Shan J, Ng KF, Pang P: Morphine and methadone have different effects on calcium channel currents in neuroblastoma cells. Brain Res 2000;870:199–203.

23 Sternini C: Receptors and transmission in the brain-gut axis: potential for novel therapies. III. μ-Opioid receptors in the enteric nervous system. Am J Physiol Gastrointert Liver Physiol 2001;281:G8–G15.

24 Daniel C: Molecular and integrative physiology of intestinal peptide transport. Annu Rev Physiol 2004;66:361–384.

25 Boll M, Markovich D, Weber WM, Korte H, Daniel H, Murer H: Expression cloning of a cDNA from rabbit small intestine related to proton-coupled transport of peptides, β-lactam antibiotics and ACE inhibitors. Pflugers Arch 1994;429:146–149.

26 Nielsen CU, Brodin B: Di-/tri-peptide transporters as drug delivery targets: regulation of transportation under physiological and pathophysiological conditions. Curr Drug Targets 2003;4:373–388.

27 Lee VH: Membrane transporters. Eur J Pharm Sci 2000;11(suppl 2):S41–S50.

28 Booth DA, Chase A, Campbell AT: Relative effectiveness of protein in the late stages of appetite suppression in man. Physiol Behav 1970;5:1299–1302.

29 Rolls BJ, Hetherington M, Burley VJ: The specificity of satiety: the impact of foods of different macronutrient happy on the development of satiety. Physiol Behav 1988;43:145–153.

Gilles Mithieux, PhD
UMR INSERM U855, Faculty of Medicine Laennec Lyon-East
7–11, rue Guillaume Paradin
FR–69372 Lyon Cedex 08 (France)
E-Mail gilles.mithieux@inserm.fr

Delhanty PJD, van der Lely AJ (eds): How Gut and Brain Control Metabolism.
Front Horm Res. Basel, Karger, 2014, vol 42, pp 163–174 (DOI: 10.1159/000358345)

Should We Consider Des-Acyl Ghrelin as a Separate Hormone and If So, What Does It Do?

Patric J.D. Delhanty · Sebastian J. Neggers · Aart J. van der Lely

Department of Internal Medicine, Erasmus MC, Rotterdam, The Netherlands

Abstract

The peptides ghrelin (or acyl ghrelin; AG), des-acyl ghrelin (DAG) and obestatin are all encoded by the prepro-ghrelin gene that is expressed predominantly in the stomach. Compared with ghrelin and obestatin, DAG has not received a great amount of attention. DAG has long been considered an inert degradation product of AG. Recent evidence, however, indicates that DAG behaves like a separate hormone. Therefore, it is believed that DAG must activate its own receptor, and that it may also interact with AG at this receptor. DAG can act together with AG, can antagonize AG and seems to have AG-independent effects. Of potential clinical importance is that an increasing number of studies suggest that DAG is a functional inhibitor of AG. Therefore, DAG or DAG analogs are being trialed in early clinical studies for treatment of metabolic disorders such as diabetes, obesity and Prader-Willi syndrome. © 2014 S. Karger AG, Basel

Ghrelin (or acylated ghrelin (AG)) and des-acyl ghrelin (DAG) were first described in 1999 by Kojima et al. [1]. They are both products of the prepro-ghrelin gene, which also encodes obestatin (fig. 1). AG is mainly produced by the stomach and exerts its central and peripheral effects through the growth hormone secretagogue receptor (GHSR) [1]. Ghrelin is acylated by ghrelin O-acyltransferase, or GOAT [2–4], a member of the membrane-bound O-acyltransferase family of enzymes. GOAT is predominantly co-expressed with the prepro-ghrelin gene in the stomach, but also at other sites [5, 6]. DAG is unable to bind and activate the GHSR in the sub-micromolar, physiological range [1, 7] and is therefore is considered by many to be physiologically inactive.

This chapter will however try and convince the reader that DAG does have many interesting and AG-independent actions in a multitude of (patho)physiological processes, as suggested by a number of recent studies [e.g. 8].

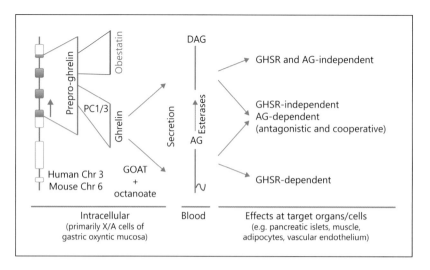

Fig. 1. Overview of mechanisms of AG and DAG synthesis and cellular actions. Ghrelin is translated as a prepro-hormone and is processed to form mature ghrelin (and obestatin) by prohormone convertases, including prohormone convertase 1/3 (PC1/3). The ghrelin peptide is also acylated by GOAT, a membrane-spanning enzyme, likely in the endoplasmic reticulum. The posttranslationally modified peptides are then secreted to have either local or endocrine actions at their target organs and cells. These effects can be independent of the ghrelin receptor (GHSR), possibly via an uncharacterized receptor.

Interaction between AG and DAG in Humans

There are only limited data on the pharmacokinetics and physiological interaction between AG and DAG. This inspired Tong et al. [9] to investigate key pharmacokinetic parameters of AG, DAG, and total ghrelin in healthy men and women. In this paper they performed two studies. In the first study, AG (1, 3, and 5 µg/kg·h) was infused for 65 min into 12 healthy (8 F/4 M) subjects in randomized order. In the second study, AG (1 µg/kg·h), DAG (4 µg/kg·h), or both were infused for 210 min into 10 healthy individuals (5 F/5 M). Plasma AG and DAG were measured using specific two-site ELISAs (studies 1 and 2), and total ghrelin with a commercial RIA (study 1). They found that after the 1, 3, and 5 µg/kg·h doses of AG, there was a dose-dependent increase in the maximum concentration and area under the curve of AG and total ghrelin [9]. Among the different AG doses, there was no difference in the elimination half-life (~10 min), systemic clearance, and volume of distribution. DAG had a decreased clearance relative to AG. The plasma DAG/AG ratio was ~2:1 during steady-state infusion of AG. Tong et al. [9] also reported that in their studies the infusion of AG caused an increase in DAG, but DAG administration did not change plasma AG. Finally, they observed deacylation of AG in the plasma but no evidence of acylation [9].

In contrast to the observations by Tong et al. [9], Ozcan et al. [10] recently reported the effects of continuous overnight infusion of DAG on AG levels and glucose and insulin responses to a standard breakfast meal in 8 overweight patients with type 2 diabetes. In addition to this, they investigated in the same patients plus 2 additional subjects, the effects of DAG infusion on AG concentrations and insulin sensitivity during a hyperinsulinemic-euglycemic clamp (HEC). In their double-blind placebo-controlled cross-over study, they used overnight continuous DAG infusions of 3 and 10 µg/kg·h and placebo to study the effects on a standard breakfast meal. They reported overnight DAG administration significantly decreased postprandial glucose levels, both during continuous glucose monitoring and in peak serum glucose levels [10]. The degree of improvement in glycemia was correlated with baseline plasma AG concentrations in their series. Concurrently, DAG infusion significantly decreased fasting and postprandial AG levels. During the HEC, 2.5 h of DAG infusion markedly decreased AG levels, and the M-index, a measure of insulin sensitivity, was significantly improved in the 6 subjects in which we were able to attain steady-state euglycemia [10].

Blijdorp et al. [11] reported on a study in which they assessed changes in DAG in response to the rapid increase in insulin concentration during an insulin tolerance test in normal weight and obese subjects. Median DAG levels decreased after insulin infusion, especially in normal weight subjects. Baseline DAG was lower in subjects with higher BMI and higher fasting insulin. DAG changes correlated with fasting insulin levels, BMI and waist circumference. Apparently, DAG levels rapidly decrease in response to insulin administration in normal subjects, but not in insulin-resistant obese subjects who are in a state of relative DAG deficiency [11].

Occurrence of High and Low AG and DAG Levels

Obesity might reflect a relative DAG deficiency, and DAG levels might be regulated by body weight as several studies have indicated that obese mice and humans have lower DAG levels than normal weight subjects whereas AG levels are similar [12–14]. Also, insulin-resistant obese subjects have an elevated AG/DAG ratio when compared to insulin-sensitive obese subjects [15, 16]. St-Pierre et al. [15] reported that the dysregulation of ghrelin secretion profiles during a HEC is associated with insulin resistance.

Rodriguez et al. [17] found that AG levels were increased in obesity and obesity-associated type 2 diabetes, whereas DAG levels were decreased. Body mass index, waist circumference, insulin and HOMA (homeostasis model assessment) index were positively correlated with AG levels [17].

Barazzoni et al. [16] reported on differential associations of ghrelin isoforms with insulin resistance and the impact of obesity on their plasma concentrations in 45 subjects with metabolic syndrome. Plasma insulin and HOMA-IR were negatively associated with DAG but positively with AG and AG/DAG ratios. Compared with the non-obese subjects, obese metabolic syndrome patients had a lower DAG but comparable AG and higher AG/DAG ratios. These data together indicate that obesity can alter circulating ghrelin profiles, and a relative AG excess or DAG deficiency can contribute to obesity-associated insulin resistance in metabolic syndrome.

The concept that low AG/DAG ratios are accompanied by an improved metabolic state was supported by Cederberg et al. [18]. They reported that after 6 months of an intensive long-term physical exercise by 552 young men undergoing military service, improvements in body weight and body composition were associated with an increase in DAG.

In support of these findings in humans, specific suppression AG, but not DAG, production by inhibition of GOAT activity with the ghrelin analog GO-CoA-TAT improves glucose homeostasis and reduces weight gain in mice [19].

However, genetic manipulation of AG levels in mouse models of obesity in which GOAT levels have been manipulated genetically seem to contradict these findings. In a recent study by Kirchner et al. [20] using extremely obese leptin-deficient *ob/ob* mice, specific removal of AG but not DAG, through deletion of the GOAT gene, did not improve glucose homeostasis. It was concluded that neither AG nor the decreased AG/DAG ratio is crucial for regulating glucose homeostasis [20], although this outcome may have been influenced by the extreme nature of this leptin-deficient model of obesity.

The AG/DAG ratio is highly dependent on the quality of the method of stabilization of acylation of ghrelin in blood samples, particularly in human blood [21]. Use of validated techniques for ghrelin stabilization are essential in any future studies of the effects of altered metabolism on circulating levels of AG and DAG.

Prader-Willi Syndrome: An Example of High Ghrelin Levels

Prader-Willi syndrome (PWS) is a leading genetic cause of obesity, characterized by hyperphagia, endocrine and developmental disorders. Many groups have reported that the hyperphagia results from impaired gut hormone signaling. For example, Purtell et al. [22] reported that hyperphagia in PWS is not related to a lower postprandial glucagon-like peptide-1 (GLP-1) or peptide YY (PYY) response. However, elevated ghrelin levels in PWS are linked with increased hunger.

Goldstone et al. [23] investigated whether differences in appetite hormones may explain the development of abnormal eating behavior in 42 young (<5 years) children with PWS. They found no significant relationships between eating behavior and the levels of any of the hormones measured. However, even in these young children, PWS was associated with low levels of the anorexigenic pancreatic polypeptide, as has been described in older children and adults. Only later in life did hyperghrelinemia or hypoinsulinemia begin to contribute to the hyperphagia of PWS [23].

DAG as an AG Antagonist

The findings of a study by Broglio et al. [24], in which they examined the interaction of AG and DAG administered to 6 normal young volunteers, caused a shift in the existing paradigm by suggesting that DAG should be considered a separate hormone. As expected, AG administration markedly increased circulating growth hormone (GH), prolactin, adrenocorticotropin and cortisol levels. Ghrelin administration was also followed by a decrease in insulin levels and an increase in plasma glucose levels. However, co-administration of DAG and AG diminished the insulin and glucose response to AG, while DAG administration alone had no effects [24]. These findings indicated that DAG has metabolic activity, and was later confirmed and extended by Gauna et al. [25] who reported that administration of AG in humans reduces insulin sensitivity, whereas co-infusion with DAG blocked this effect. They studied the effects of acute administration of AG and DAG, separately and together, in 8 adult-onset GH-deficient patients. AG, which was rapidly cleared from the circulation, induced a rapid rise in glucose and insulin levels. AG and DAG co-administration, however, prevented the AG-induced rise in insulin and glucose. Moreover, co-treatment with DAG prevented AG-induced insulin resistance for at least 6 h after administration [25].

Similar effects have been observed in animal studies. For example, Inhoff et al. [26] showed that the metabolic effects of AG (administered intraperitoneally) could be abrogated by co-administered DAG in non-fasted rats. DAG alone did not alter food intake, as has been reported by others, for example Neary et al. [27].

In vitro Interactions between AG and DAG

Granata et al. [28] reported on the effects of AG on pancreatic β-cell proliferation as well as apoptosis induced by serum starvation or cytokine (interferon-γ/TNF-α) treatment. Interestingly, both DAG and AG induced cell survival and protected against apoptosis in hamster insulinoma cell line HIT-T15 and isolated human islets of Langerhans. Despite not expressing GHSR mRNA, both DAG and AG recognized common high-affinity binding sites on these cells, suggesting that the effects of DAG and AG occur via mechanisms independent of the GHSR [28].

Gauna et al. [29] reported that AG stimulates, whereas DAG inhibits glucose output by primary hepatocytes. Interestingly, GHSR gene expression was not detectable in the hepatocyte preparations. The effects of DAG, in the absence of GHSR expression and lack of a response to hexarelin treatment, again indicate the involvement of an uncharacterized ghrelin receptor (sub)type [29].

More recently, Miegueu et al. [30] reported the direct effects of ghrelin gene family peptides on preadipocyte proliferation, differentiation and adipocyte lipid and glucose metabolism in 3T3-L1 adipocytes. Interestingly, DAG stimulation of FA uptake was blocked by the GHSR antagonist [D-Lys3]-GHRP-6, which suggests that [D-Lys3]-GHRP-6 can also block the hypothetical DAG receptor [30]. An independent report on the effects of AG and DAG in adipocytes by Rodriguez et al. [17] also shows that AG and DAG can stimulate lipid accumulation in human visceral adipocytes.

Baragli et al. [31] reported that AG and DAG block isoproterenol and forskolin-induced lipolysis; a process in which phosphodiesterase seems to be involved. In particular, selective inhibition of PI3K iso-enzyme-γ (PI3K-γ) prevented AG and DAG effects on isoproterenol-stimulated lipolysis, impeding AKT phosphorylation [31].

Lear et al. [32] also reported that DAG has specific binding sites and different metabolic effects in the murine HL-1 adult cardiomyocyte cell line. They compared the effects of AG and DAG on glucose and FA uptake and attempted to identify DAG-specific binding sites in cardiomyocytes. AG and DAG had opposing metabolic effects: DAG increased medium-chain FA uptake, whereas neither AG alone nor in combination with DAG did so. In these HL-1 cells, DAG binds to specific receptors and has effects on glucose and medium-chain fatty acid uptake that are distinct from those of AG [32].

Finally, Kumar et al. [33] have demonstrated a direct antagonistic effect of DAG on AG. They used isolated mouse pancreatic islets to study the suppression of the spontaneous secretion of pancreatic polypeptide by AG. This modulation of pancreatic polypeptide release by AG was dose-dependently counteracted by DAG. They conclude that DAG acts as a competitive inhibitor of AG. Since DAG does not antagonize AG at the GHSR, it is likely that it is acting via a non-GHSR-mediated mechanism in the islets [7].

Effects of DAG in Rodents; in vivo Studies

In 2005, Asakawa et al. [34] reported that DAG appeared to decrease food intake and the gastric emptying rate through actions on the hypothalamus. DAG transgenic mice exhibit a decrease in body weight, food intake, and fat pad mass accompanied by moderately decreased linear growth, along with a decrease in gastric emptying [34].

Zhang et al. [35] studied the effects of overexpressing DAG in the fat depots of mice on adiposity and glucose metabolism using the fatty acid-binding protein-4 (FABP4) promoter to drive expression of a murine prepro-ghrelin transgene. FABP4-ghrelin transgenic mice exhibited markedly raised circulating DAG levels and were resistant to obesity induced by high-fat diet. Glucose-tolerance tests showed significantly faster clearance of glucose in FABP4-ghrelin transgenic mice than in controls. Insulin-sensitivity testing showed that FABP4-ghrelin transgenic mice had a significantly greater hypoglycemic response to insulin, indicating markedly improved insulin sensitivity [35]. As the FABP4 promoter is also active in the hypothalamus [36], it is very likely that FABP4-ghrelin transgenic mice overexpress DAG in the hypothalamus as well, and that part of the effect may be through actions of DAG at a central level.

Effects of DAG Administration in Humans

Benso et al. [37] reported that intravenous DAG administration improves glucose metabolism and inhibits lipolysis in healthy volunteers. Apparently, and in contrast to the diabetogenic action of AG, DAG displays hypoglycemic properties. They studied the effects of a 16-hour overnight infusion of DAG or saline in 8 normal subjects. Postprandial insulin levels after both dinner and breakfast were significantly increased following DAG treatment compared with placebo.

Ozcan et al. [10] recently reported the results of a clinical study in 8 overweight patients with controlled type 2 diabetes in whom the effects of a continuous overnight infusion of two doses of DAG versus placebo in a double-blind cross-over study on AG concentrations, and the glucose and insulin responses to a standard breakfast meal were studied. DAG administration markedly decreased AG levels following breakfast. Moreover, overnight infusions of DAG significantly decreased postprandial glucose levels [10].

DAG Actions That Are GHSR-Independent

Gauna et al. [38] reported the results of a study on the interactions between AG and DAG on ghrelin receptors in INS-1E rat insulinoma cells. Their data strongly suggest the existence of a specific receptor for DAG, other than the GHS-R1a that DAG might share with AG, as both DAG and AG dose-dependently stimulated insulin release in the nanomolar range. As expected, the AG-induced insulin output was antagonized by the two GHSR antagonists [D-Lys3]-GHRP-6 and BIM28163. These GHSR blockers, however, did not block DAG-induced insulin secretion.

Halem et al. [39] demonstrated that this GHSR-blocker BIM-28163 blocked AG activation of the GHSR receptor, and inhibited AG-induced GH secretion in vivo. Interestingly, they observed that BIM-28163 also acted as an agonist with regard to stimulating weight gain. Their results again suggest the presence of an unknown ghrelin receptor that modulates ghrelin actions on weight gain [39].

Delhanty et al. [4] studied the GHSR-independent effects of DAG in mice in vivo. Using microarrays, they examined rapid effects of DAG on genome-wide expression patterns in fat, muscle and liver of GHSR-deficient mice. They found that DAG acutely regulated clusters of genes involved in glucose and lipid metabolism. These results strongly indicate a direct, GHSR-independent, action of DAG that improves insulin-sensitivity and metabolic profile [4].

Moazed et al. [40] suggested the presence of a non-GHSR receptor that can be activated by DAG. In their studies performed on the perfused mesenteric vascular bed in rats, DAG evoked endothelium-dependent vasodilatation via activation of potassium channels. However, this vasodilator response was not mediated by the classical GHSR [40].

Rodriguez et al. [41] evaluated the effects of obesity and obesity-associated type 2 diabetes on AG, DAG and their association with TNF-α levels. They also assessed the roles of AG and DAG in the control of apoptosis and autophagy in isolated human fat tissue and adipocytes. In subjects with obesity-associated type 2 diabetes, circulating AG and TNF-α levels were increased, whereas DAG was decreased [41]. Ghrelin and GOAT were produced in omental and subcutaneous adipose tissue. Visceral adipose tissue from obese patients with type 2 diabetes showed higher levels of GOAT, increased adipocyte apoptosis and increased expression of the autophagy-related genes ATG5, BECN1 and ATG7. In differentiating human omental adipocytes in vitro, incubation with AG and DAG reduced TNF-α-induced activation of caspase-8 and caspase-3, and cell death [41]. In addition, AG reduced the basal expression of the autophagy-related genes ATG5 and ATG7, while DAG inhibited the TNF-α-induced increase of ATG5, BECN1 and ATG7 expression. Therefore, apoptosis and autophagy are upregulated in human visceral adipose tissue of patients with type 2 diabetes, and AG and DAG may act to suppress these processes [41].

DAG Effects on Non-Metabolic Tissues

Togliatto et al. [42] investigated the potential of DAG to reverse diabetes-associated pathologies in individuals with type 2 diabetes, and *ob/ob* mice. They observed that DAG can rescue endothelial progenitor cell function [42]. In addition, unlike AG, DAG facilitated the recovery of bone marrow endothelial progenitor cell mobilization [42].

Zhang et al. [43] reported that low (total) ghrelin levels are closely associated with severity and morphology of angiographically-detected coronary atherosclerosis in patients with diabetes mellitus.

Wu et al. [44] reported that ghrelin maintains the cardiovascular stability in severe sepsis. In their study, male adult rats were made septic by cecal ligation and puncture (CLP). At 5 h after CLP, a bolus intravenous injection of ghrelin was followed by continuous infusion of 12 nmol ghrelin via a primed mini-pump for 15 h. Treatment with ghrelin significantly augmented the maximal rates of ventricular pressure increase and decrease by 36 and 35%, respectively. Ghrelin treatment also reversed the suppression of norepinephrine-induced vascular contraction and acetylcholine-induced endothelium-dependent vascular relaxation caused by CLP [44].

Sheriff et al. [45] observed that DAG exhibits pro-anabolic and anti-catabolic effects on C2C12 myotubes exposed to cytokines and reduces burn-induced muscle proteolysis in rats. In an extensive related study, Porporato et al. [46] convincingly show that AG and DAG can protect against skeletal muscle atrophy independent of the GHSR. AG and DAG were found to inhibit dexamethasone-induced skeletal muscle atrophy and atrogene expression through PI3K-β-, mTORC2-, and p38-mediated pathways in myotubes. Increasing the level of DAG in mice, either by peptide

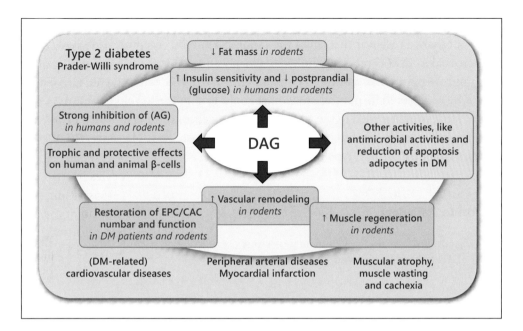

Fig. 2. Overview of reported DAG ghrelin actions.

treatment or muscle-specific transgenesis, reduced skeletal muscle atrophy induced by either fasting or denervation, without stimulating muscle hypertrophy. In GHSR-deficient mice, both AG and DAG treatment prevent fasting-induced skeletal muscle atrophy, possibly via an Akt-dependent pathway, demonstrating a GHSR-independent mechanism of action.

Even antimicrobial activities have been reported of AG and DAG. Min et al. [47] demonstrated that AG and DAG have the same degree of bactericidal activity against Gram-negative *Escherichia coli* and *Pseudomonas aeruginosa*, while bactericidal effects against Gram-positive *Staphylococcus aureus* and *Enterococcus faecalis* were minimal or absent, respectively. They showed that AG and DAG similarly quenched the negative surface charge of *E. coli*, suggesting that ghrelin-mediated bactericidal effects are influenced by charge-dependent binding and not by acyl modification [47]. Although, like most cationic antimicrobial peptides, the antibacterial activity of AG was attenuated by physiological salt concentrations, their findings indicate that both AG and DAG can act against Gram-negative bacteria.

Conclusion

In this chapter we have tried to convince the reader that DAG is more than just a degradation product of ghrelin. DAG should be considered as a separate hormone, independent of AG, and that it has a number of biological activities (fig. 2). In certain cases, DAG seems to act on its own receptor, while other data suggest that AG and DAG can share a receptor that is not the canonical ghrelin receptor, GHSR-1a.

Increased AG/DAG ratios are linked to obesity and diabetes and DAG administration improves glycemic control. The paradigm that DAG can antagonize AG and should be considered its natural antagonist could lead to the development of AG inhibitors that could be used in the treatment of clinical conditions in which raised AG activity and/or levels are linked with severity of disease. Possible examples of such diseases include PWS and type 2 diabetes of obesity.

Disclosure Statement

P.J.D.D. and S.J.N. have no conflicts of interest to disclose. A.J.v.d.L. is scientific advisor and shareholder of Alizé Pharma SAS, Lyon, France.

References

1 Kojima M, Hosoda H, Date Y, Nakazato M, Matsuo H, Kangawa K: Ghrelin is a growth-hormone-releasing acylated peptide from stomach. Nature 1999;402: 656–660.

2 Gutierrez JA, Solenberg PJ, Perkins DR, Willency JA, Knierman MD, Jin Z, Witcher DR, Luo S, Onyia JE, Hale JE: Ghrelin octanoylation mediated by an orphan lipid transferase. Proc Natl Acad Sci USA 2008; 105:6320–6325.

3 Yang J, Brown MS, Liang G, Grishin NV, Goldstein JL: Identification of the acyltransferase that octanoylates ghrelin, an appetite-stimulating peptide hormone. Cell 2008;132:387–396.

4 Delhanty PJ, Sun Y, Visser JA, van Kerkwijk A, Huisman M, van Ijcken WF, Swagemakers S, Smith RG, Themmen AP, van der Lely AJ: Unacylated ghrelin rapidly modulates lipogenic and insulin signaling pathway gene expression in metabolically active tissues of GHSR deleted mice. PLoS One 2010;5:e11749.

5 Kang K, Schmahl J, Lee JM, Garcia K, Patil K, Chen A, Keene M, Murphy A, Sleeman MW: Mouse ghrelin-O-acyltransferase (GOAT) plays a critical role in bile acid reabsorption. FASEB J 2012;26:259–271.

6 Seim I, Jeffery PL, de Amorim L, Walpole CM, Fung J, Whiteside EJ, Lourie R, Herington AC, Chopin LK: Ghrelin O-acyltransferase (GOAT) is expressed in prostate cancer tissues and cell lines and expression is differentially regulated in vitro by ghrelin. Reprod Biol Endocrinol 2013;11:70.

7 Gauna C, van de Zande B, van Kerkwijk A, Themmen AP, van der Lely AJ, Delhanty PJ: Unacylated ghrelin is not a functional antagonist but a full agonist of the type 1a growth hormone secretagogue receptor (GHS-R). Mol Cell Endocrinol 2007;274:30–34.

8 Delhanty PJ, Neggers SJ, van der Lely AJ: Mechanisms in endocrinology: ghrelin: the differences between acyl- and des-acyl ghrelin. Eur J Endocrinol 2012;167:601–608.

9 Tong J, Dave N, Mugundu GM, Davis HW, Gaylinn BD, Thorner MO, Tschöp MH, D'Alessio D, Desai PB: The pharmacokinetics of acyl, des-acyl, and total ghrelin in healthy human subjects. Eur J Endocrinol 2013;168:821–828.

10 Ozcan B, Neggers SJ, Miller AR, Yang HC, Lucaites V, Abribat T, Allas S, Huisman M, Visser JA, Themmen AP, Sijbrands E, Delhanty P, van der Lely AJ: Does des-acyl ghrelin improve glycemic control in obese diabetic subjects by decreasing acylated ghrelin levels? Eur J Endocrinol 2013, Epub ahead of print.

11 Blijdorp K, van der Lely AJ, van den Heuvel-Eibrink MM, Huisman TM, Themmen AP, Delhanty PJ, Neggers SJ: Desacyl ghrelin is influenced by changes in insulin concentration during an insulin tolerance test. Growth Horm IGF Res 2013;23:193–195.

12 Longo KA, Charoenthongtrakul S, Giuliana DJ, Govek EK, McDonagh T, Qi Y, DiStefano PS, Geddes BJ: Improved insulin sensitivity and metabolic flexibility in ghrelin receptor knockout mice. Regul Pept 2008;150:55–61.

13 Nonogaki K, Nozue K, Oka Y: Hyperphagia alters expression of hypothalamic 5-HT_{2C} and 5-HT_{1B} receptor genes and plasma des-acyl ghrelin levels in Ay mice. Endocrinology 2006;147:5893–5900.

14 Pacifico L, Poggiogalle E, Costantino F, Anania C, Ferraro F, Chiarelli F, Chiesa C: Acylated and non-acylated ghrelin levels and their associations with insulin resistance in obese and normal weight children with metabolic syndrome. Eur J Endocrinol 2009; 161:861–870.

15 St-Pierre DH, Karelis AD, Coderre L, Malita F, Fontaine J, Mignault D, Brochu M, Bastard JP, Cianflone K, Doucet E, Imbeault P, Rabasa-Lhoret R: Association of acylated and nonacylated ghrelin with insulin sensitivity in overweight and obese postmenopausal women. J Clin Endocrinol Metab 2007;92:264–269.

16 Barazzoni R, Zanetti M, Ferreira C, Vinci P, Pirulli A, Mucci M, Dore F, Fonda M, Ciocchi B, Cattin L, Guarnieri G: Relationships between desacylated and acylated ghrelin and insulin sensitivity in the metabolic syndrome. J Clin Endocrinol Metab 2007;92:3935–3940.

17 Rodriguez A, Gomez-Ambrosi J, Catalan V, Gil MJ, Becerril S, Sainz N, Silva C, Salvador J, Colina I, Fruhbeck G: Acylated and desacyl ghrelin stimulate lipid accumulation in human visceral adipocytes. Int J Obes 2009;33:541–552.

18 Cederberg H, Rajala U, Koivisto VM, Jokelainen J, Surcel HM, Keinanen-Kiukaanniemi S, Laakso M: Unacylated ghrelin is associated with changes in body composition and body fat distribution during long-term exercise intervention. Eur J Endocrinol 2011;165:243–248.

19 Barnett BP, Hwang Y, Taylor MS, Kirchner H, Pfluger PT, Bernard V, Lin Y, Bowers EM, Mukherjee C, Song W-J, Longo PA, Leahy DJ, Hussain MA, Tschöp MH, Boeke JD, Cole PA: Glucose and weight control in mice with a designed ghrelin O-acyltransferase inhibitor. Science 2010;330:1689–1692.

20 Kirchner H, Heppner KM, Holland J, Kabra D, Chop MH, Pfluger PT: Ablation of ghrelin O-acyltransferase does not improve glucose intolerance or body adiposity in mice on a leptin-deficient *ob/ob* background. PLoS One 2013;8:e61822.

21 Blatnik M, Soderstrom CI: A practical guide for the stabilization of acyl ghrelin in human blood collections. Clin Endocrinol (Oxf) 2011;74:325–331.

22 Purtell L, Sze L, Loughnan G, Smith E, Herzog H, Sainsbury A, Steinbeck K, Campbell LV, Viardot A: In adults with Prader-Willi syndrome, elevated ghrelin levels are more consistent with hyperphagia than high PYY and GLP-1 levels. Neuropeptides 2011;45: 301–307.

23 Goldstone JV, Holland AJ, Butler JV, Whittington JE: Appetite hormones and the transition to hyperphagia in children with Prader-Willi syndrome. Int J Obes 2012;36:1564–1570.

24 Broglio F, Gottero C, Prodam F, Gauna C, Muccioli G, Papotti M, Abribat T, van der Lely AJ, Ghigo E: Non-acylated ghrelin counteracts the metabolic but not the neuroendocrine response to acylated ghrelin in humans. J Clin Endocrinol Metab 2004;89:3062–3065.

25 Gauna C, Meyler FM, Janssen JA, Delhanty PJ, Abribat T, van Koetsveld P, Hofland LJ, Broglio F, Ghigo E, van der Lely AJ: Administration of acylated ghrelin reduces insulin sensitivity, whereas the combination of acylated plus unacylated ghrelin strongly improves insulin sensitivity. J Clin Endocrinol Metab 2004;89:5035–5042.

26 Inhoff T, Monnikes H, Noetzel S, Stengel A, Goebel M, Dinh QT, Riedl A, Bannert N, Wisser AS, Wiedenmann B, Klapp BF, Tache Y, Kobelt P: Desacyl ghrelin inhibits the orexigenic effect of peripherally injected ghrelin in rats. Peptides 2008;29:2159–2168.

27 Neary NM, Druce MR, Small CJ, Bloom SR: Acylated ghrelin stimulates food intake in the fed and fasted states but desacylated ghrelin has no effect. Gut 2006; 55:135.

28 Granata R, Settanni F, Biancone L, Trovato L, Nano R, Bertuzzi F, Destefanis S, Annunziata M, Martinetti M, Catapano F, Ghè C, Isgaard J, Papotti M, Ghigo E, Muccioli G: Acylated and unacylated ghrelin promote proliferation and inhibit apoptosis of pancreatic β-cells and human islets: involvement of 3′,5′-cyclic adenosine monophosphate/protein kinase A, extracellular signal-regulated kinase 1/2, and phosphatidylinositol 3-Kinase/Akt signaling. Endocrinology 2007;148:512–529.

29 Gauna C, Delhanty PJD, Hofland LJ, Janssen J, Broglio F, Ross RJM, Ghigo E, van der Lely AJ: Ghrelin stimulates, whereas des-octanoyl ghrelin inhibits, glucose output by primary hepatocytes. J Clin Endocrinol Metab 2005;90:1055–1060.

30 Miegueu P, St Pierre D, Broglio F, Cianflone K: Effect of desacyl ghrelin, obestatin and related peptides on triglyceride storage, metabolism and GHSR signaling in 3T3-L1 adipocytes. J Cell Biochem 2011;112:704–714.

31 Baragli A, Ghè C, Arnoletti E, Granata R, Ghigo E, Muccioli G: Acylated and unacylated ghrelin attenuate isoproterenol-induced lipolysis in isolated rat visceral adipocytes through activation of phosphoinositide 3-kinase γ and phosphodiesterase 3B. Biochim Biophys Acta 2011;1811:386–396.

32 Lear PV, Iglesias MJ, Feijoo-Bandin S, Rodriguez-Penas D, Mosquera-Leal A, Garcia-Rua V, Gualillo O, Ghè C, Arnoletti E, Muccioli G, Dieguez C, Gonzalez-Juanatey JR, Lago F: Des-acyl ghrelin has specific binding sites and different metabolic effects from ghrelin in cardiomyocytes. Endocrinology 2010;151:3286–3298.

33 Kumar R, Salehi A, Rehfeld JF, Hoglund P, Lind-strom E, Hakanson R: Proghrelin peptides: desacyl ghrelin is a powerful inhibitor of acylated ghrelin, likely to impair physiological effects of acyl ghrelin but not of obestatin. A study of pancreatic polypeptide secretion from mouse islets. Regul Pept 2010; 164:65–70.

34 Asakawa A, Inui A, Fujimiya M, Sakamaki R, Shinfuku N, Ueta Y, Meguid MM, Kasuga M: Stomach regulates energy balance via acylated ghrelin and desacyl ghrelin. Gut 2005;54:18–24.

35 Zhang W, Chai B, Li JY, Wang H, Mulholland MW: Effect of des-acyl ghrelin on adiposity and glucose metabolism. Endocrinology 2008;149:4710–4716.

36 Martens K, Bottelbergs A, Baes M: Ectopic recombination in the central and peripheral nervous system by aP2/FABP4-Cre mice: implications for metabolism research. FEBS Lett 2010;584:1054–1058.

37 Benso A, St-Pierre DH, Prodam F, Gramaglia E, Granata R, van der Lely AJ, Ghigo E, Broglio F: Metabolic effects of overnight continuous infusion of unacylated ghrelin in humans. Eur J Endocrinol 2012;166:911–916.

38 Gauna C, Delhanty PJ, van Aken MO, Janssen JA, Themmen AP, Hofland LJ, Culler M, Broglio F, Ghigo E, van der Lely AJ: Unacylated ghrelin is active on the INS-1E rat insulinoma cell line independently of the growth hormone secretagogue receptor type 1a and the corticotropin-releasing factor 2 receptor. Mol Cell Endocrinol 2006;251:103–111.

39 Halem HA, Taylor JE, Dong JZ, Shen Y, Datta R, Abizaid A, Diano S, Horvath TL, Culler MD: A novel growth hormone secretagogue-1a receptor antagonist that blocks ghrelin-induced growth hormone secretion but induces increased body weight gain. Neuroendocrinology 2005;81:339–349.

40 Moazed B, Quest D, Gopalakrishnan V: Des-acyl ghrelin fragments evoke endothelium-dependent vasodilatation of rat mesenteric vascular bed via activation of potassium channels. Eur J Pharmacol 2009;604:79–86.

41 Rodriguez A, Gomez-Ambrosi J, Catalan V, Rotellar F, Valenti V, Silva C, Mugueta C, Pulido MR, Vazquez R, Salvador J, Malagon MM, Colina I, Fruhbeck G: The ghrelin O-acyltransferase-ghrelin system reduces TNF-α-induced apoptosis and autophagy in human visceral adipocytes. Diabetologia 2012; 55:3038–3050.

42 Togliatto G, Trombetta A, Dentelli P, Baragli A, Rosso A, Granata R, Ghigo D, Pegoraro L, Ghigo E, Brizzi MF: Unacylated ghrelin rescues endothelial progenitor cell function in individuals with type 2 diabetes. Diabetes 2010;59:1016–1025.

43 Zhang M, Fang WY, Yuan F, Qu XK, Liu H, Xu YJ, Chen H, Yu YF, Shen Y, Zheng ZC: Plasma ghrelin levels are closely associated with severity and morphology of angiographically-detected coronary atherosclerosis in Chinese patients with diabetes mellitus. Acta Pharmacol Sin 2012;33:452–458.

44 Wu R, Chaung WW, Dong W, Ji Y, Barrera R, Nicastro J, Molmenti EP, Coppa GF, Wang P: Ghrelin maintains the cardiovascular stability in severe sepsis. J Surg Res 2012;178:370–377.

45 Sheriff S, Kadeer N, Joshi R, Friend LA, James JH, Balasubramaniam A: Des-acyl ghrelin exhibits pro-anabolic and anti-catabolic effects on C2C12 myotubes exposed to cytokines and reduces burn-induced muscle proteolysis in rats. Mol Cell Endocrinol 2012;351:286–295.

46 Porporato PE, Filigheddu N, Reano S, Ferrara M, Angelino E, Gnocchi VF, Prodam F, Ronchi G, Fagoonee S, Fornaro M, Chianale F, Baldanzi G, Surico F, Sinigaglia F, Perroteau I, Smith RG, Sun Y, Geuna S, Graziani A: Acylated and unacylated ghrelin impair skeletal muscle atrophy in mice. J Clin Invest 2013;123:611–622.

47 Min C, Ohta M, Kajiya M, Zhu T, Sharma K, Shin J, Mawardi H, Howait M, Hirschfeld J, Bahammam L, Ichimonji I, Ganta S, Amiji M, Kawai T: The antimicrobial activity of the appetite peptide hormone ghrelin. Peptides 2012;36:151–156.

Aart J. van der Lely, MD, PhD
Department of Internal Medicine
Erasmus MC, PO Box 2040
NL–3000 CA Rotterdam (The Netherlands)
E-Mail a.vanderlelij@erasmusmc.nl

Delhanty · Neggers · van der Lely

Delhanty PJD, van der Lely AJ (eds): How Gut and Brain Control Metabolism.
Front Horm Res. Basel, Karger, 2014, vol 42, pp 175–185 (DOI: 10.1159/000358346)

Obestatin: Is It Really Doing Something?

Letizia Trovato · Davide Gallo · Fabio Settanni · Iacopo Gesmundo ·
Ezio Ghigo · Riccarda Granata

Division of Endocrinology, Diabetology and Metabolism, Department of Medical Sciences,
University of Turin, Turin, Italy

Abstract

Obestatin was identified in 2005 by Zhang and colleagues as a ghrelin-associated peptide, derived from posttranslational processing of the prepro-ghrelin gene. Initially, obestatin was reported to activate the G-protein-coupled receptor GPR39 and to reduce food intake and gastric emptying. However, obestatin remains a controversial peptide, as these findings have been questioned and its receptor is still a matter of debate, as well as its effects on feeding behavior. Recently, interaction with the glucagon-like peptide 1 receptor has been suggested, in line with obestatin-positive effects on glucose and lipid metabolism. In addition, obestatin displays a variety of cellular effects, by regulating metabolic cell functions, increasing cell survival and proliferation, and inhibiting apoptosis and inflammation in different cell types. Finally, like ghrelin, obestatin is produced in the gastrointestinal tract, including the pancreas and adipose tissue, and exerts both local actions in peripheral tissues, and distant effects at the central level. Therefore, obestatin may indeed be considered a hormone, although additional studies are required to clarify its physiopathological role and to definitely identify its receptor.   © 2014 S. Karger AG, Basel

Ghrelin, a 28-amino-acid octanoylated peptide, was isolated from the stomach as the endogenous ligand of the type 1 growth hormone (GH) secretagogue receptor (GHS-R1a) [1]. Ghrelin acylation on serine 3, by ghrelin O-acyltransferase (GOAT) is essential for receptor binding and for ghrelin endocrine activities, including stimulation of GH release and food intake [2]. Des-acyl ghrelin, the major circulating form of ghrelin, although unable to bind to GHS-R1a and devoid of GH-releasing activity, displays many peripheral functions, which are either equal or opposed to those of acylated ghrelin, through binding to a yet unknown receptor [3].

In 2005, Zhang et al. [4], on the basis of bioinformatic searches, identified obestatin, a 23-amino-acid amidated peptide encoded by the ghrelin precursor (prepro-ghrelin). The term obestatin originated from the Latin verb 'obedere', meaning 'to devour', and 'statin', denoting suppression. Indeed, obestatin was initially claimed to behave as a physiological opponent of ghrelin, inhibiting either ghrelin orexigenic action or the stimulatory effect on GH secretion [4]. Interestingly, ghrelin, as well as des-acyl ghrelin and obestatin, have been shown to play a role in glucose and lipid homeostasis and, whereas ghrelin effects are mainly diabetogenic, both des-acyl ghrelin and obestatin behave as antidiabetogenic peptides by positively influencing glucose and lipid metabolism [5].

Obestatin was initially discovered as the cognate ligand for the orphan G-protein-coupled receptor GPR39 [4, 6]. However, these findings were later challenged by several independent groups that were unable to confirm that obestatin has agonist properties on GPR39 [5, 7, 8]. More recently, obestatin binding to the glucagon-like peptide 1 receptor (GLP-1R) in pancreatic β-cells and adipocytes has been proposed, in line with the effects of GLP-1 and its analogs in these cells [9, 10]. Furthermore, different cell types have shown specific binding sites for obestatin, suggesting biological responses of the peptide at different levels [6, 10, 11]. At present, the identification of obestatin receptor is still an open issue, although the many existing studies seem to exclude GPR39 from the possible candidates.

With regard to its distribution, obestatin, like ghrelin, was found to be mainly produced by the rat stomach [4], in cells of rat and human gastric mucosa, as well as in gastric myenteric cholinergic neurons [12]. However, other studies found little or no immunoreactivity in the stomach [13, 14], therefore additional studies will be required to confirm obestatin presence at the gastric level. Obestatin expression has been also shown in the endocrine pancreas, adipose tissue, skeletal muscle, liver, lung, thyroid, mammary gland and male reproductive system, suggesting autocrine/paracrine activities in peripheral tissues and organs [5, 10, 12, 15–19].

Like ghrelin, plasma obestatin is increased in anorexia nervosa and reduced in obesity; therefore, its levels may reflect body adiposity and insulin resistance, and obestatin may be a good nutritional marker and a potential target for the diagnosis and treatment of anorexia nervosa [20]. Furthermore and differently from ghrelin, whose levels were found unchanged, plasma obestatin and autonomic function were increased in orexin-deficient narcolepsy, suggesting a role for obestatin in the disrupted sleep-state control in narcolepsy [21].

Serum obestatin also decreased with metabolic syndrome, and further decreased with TRIB3 Q84R polymorphism, which has been associated with carotid atherosclerosis [22]. Therefore, it was proposed that obestatin would exert protective effects against insulin resistance and carotid atherosclerosis. Obestatin, like ghrelin, is expressed in human neuroendocrine tumors and exerts antiproliferative effects in neuroendocrine cell lines [16, 23]. However, in healthy controls, obestatin levels were reduced by food intake, and no variation was observed in patients with pancreatic neuroendocrine tumors [23]. Moreover, the ghrelin/obestatin ratio is reduced in inflammatory bowel disease [24], chronic atrophic gastritis [25] and following *Helicobacter pylori* eradication [26], suggesting obestatin involvement in the pathogenesis of these diseases.

With regard to its central activities, besides counteracting ghrelin effects on food intake and GH secretion, obestatin was found to exert its own effects, by suppressing food intake, slowing gastric emptying and jejunal motility and reducing body weight gain in rodents [4, 6, 27]. Despite these findings, obestatin central effects are still controversial, as studies in rats and mice also showed no inhibitory effect on food intake and body weight gain, in both the absence or presence of ghrelin [7, 8]. In addition, obestatin inhibits thirst and influences memory, anxiety, and sleep likely through indirect action on vagal neurons or by regulating secretion of other hormones that may reach the target cells [28–30]. In peripheral cells and tissues, obestatin promotes cell proliferation [10, 31, 32], prevents apoptosis, regulates cell function and differentiation, reduces inflammation, promotes cardioprotection and myogenesis and regulates atherogenesis and immune cell function [5, 8–11, 33–41]. These effects were found to either involve GPR39 [18, 36], GLP-1R [9, 10] or specific but yet unknown receptors [11].

This is an overview of obestatin biological effects, particularly at the peripheral level and with major attention on its metabolic functions. Whether obestatin may or not be considered a hormone, it is certainly a biologically active peptide, showing unexpected effects which makes it appealing both from a scientific point of view and as a possible therapeutic candidate in conditions such as metabolic dysfunctions.

Obestatin Effects in Adipocyte Function

The role of obestatin in adipocyte function has been addressed by different groups and the findings, which in most cases go in the same direction, have evidenced novel and unexpected biological effects of the peptide (fig. 1).

Indeed, obestatin plays a relevant role in adipocytes, regulating cell survival, adipogenesis, glucose and lipid metabolism and adipokine release.

Obestatin was found to increase c-fos staining in adipocytes from mouse white adipose tissue, and to increase c-fos protein expression in 3T3-L1 preadipocytes [6]. These effects involved activation of GPR39, as demonstrated by binding studies and by lack of obestatin-induced c-fos upregulation in GPR39 null mice [6]. In 3T3-L1 cells and human adipocytes, obestatin even increased extracellular signal-related kinase (ERK1/2) and phosphatidylinositol 3-kinase (PI3K)/Akt phosphorylation [6, 9], in line with the survival and metabolic effects observed in these cells, and the survival and proliferative effects in other cell types [9, 10, 31, 32, 37]. Apart from GPR39, obestatin has demonstrated binding specificity in 3T3-L1 preadipocytes, human subcutaneous (SC) preadipocytes and differentiated adipocytes [9]. Interestingly, obestatin binding is displaced by the GLP-1R agonist Ex-4 and by the antagonist Ex-9, and prevented by small interfering RNA (siRNA) against GLP-1R, suggesting possible interaction with GLP-1R [9]. Besides the debated role of GPR39, additional studies in these and other cell types are needed to clarify whether GLP-1R may be or not a putative obestatin receptor [7].

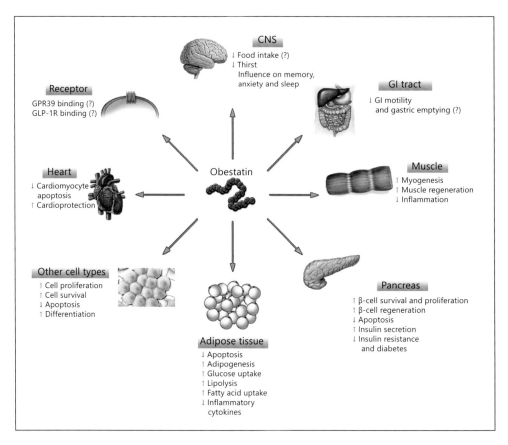

Fig. 1. Simplified representation of obestatin biological effects. Question marks indicate controversial data. GLP-1R = Glucagon-like peptide-1 receptor; GPR39 = G-protein-coupled receptor 39; CNS = central nervous system; GI = gastro-intestinal.

With regard to adipogenic signaling, obestatin has been shown to increase the expression of key regulators of adipogenesis, such as the CCAAT-enhancer-binding proteins (C-EBP) C/EBPα, C/EBPβ, C/EBPδ and peroxisome proliferator-activated receptor-γ (PPAR-γ) [36]. The adipogenic role of obestatin was further confirmed in vivo, in white adipose tissues of rats infused with obestatin and in obestatin-treated mice fed with either a low-fat diet (LFD) or a high-fat diet (HFD) [9, 36]. Interestingly, obestatin also regulates lipid metabolism by inhibiting lipolysis, as observed in 3T3-L1 and human SC and omental (OM) adipocytes isolated from both lean and obese individuals, and from HFD-treated mice [9, 37]. Moreover, AMP kinase (AMPK) phosphorylation, whose increase has been associated with inhibition of lipolysis, was found enhanced by obestatin in both 3T3-L1 and human adipocytes [9]. In vivo studies also showed that in rat, plasma triglyceride levels were significantly reduced by a chronic 14-day treatment with a stable obestatin analog, N-terminally PEGylated obestatin [42], suggestive of a possible role of obestatin in lipid

Trovato · Gallo · Settanni · Gesmundo · Ghigo · Granata

homeostasis. Furthermore, in cow WAT, obestatin infusion decreased the expression levels of ABCA1 (ATP-binding cassette A1), a key cholesterol transporter [43].

Besides lipid metabolism, obestatin also regulates glucose homeostasis in adipocytes. In fact, obestatin promotes glucose uptake in both 3T3-L1 and human SC adipocytes, and induces the translocation of glucose transporter GLUT4 [9, 36]. The NAD-dependent deacetylase sirtuin 1 (SIRT1) [44], a positive regulator of glucose transport and insulin signaling in adipocytes, was found involved in these effects as its downregulation, by means of specific siRNA, blocked obestatin-induced glucose uptake in 3T3-L1 adipocytes [9]. PI3K/Akt plays a major role in insulin-stimulated glucose transport and GLUT4 translocation to the cell membrane, and obestatin was found to promote Akt phosphorylation in 3T3-L1 and human SC adipocytes and to activate Akt downstream pathways such as GSK-3β, mTOR and S6K1 [9, 36].

Akt activation was also shown in vivo, in fat, muscle and liver of obestatin-treated mice fed a HFD, and in WAT of obestatin-infused rats [9, 36]. In 3T3-L1 and human SC adipocytes, obestatin even increased the secretion of adiponectin and inhibited that of leptin, which exert either a positive or negative role on glucose metabolism, respectively [9, 45, 46].

In vivo studies showed positive effects of obestatin in regulating glucose and lipid homeostasis. Indeed, obestatin reduces insulin resistance and inflammation in mice fed a HFD, by improving glucose levels and increasing both plasma and pancreatic insulin levels, likely because of its insulinotropic action [9]. Accordingly, obestatin was found to preserve islet area and to increase glucose-induced insulin secretion in islets from mice fed with both LFD and HFD. Furthermore, obestatin counteracted the effect of HFD on lipolysis, apoptosis and reduction of glucose uptake in epididymal fat. Interestingly, obestatin-treated mice showed increased number of small, likely insulin-sensitive adipocytes in epididymal and particularly SC fat, as compared to untreated animals, suggesting WAT expansion and increased protection against diet-induced insulin resistance [9]. In addition, and in agreement with the results obtained in cultured adipocytes, mice treated with obestatin showed increased plasma adiponectin and reduced leptin levels, in both epididymal and SC adipose tissue of HFD mice. In these mice, obestatin even reduced inflammation, a hallmark of insulin resistance and diabetes, by inhibiting proinflammatory cytokine release in fat, muscle and liver, through activation of signaling pathways involved in glucose metabolism and insulin signaling [9].

Obestatin and Pancreatic Functions

Obestatin expression has been demonstrated in the endocrine pancreas, where it co-localizes with ghrelin in both fetal and adult human pancreas, suggesting that these hormones may act together as local regulators of β-cell fate and function [10, 15–17,

47, 48]. Obestatin is also secreted by pancreatic β-cell lines and human pancreatic islets, and incubation of both INS-1E β-cells and human islets with an anti-obestatin antibody was found to reduce cell viability, suggesting autocrine/paracrine survival effects of the peptide [10].

Obestatin has been shown to reduce apoptosis and to promote proliferation of β-cells and human pancreatic islets cultured in either serum-starved conditions or with inflammatory cytokines [10]. Indeed, identifying molecules improving β-cell survival and function is of major importance for designing new therapeutic strategies in diabetes, and for improving islet transplantation, which are both characterized by increased inflammation and β-cell loss [49]. Obestatin survival effects in β-cells involved cAMP increase and activation of survival pathways such as PI3K/Akt and extracellular signal-related kinase (ERK)1/2. In addition, obestatin upregulated the expression of genes which play a key role in insulin signaling, glucose homeostasis and β-cell survival and differentiation, such as insulin receptor substrate 2 (IRS-2), cAMP response element-binding protein (CREB), pancreatic and duodenal homeobox 1 (PDX-1) and glucokinase [10]. Obestatin effects in β-cells and underlying signaling pathways were found to be very similar to those of GLP-1; therefore, it was hypothesized that obestatin would interact with GLP-1R. In fact, obestatin-induced survival in β-cells was lost in the presence of the GLP-1R antagonist exendin-9 and, besides recognizing specific binding sites in β-cells, obestatin showed specific binding to GLP-1R and upregulated GLP-1R mRNA [10]. Apart from GLP-1R, obestatin also interacted with ghrelin and des-acyl ghrelin-binding sites, and obestatin survival effects in β-cells were blunted by the ghrelin receptor antagonist [D-Lys3]-GHRP-6, suggesting cross-talk between the different ghrelin gene-derived peptides [10].

Obestatin, like ghrelin and des-acyl ghrelin, was shown to display antiapoptotic effects in human pancreatic islet microendothelial cells (MECs) exposed to chronic hyperglycemia. These effects were similar to those induced by the GLP-1R agonist exendin-4 (Ex-4); moreover, the signaling pathways involved were the same as those elicited in pancreatic β-cells [34]. On the basis of these findings, it was suggested that all the ghrelin gene peptides may improve islet vascularization and, by consequence, islet cell function [34].

Obestatin ability to promote in vitro β-cell generation from mouse pancreatic islet-derived precursors has been recently investigated [35]. In cultured mouse pancreatic islets, obestatin induced the generation of islet-like cell clusters (ICCs), that showed increased insulin gene expression and C-peptide secretion, as compared to untreated ICCs. This effect was likely due to obestatin-induced regulation of developmental pathways, such as downregulation of fibroblast growth factor receptors (FGFRs), modulation of Notch receptors and induction of neurogenin 3 (Ngn3) [35]. These findings, together with its early expression in the developing pancreas [50], suggest a role of obestatin in pancreas regeneration and formation and its potential implication for cell-based replacement therapy in diabetes.

In newborn rats treated with streptozotocin (STZ), obestatin, like ghrelin and des-acyl ghrelin, reduced diabetes at adult age, by preventing β-cell loss, reducing glucose levels and increasing insulin expression and secretion in pancreatic islets [33]. Obestatin has been also shown to inhibit the development of cerulein-induced pancreatitis in rats, by reducing pancreatitis-evoked activity of digestive enzymes, improving pancreatic blood flow and decreasing serum levels of proinflammatory interleukin-1β [41]. Moreover, intravenous administration of obestatin stimulates pancreatic protein output in anesthetized rats, via a cholecystokinin- and vagal-dependent mechanism [39, 40].

The role of obestatin on insulin secretion is still controversial, as both stimulatory and inhibitory effects have been described. Obestatin was found to inhibit insulin secretion even more effectively than ghrelin, to inhibit somatostatin and pancreatic polypeptide (PP) secretion, and to stimulate glucagon secretion in isolated mouse islets [51]. Obestatin was also shown to either inhibit insulin release in vivo in rats and in isolated rat pancreatic islets [52], or to have no effect on glucose and insulin levels, in both basal or fasting conditions in rats and mice [27]. Conversely, in perfused rat pancreas, obestatin either potentiated or inhibited insulin secretion, when used at low or at high concentrations, respectively [53], and increased the stimulatory effects of arginine and tolbutamide [53]. Obestatin-induced insulin release in response to glucose has been also described in vitro, in β-cell lines and human pancreatic islets [10], as well as in vivo and in pancreatic islets of mice fed with both LFD and HFD [9]. Obestatin insulinotropic action is further supported by studies showing GLP-1R involvement in obestatin survival and metabolic effects in β-cells and adipocytes, as well as obestatin ability to interact with GLP-1R [5, 9, 10].

Obestatin Effects in Cardiovascular System and Skeletal Muscle

Besides the effects on cell survival and glucose/lipid metabolism in the endocrine pancreas and adipocytes, different groups have investigated the cardiovascular effects of obestatin and its role on myogenesis. In humans, fasting plasma obestatin levels have been found to negatively correlate with systolic blood pressure [54]; however, obestatin levels were increased in hypertensive rats [55]. Moreover, obestatin may have a role in blood pressure regulation, as its concentrations have been shown to positively correlate with systemic blood pressure in normal pregnant women and in those with pregnancy-induced hypertension [56].

In the isolated heart, the addition of rat obestatin before ischemia reduced infarct size and contractile dysfunction in a concentration-dependent manner. Moreover, in rat H9c2 cardiac cells or isolated ventricular myocytes subjected to ischemia/reperfusion, obestatin reduced cardiomyocyte apoptosis and reduced caspase-3 activation [11]. Obestatin also preserved papillary muscle contractility, β-adrenergic response, as well as β_1-adrenoreceptors and α-myosin heavy chain (α-MHC) levels in rat diabetic myocardial tissue [39]. However, obestatin was also found unable to prevent arabinoside-induced apoptosis or to modify the cell cycle or viability of HL-1 cardiomyocytes [57].

A role for obestatin/GPR39 has been also demonstrated in muscle regeneration, in which obestatin was found to exert an autocrine function to control the myogenic differentiation program, through involvement of GPR39 [18]. Obestatin infusion in rats also increased the expression of myogenic genes, further supporting its role in muscle regeneration [18].

Conclusions

Obestatin is still a debated peptide, particularly because of its controversial effects at the central level and the yet unknown identity of the receptor involved in its activities. Although GLP-1R has been suggested as a possible candidate receptor, this possibility needs to be sustained by additional studies, and the role of GPR39 cannot be completely excluded. Notably, obestatin exerts survival effects in different cell types, positively regulates glucose and lipid metabolism, reduces inflammation and promotes cardioprotection and muscle regeneration. Obestatin secretion has been also demonstrated in different tissues and cells, where autocrine/paracrine effects were demonstrated. Therefore, on this basis, obestatin may be considered a hormone and hopefully, future studies and results will help to convince the more skeptical groups on the potential biological and therapeutic importance of this peptide.

References

1 Kojima M, Hosoda H, Date Y, Nakazato M, Matsuo H, Kangawa K: Ghrelin is a growth-hormone-releasing acylated peptide from stomach. Nature 1999;402:656–660.
2 Mohan H, Unniappan S: Discovery of ghrelin O-acyltransferase. Endocr Dev 2013;25:16–24.
3 Delhanty PJ, Neggers SJ, van der Lely AJ: Des-acyl ghrelin: a metabolically active peptide. Endocr Dev 2013;25:112–121.
4 Zhang JV, Ren PG, Avsian-Kretchmer O, Luo CW, Rauch R, Klein C, Hsueh AJ: Obestatin, a peptide encoded by the ghrelin gene, opposes ghrelin's effects on food intake. Science 2005;310:996–999.
5 Granata R, Baragli A, Settanni F, Scarlatti F, Ghigo E: Unraveling the role of the ghrelin gene peptides in the endocrine pancreas. J Mol Endocrinol 2010;45:107–118.
6 Zhang JV, Jahr H, Luo CW, Klein C, Van Kolen K, Ver Donck L, De A, Baart E, Li J, Moechars D, Hsueh AJ: Obestatin induction of early-response gene expression in gastrointestinal and adipose tissues and the mediatory role of G-protein-coupled receptor, GPR39. Mol Endocrinol 2008;22:1464–1475.
7 Zhang JV, Li L, Huang Q, Ren PG: Obestatin receptor in energy homeostasis and obesity pathogenesis. Prog Mol Biol Transl Sci 2013;114:89–107.
8 Ren G, He Z, Cong P, Chen H, Guo Y, Yu J, Liu Z, Ji Q, Song Z, Chen Y: Peripheral administration of TAT-obestatin can influence the expression of lipo-regulatory genes but fails to affect food intake in mice. Peptides 2013;42C:8–14.

9 Granata R, Gallo D, Luque RM, Baragli A, Scarlatti F, Grande C, Gesmundo I, Cordoba-Chacon J, Bergandi L, Settanni F, Togliatto G, Volante M, Garetto S, Annunziata M, Chanclon B, Gargantini E, Rocchietto S, Matera L, Datta G, Morino M, Brizzi MF, Ong H, Camussi G, Castano JP, Papotti M, Ghigo E: Obestatin regulates adipocyte function and protects against diet-induced insulin resistance and inflammation. FASEB J 2012;26:3393–3411.

10 Granata R, Settanni F, Gallo D, Trovato L, Biancone L, Cantaluppi V, Nano R, Annunziata M, Campiglia P, Arnoletti E, Ghè C, Volante M, Papotti M, Muccioli G, Ghigo E: Obestatin promotes survival of pancreatic β-cells and human islets and induces expression of genes involved in the regulation of β-cell mass and function. Diabetes 2008;57:967–979.

11 Alloatti G, Arnoletti E, Bassino E, Penna C, Perrelli MG, Ghè C, Muccioli G: Obestatin affords cardioprotection to the ischemic-reperfused isolated rat heart and inhibits apoptosis in cultures of similarly stressed cardiomyocytes. Am J Physiol Heart Circ Physiol 2010;299:H470–H481.

12 Dun SL, Brailoiu GC, Brailoiu E, Yang J, Chang JK, Dun NJ: Distribution and biological activity of obestatin in the rat. J Endocrinol 2006;191:481–489.

13 Chanoine JP, Wong AC, Barrios V: Obestatin, acylated and total ghrelin concentrations in the perinatal rat pancreas. Horm Res 2006;66:81–88.

14 Bang AS, Soule SG, Yandle TG, Richards AM, Pemberton CJ: Characterisation of proghrelin peptides in mammalian tissue and plasma. J Endocrinol 2007;192:313–323.

15 Gronberg M, Tsolakis AV, Magnusson L, Janson ET, Saras J: Distribution of obestatin and ghrelin in human tissues: immunoreactive cells in the gastrointestinal tract, pancreas, and mammary glands. J Histochem Cytochem 2008;56:793–801.

16 Volante M, Rosas R, Ceppi P, Rapa I, Cassoni P, Wiedenmann B, Settanni F, Granata R, Papotti M: Obestatin in human neuroendocrine tissues and tumours: expression and effect on tumour growth. J Pathol 2009;218:458–466.

17 Zhao CM, Furnes MW, Stenstrom B, Kulseng B, Chen D: Characterization of obestatin- and ghrelin-producing cells in the gastrointestinal tract and pancreas of rats: an immunohistochemical and electron-microscopic study. Cell Tissue Res 2008;331:575–587.

18 Gurriaran-Rodriguez U, Santos-Zas I, Al-Massadi O, Mosteiro CS, Beiroa D, Nogueiras R, Crujeiras AB, Seoane LM, Senaris J, Garcia-Caballero T, Gallego R, Casanueva FF, Pazos Y, Camina JP: The obestatin/GPR39 system is upregulated by muscle injury and functions as an autocrine regenerative system. J Biol Chem 2012;287:38379–38389.

19 Moretti E, Vindigni C, Tripodi SA, Mazzi L, Nuti R, Figura N, Collodel G: Immunolocalisation of ghrelin and obestatin in human testis, seminal vesicles, prostate and spermatozoa. Andrologia 2013, Epub ahead of print.

20 Seim I, Walpole C, Amorim L, Josh P, Herington A, Chopin L: The expanding roles of the ghrelin-gene derived peptide obestatin in health and disease. Mol Cell Endocrinol 2012;340:111.

21 Huda MS, Mani H, Durham BH, Dovey TM, Halford JC, Aditya BS, Pinkney JH, Wilding JP, Hart IK: Plasma obestatin and autonomic function are altered in orexin-deficient narcolepsy, but ghrelin is unchanged. Endocrine 2013;43:696–704.

22 Cui AD, Gai NN, Zhang XH, Jia KZ, Yang YL, Song ZJ: Decreased serum obestatin consequent upon TRIB3 Q84R polymorphism exacerbates carotid atherosclerosis in subjects with metabolic syndrome. Diabetol Metab Syndr 2012;4:52.

23 Gronberg M, Tsolakis AV, Holmback U, Stridsberg M, Grimelius L, Janson ET: Ghrelin and obestatin in human neuroendocrine tumors: expression and effect on obestatin levels after food intake. Neuroendocrinology 2013;97:291–299.

24 Alexandridis E, Zisimopoulos A, Liratzopoulos N, Katsos I, Manolas K, Kouklakis G, Obestatin/ghrelin ratio: a new activity index in inflammatory bowel diseases. Inflamm Bowel Dis 2009;15:1557–1561.

25 Gao XY, Kuang HY, Liu XM, Ma ZB, Nie HJ, Guo H: Plasma obestatin levels in men with chronic atrophic gastritis. Peptides 2008;29:1749–1754.

26 Ulasoglu C, Isbilen B, Doganay L, Ozen F, Kiziltas S, Tuncer I: Effect of *Helicobacter pylori* eradication on serum ghrelin and obestatin levels. World J Gastroenterol 2013;19:2388–2394.

27 Green BD, Irwin N, Flatt PR: Direct and indirect effects of obestatin peptides on food intake and the regulation of glucose homeostasis and insulin secretion in mice. Peptides 2007;28:981–987.

28 Samson WK, White MM, Price C, Ferguson AV: Obestatin acts in brain to inhibit thirst. Am J Physiol Regul Integr Comp Physiol 2007;292:R637–R643.

29 Carlini VP, Schioth HB, Debarioglio SR: Obestatin improves memory performance and causes anxiolytic effects in rats. Biochem Biophys Res Commun 2007;352:907–912.

30 Szentirmai E, Krueger JM: Obestatin alters sleep in rats. Neurosci Lett 2006;404:222–226.

31 Camina JP, Campos JF, Caminos JE, Dieguez C, Casanueva FF: Obestatin-mediated proliferation of human retinal pigment epithelial cells: regulatory mechanisms. J Cell Physiol 2007;211:1–9.

32 Pazos Y, Alvarez CJ, Camina JP, Casanueva FF: Stimulation of extracellular signal-regulated kinases and proliferation in the human gastric cancer cells KATO-III by obestatin. Growth Factors 2007;25: 373–381.

33 Granata R, Volante M, Settanni F, Gauna C, Ghè C, Annunziata M, Deidda B, Gesmundo I, Abribat T, van der Lely AJ, Muccioli G, Ghigo E, Papotti M: Unacylated ghrelin and obestatin increase islet cell mass and prevent diabetes in streptozotocin-treated newborn rats. J Mol Endocrinol 2010;45: 9–17.

34 Favaro E, Granata R, Miceli I, Baragli A, Settanni F, Cavallo Perin P, Ghigo E, Camussi G, Zanone MM, The ghrelin gene products and exendin-4 promote survival of human pancreatic islet endothelial cells in hyperglycaemic conditions, through phosphoinositide 3-kinase/Akt, extracellular signal-related kinase (ERK)1/2 and cAMP/protein kinase A (PKA) signalling pathways. Diabetologia 2012;55:1058–1070.

35 Baragli A, Grande C, Gesmundo I, Settanni F, Taliano M, Gallo D, Gargantini E, Ghigo E, Granata R: Obestatin enhances in vitro generation of pancreatic islets through regulation of developmental pathways. PLoS One 2013;8:e64374.

36 Gurriaran-Rodriguez U, Al-Massadi O, Roca-Rivada A, Crujeiras AB, Gallego R, Pardo M, Seoane LM, Pazos Y, Casanueva FF, Camina JP: Obestatin as a regulator of adipocyte metabolism and adipogenesis. J Cell Mol Med 2011;15:1927–1940.

37 Miegueu P, St Pierre D, Broglio F, Cianflone K: Effect of desacyl ghrelin, obestatin and related peptides on triglyceride storage, metabolism and GHSR signaling in 3T3-L1 adipocytes. J Cell Biochem 2011;112: 704–714.

38 Pruszynska-Oszmalek E, Szczepankiewicz D, Hertig I, Skrzypski M, Sassek M, Kaczmarek P, Kolodziejski PA, Mackowiak P, Nowak KW, Strowski MZ, Wojciechowicz T: Obestatin inhibits lipogenesis and glucose uptake in isolated primary rat adipocytes. J Biol Regul Homeost Agents 2013;27:23–33.

39 Aragno M, Mastrocola R, Ghè C, Arnoletti E, Bassino E, Alloatti G, Muccioli G: Obestatin-induced recovery of myocardial dysfunction in type 1 diabetic rats: underlying mechanisms. Cardiovasc Diabetol 2012;11:129.

40 Kellokoski E, Kunnari A, Jokela M, Makela S, Kesaniemi YA, Horkko S: Ghrelin and obestatin modulate early atherogenic processes on cells: enhancement of monocyte adhesion and oxidized low-density lipoprotein binding. Metabolism 2009; 58:1572–1580.

41 Ceranowicz P, Warzecha Z, Dembinski A, Cieszkowski J, Dembinski M, Sendur R, Kusnierz-Cabala B, Tomaszewska R, Kuwahara A, Kato I: Pretreatment with obestatin inhibits the development of cerulein-induced pancreatitis. J Physiol Pharmacol 2009;60:95–101.

42 Agnew A, Calderwood D, Chevallier OP, Greer B, Grieve DJ, Green BD: Chronic treatment with a stable obestatin analog significantly alters plasma triglyceride levels but fails to influence food intake; fluid intake; body weight; or body composition in rats. Peptides 2011;32:755–762.

43 Grala TM, Kay JK, Walker CG, Sheahan AJ, Littlejohn MD, Lucy MC, Roche JR, Expression analysis of key somatotropic axis and liporegulatory genes in ghrelin- and obestatin-infused dairy cows. Domest Anim Endocrinol 2010;39:76–83.

44 Yoshizaki T, Milne JC, Imamura T, Schenk S, Sonoda N, Babendure JL, Lu JC, Smith JJ, Jirousek MR, Olefsky JM: SIRT1 exerts anti-inflammatory effects and improves insulin sensitivity in adipocytes. Mol Cell Biol 2009;29:1363–1374.

45 Kadowaki T, Yamauchi T, Kubota N, Hara K, Ueki K, Tobe K: Adiponectin and adiponectin receptors in insulin resistance, diabetes, and the metabolic syndrome. J Clin Invest 2006;116:1784–1792.

46 Siegrist-Kaiser CA, Pauli V, Juge-Aubry CE, Boss O, Pernin A, Chin WW, Cusin I, Rohner-Jeanrenaud F, Burger AG, Zapf J, Meier CA: Direct effects of leptin on brown and white adipose tissue. J Clin Invest 1997;100:2858–2864.

47 Walia P, Asadi A, Kieffer TJ, Johnson JD, Chanoine JP: Ontogeny of ghrelin, obestatin, preproghrelin, and prohormone convertases in rat pancreas and stomach. Pediatr Res 2009;65:39–44.

48 Turk N, Dagistanli FK, Sacan O, Yanardag R, Bolkent S: Obestatin and insulin in pancreas of newborn diabetic rats treated with exogenous ghrelin. Acta Histochem 2012;114:349–357.

49 Donath MY, Halban PA: Decreased β-cell mass in diabetes: significance, mechanisms and therapeutic implications. Diabetologia 2004;47:581–589.

50 Wierup N, Svensson H, Mulder H, Sundler F: The ghrelin cell: a novel developmentally regulated islet cell in the human pancreas. Regul Pept 2002;107: 63–69.

51 Qader SS, Hakanson R, Rehfeld JF, Lundquist I, Salehi A: Proghrelin-derived peptides influence the secretion of insulin, glucagon, pancreatic polypeptide and somatostatin: a study on isolated islets from mouse and rat pancreas. Regul Pept 2008;146:230–237.

52 Ren AJ, Guo ZF, Wang YK, Wang LG, Wang WZ, Lin L, Zheng X, Yuan WJ: Inhibitory effect of obestatin on glucose-induced insulin secretion in rats. Biochem Biophys Res Commun 2008;369:969–972.

Trovato · Gallo · Settanni · Gesmundo · Ghigo · Granata

53 Egido EM, Hernandez R, Marco J, Silvestre RA: Effect of obestatin on insulin, glucagon and somatostatin secretion in the perfused rat pancreas. Regul Pept 2009.

54 Anderwald-Stadler M, Krebs M, Promintzer M, Mandl M, Bischof MG, Nowotny P, Kastenbauer T, Luger A, Prager R, Anderwald C: Plasma obestatin is lower at fasting and not suppressed by insulin in insulin-resistant humans. Am J Physiol Endocrinol Metab 2007;293:E1393–E1398.

55 Li ZF, Guo ZF, Cao J, Hu JQ, Zhao XX, Xu RL, Huang XM, Qin YW, Zheng X: Plasma ghrelin and obestatin levels are increased in spontaneously hypertensive rats. Peptides 2010;31:297–300.

56 Ren AJ, He Q, Shi JS, Guo ZF, Zheng X, Lin L, Wang YK, Xia SY, Sun LL, Du X, Sun Y, Zhang LM, Yuan WJ: Association of obestatin with blood pressure in the third trimesters of pregnancy. Peptides 2009;30: 1742–1745.

57 Iglesias MJ, Salgado A, Pineiro R, Rodino BK, Otero MF, Grigorian L, Gallego R, Dieguez C, Gualillo O, Gonzalez-Juanatey JR, Lago F: Lack of effect of the ghrelin gene-derived peptide obestatin on cardiomyocyte viability and metabolism. J Endocrinol Invest 2007;30:470–476.

Riccarda Granata, PhD
Laboratory of Molecular and Cellular Endocrinology
Division of Endocrinology, Diabetology and Metabolism
Department of Medical Sciences, University of Turin
Corso Dogliotti, 14, IT–10126 Turin (Italy)
E-Mail riccarda.granata@unito.it

Author Index

Subject Index